Rheumatoid Arthritis: Diagnosis, Pathophysiology and Treatment

Editor: Travis Reagan

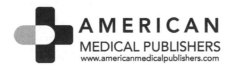
AMERICAN
MEDICAL PUBLISHERS
www.americanmedicalpublishers.com

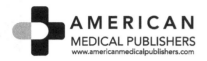

Cataloging-in-Publication Data

Rheumatoid arthritis : diagnosis, pathophysiology and treatment / edited by Travis Reagan.
      p. cm.
Includes bibliographical references and index.
ISBN 979-8-88740-440-0
1. Rheumatoid arthritis. 2. Rheumatoid arthritis--Diagnosis. 3. Rheumatoid arthritis--Pathophysiology.
4. Rheumatoid arthritis--Treatment. 5. Arthritis. 6. Rheumatism. I. Reagan, Travis.
RC933 .R44 2023
616.722--dc23

American Medical Publishers,
41 Flatbush Avenue,
1st Floor, New York,
NY 11217, USA

ISBN 979-8-88740-440-0 (Hardback)

Rheumatoid Arthritis: Diagnosis, Pathophysiology and Treatment

Contents

Preface

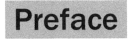

Rheumatoid arthritis (RA) refers to an autoimmune disorder that affects the joints. It usually causes painful, swollen and warm joints. The joints of knees, hands and wrists are affected by RA. In addition to damaging the joint tissues, RA can also affect other organs, including the eyes, heart and lungs, as well as other tissues all over the body. There are various signs and symptoms of RA, which includes fever, stiffness in several joints, weight loss, tiredness or fatigue. Smoking, aging, obesity and genetics are its major risk factors. The diagnosis of this disorder is done through assessing symptoms, physical examination and by performing lab tests and X-rays. The objectives of treatment are to reduce inflammation, alleviate pain and enhance overall functioning. Self-management techniques as well as medications can effectively manage and treat RA. This book unravels the recent studies on rheumatoid arthritis. It elucidates the diagnosis, pathophysiology and treatment of this disease. The readers would gain knowledge that would broaden their perspective in this area.

The information contained in this book is the result of intensive hard work done by researchers in this field. All due efforts have been made to make this book serve as a complete guiding source for students and researchers. The topics in this book have been comprehensively explained to help readers understand the growing trends in the field.

I would like to thank the entire group of writers who made sincere efforts in this book and my family who supported me in my efforts of working on this book. I take this opportunity to thank all those who have been a guiding force throughout my life.

Editor

Ultrasound and its clinical use in rheumatoid arthritis: Where do we stand?

Aline Defaveri do Prado[1,2*], Henrique Luiz Staub[2], Melissa Cláudia Bisi[2], Inês Guimarães da Silveira[2], José Alexandre Mendonça[3], Joaquim Polido-Pereira[4,5] and João Eurico Fonseca[4,5]

Abstract

High-resolution musculoskeletal ultrasound (MSUS) has been increasingly employed in daily rheumatological practice and in clinical research. In rheumatoid arthritis (RA), MSUS can be now considered a complement to physical examination. This method evaluates synovitis through gray-scale and power Doppler and it is also able to identify bone erosions. The utilization of MSUS as a marker of RA activity has received attention in recent literature. Current data account for good correlation of MSUS with classical measures of clinical activity; in some instances, MSUS appears to perform even better. Diagnosis of subclinical synovitis by MSUS might help the physician in RA management. With some variation, interobserver MSUS agreement seems excellent for erosion and good for synovitis. However, lack of MSUS score standardization is still an unmet need. In this review, we describe several MSUS scores, as well as their correlation with clinical RA activity and response to therapy. Finally, we look at the relationship of MSUS with synovial tissue inflammation and discuss future perspectives for a better interpretation and integration of this imaging method into clinical practice.

Keywords: Musculoskeletal ultrasound, Gray-scale, Power Doppler, Cytokines, Rheumatoid arthritis

Background

Rheumatoid arthritis (RA) is a chronic inflammatory immune mediated disorder where synovial proliferation, pannus formation and bone erosions are histological hallmarks [1]. Proinflammatory cytokines play a major role in development of disease and clinical progression. Anti-cytokine therapy has brought a major impact in RA management [2].

Clinical assessment of RA patients includes history, physical examination, scores of disease activity and questionnaires addressing quality of life. As far as imaging is concerned, conventional radiograms and magnetic resonance imaging (MRI) are well-recognized support methods for clinical assessment and response to therapy. They have intrinsic problems, nevertheless. Radiograms cannot evaluate joint inflammation and show low sensitivity for damage; MRI, although sensitive, is expensive and not widely available [1, 2].

In recent years, high-resolution musculoskeletal ultrasound (MSUS) has been increasingly used in rheumatological practice worldwide [3]. While MSUS gray-scale (GS) usually identifies synovial proliferation, power Doppler (pD) may recognize active inflammation and neoangiogenesis. Both parameters seem worthy of utilization in the follow-up of RA patients [4]. In addition, MSUS is also reliable for the detection of bone erosions [5] as well as for the detection of subclinical synovitis and prediction of disease relapse and structural progression [6].

Although unequivocally useful in RA, MSUS has intrinsic reproducibility issues that may be optimized through standardized training and recommendations. In 2010, a multinational group of 25 Rheumatologists from the American Continent participated in a consensus-based questionnaire and established the first recommendations and guidelines for MSUS course training in the Americas [7]. Besides, EULAR consensual advice for use of imaging techniques (MSUS included) in the management of RA has been recently proposed [8].

* Correspondence: adprado@gmail.com
[1]Rheumatology Unit, Nossa Senhora da Conceição Hospital, Porto Alegre, RS, Brazil
[2]Rheumatology Department, Sao Lucas Hospital, Faculty of Medicine of Pontifical Catholic University of Rio Grande do Sul (PUCRS), Av. Ipiranga, 6690/220, Porto Alegre 90610-000, Brazil
Full list of author information is available at the end of the article

In this paper, we review the correlation of MSUS findings with synovial tissue inflammation in RA patients and its implications for a better clinical utilization of this imaging technique. Also, we discuss MSUS clinical application as compared to classical activity parameters. Lastly, we update MSUS techniques and interobserver reliability in RA.

Ultrasound parameters and synovial tissue

Comparison of MSUS findings with features of synovial tissue allows characterizing how far this technique can capture the inflammatory activity that is actually ongoing inside joints.

Andersen et al. studied the correlation between histological synovitis and GS and pD in RA patients and found fairly good correlations between pD and histological features of inflammation and proliferation, namely synovium expression of CD3, CD68, Ki67 and von Willebrand factor (r between 0,44 and 0,57). There were areas of histological inflammation where no pD could be identified [9]. Other authors showed that 5 RA patients in DAS remission who had GS but negative pD had low likelihood of relapse after TNF inhibitor tapering and histologically had low infiltrates of macrophages (CD68+), T (CD3+) a B (CD20+) cells [10].

In a study of 14 RA patients in remission who were submitted to surgery, 15 synovial samples were collected. GS changes were found in 80% patients, pD detected in 60% of the individuals and MRI synovitis in 86%. Histologically, 4 samples had severe inflammation, 6 moderate, 3 mild and 2 minimal [11].

In another study in 20 patients with knee arthritis, pD showed better correlation with histological synovitis than contrast-enhanced MRI [12]. In the setting of rheumatoid synovium, the thickness of synovial lining and the number of vessels are increased, although it is not clear whether the angiogenesis is a cause or a consequence of the inflammatory process [13, 14].

Koski et al. found that in RA synovium there was a good correlation between the number of vessels and the inflammatory state (synovium inflammatory infiltrate), but not with pD. They concluded that chronic histological synovitis was not always related with a positive pD [15] In fact, in another study by the same authors, pD was not always translating synovial inflammation and could be related with other pathologic processes, such as fibrosis [16]. Waltheret al found a correlation between the number of vessels and pD, but did not report on the inflammatory state [17].

In healthy synovial joints, the presence of pD signal associated with serum levels of vascular endothelial growth factor (VEGF), but not with other growth factors or cytokines. This could support a role of VEGF in neo-angiogenesis in RA [18]. In a survey of 55 RA patients in clinical remission, pD correlated with VEGF levels and other angiogenesis markers [19]. On the contrary, a correlation between pD and serum vascular endothelium growth factor could not be established in RA patients according to a 2004 study [20].

Contrast-enhanced Doppler ultrasound may be superior to pD in translating a dynamic process such as synovitis in RA, in which perfusion may be determinant, but little is known about the correlation of these findings with histological features in the synovium RA. This method has proved to be superior to pD in defining active synovitis, using arthroscopy, but not MRI, as the gold standard [21–24].

Worthy of note, synovial production of IL-6 was found to associate with synovitis as detected by MRI and pD [25]. This in accordance with our own results, depicting that IL-6, but not other cytokines, correlated positively with DAS28, swollen joint count, 10-joint pD score and GS/pD of both wrists. In multiple linear regression, the association of IL-6 with 10-joint pD score was maintained even after adjustment for DAS28. There was no correlation of IL-6 with tender joint count, 10-joint GS score, or bone erosion [26].

Interestingly, Ball et al. described association of serum IL-6 with arthritis on physical examination and pD score in patients with systemic lupus erythematosus [27]. Overall, these findings [26, 27] may result from a prominent synovial production of IL-6. In fact, IL-6 stimulates angiogenesis [28], and this could eventually explain the association of IL-6 concentrations with a positive pD in RA. A recent report accounted for association of serum IL-6 with MSUS parameters of synovitis in patients with early RA; of importance, serial measurements of IL-6 were linked to structural damage [29].

In patients with established RA, a correlation of serum IL-17 with synovial hypertrophy and pD in hand MSUS was documented [30]. Interestingly, the presence of Th-17 lymphocytes in synovial tissue was associated with a persistent pD signal, according to a 2010 study [31].

As seen, the study of the relationship of MSUS parameters with synovial tissue features is clearly a field open to research, which may add new pathogenic information and help to clarify MSUS usefulness in RA management.

Correlation of MSUS with physical examination, inflammatory markers and patient reported outcomes

For many years, Rheumatologists have been using the disease activity score of 28 joints (DAS28) and other composite scores as gold standard for assessment of RA activity; these tools have clearly brought great progress in treatment monitoring. Even though they are the most extensively validated methods for measuring disease activity to date [32], the precise way of objectively defining inflammation is still lacking. MSUS can be worthwhile in this context, since it is more sensitive than physical examination for detection of arthritis according to a number of studies [33–37].

In patients with joint inflammatory symptoms lasting less than 12 months, MSUS significantly increased the classification of patients as RA (31% pretest, 61% post-test) [38]. In individuals with established RA, synovial hypertrophy and pD scores of wrists and MCP correlated significantly with physician-recorded clinical outcomes and helped the rheumatologist in clinical decision [39].

Of great importance, preliminary data indicated that the MSUS methodology improved the accuracy of the 2010 ACR/EULAR criteria for identifying patients needing methotrexate treatment. $GS \geq 2$ and $pD \geq 1$ were good indicators of synovitis [40].

According to a study published in 2001, pD scan of MCP joints was a reliable method in assessment of synovitis of RA patients, considering MRI as standard [41]. In a systematic review and metanalyis of 21 studies, MSUS was more effective than conventional radiograms for detection of bone erosions; efficacy was comparable to MRI and reproducibility was good [42]. In another systematic review, MSUS added value to clinical findings for the diagnosis of RA when studying at least MCP, wrist and MTP joints; to evaluate remission, scanning of at least wrist and MCP joints of the dominant side was advocated. In both circumstances, pD was a more reliable instrument as compared to GS [43].

Recent data suggested that both MSUS and clinical examination were relevant to appraise risk of subsequent structural damage in RA patients [44]. Subclinical joint inflammation detected by imaging techniques as MSUS probably accounts for the paradoxical structural deterioration seen in RA patients allegedly in clinical remission [45]. Of note, Peluso et al. demonstrated that remission as confirmed by pD was much more prevalent in patients with early than long-standing RA [46].

We have previously reported that pD, GS and bone erosion on MSUS were associated with swollen joint count, but not with joint tenderness [47]. Concordance of physical examinationand MSUS assessment seems poor (not more than 50% between the most affected joint and pD signal), and RA structural progression has been more associated with swollen joint count than with pain [48–50].

Correlations studies of MSUS with disease activity are a matter of debate. In a study employing pD score of 22 joints and GS score of 28 joints, a defined correlation of MSUS parameters with classical measures of RA activity (acute phase proteins, DAS28) was found. Differently, correlation of MSUS scores with health assessment questionnaires were weak to moderate [51].

In a 2014 study, concordance level of standard activity measures with MSUS was evaluated. For such, a pD score of hands, radiocarpal and MTP joints was utilized. Discrepancies between pD and DAS28 occurred in 29% of cases, promoting changes in therapeutic decision, in other words, supporting DMARD escalation in patients with continuing subclinical synovitis and preventing escalation in symptomatic patients without ultrasonographic synovitis [52]. Likewise, Gartner et al. demonstrated pD signal in up to 20% of patients in remission according to DAS28 [53].

Recently, it has been shown that the 7-joint GS/pD Backhaus score showed performance comparable to clinical and laboratory data in RA patients under various therapies. Higher score predicted bone erosions after one year. Of interest, Backhaus method was sensitive enough to demonstrate decline in bone erosions in patients who switched biological agents [54]. In patients in remission, a link of GS/pD positivity with risk of clinical flare and structural progression was demonstrated by metanalysis in 2014 [55].

A 2012 study revealed that the presence of pD signal was an accurate predictor of flare in RA patients in remission [56]. Synovitis detected by pD may predict biologic therapy tapering failure in RA patients in sustained remission, according to a very recent report [57]. Adding of pD was able to identify RA patients in DAS28 remission, with subclinically active disease. The same authors reported that the combination of clinical and pD parameters recognized patients in remission who could undergo anti-TNF dose tapering [58].

It has been observed that subclinical synovitis is long-lasting in RA patients in clinical remission [59]. In a study dated from 2012, pD, but not low-field MRI, predicted relapse and radiographic progression in RA patients with low levels of disease activity [60]. In early RA patients on conventional therapy, pD-positive synovial hypertrophy identified ongoing inflammation, even during remission and also predicted a short-term relapse [61].

In an observational study of 307 RA patients, Zufferey et al. demonstrated that many subjects in clinical remission according to classical parameters (DAS28 and ACR/EULAR criteria) showed residual synovitis on GS and pD scan [62]. Yoshimi et al. documented synovitis by pD in patients in clinical inactivity and suggested that the pD parameter is essential to confirm "true remission" of RA [63].

Recently, a group of authors originally approached the correlation of MSUS with clinical scores in RA patients with and without fibromyalgia. While GS scores correlated with classical parameters in both groups, the pD analysis was more precise by correlating with clinical scores only in patients without fibromyalgia [64].

In 68 RA patients evaluated with a six-joint pD method (two MCP, wrists, knees), the global MSUS score correlated moderately with the DAS28; in this survey, pD positivity was a sensitive-to-change method for monitoring the short-term response to anti-TNF agents [65]. In a cross-sectional study of 97 RA patients, an inactive disease status defined by a 12-joint pD score (but not clinical parameters) associated, interestingly, with decrease in complement levels in patients treated with biologics [66].

In 2015, the ARTIC trial addressed the question if MSUS could correlate with DAS28 defined RA remission criteria. In 238 patients with early RA randomized to perform or not GS/pD MSUS in addition to DAS28, both strategies (MSUS included or not) were effective to estimate remission after two years of therapy [67].

In summary, there has been plenty of recent literature looking at the role of MSUS either as a complement to physical examination or as a measure of disease activity. It seems the discrepancies between US findings and clinical findings on articular examination are more important in long standing RA and/or fibromyalgia associated RA patients, where metrics are less reliable (due to difficulties in physical examinations and on pain exacerbation). It remains an open question if MSUS would work as additional or preferential criteria for assessing RA activity. MSUS looks a promising instrument for monitoring RA disease activity, but a greater body of evidence still is required.

Intra and interobserver agreement

Another critical aspect when using MSUS in the evaluation of RA is reproductibility. Inter-reader analysis of the clinical assessment of joint inflammation can itself show some discrepancy [68, 69]. Intra and interobserver discrepancies in both acquisition of image and image interpretation have been a matter of concern.

A study dated from 2007 reported that the interobserver agreement of a 3-dimensional pD scan was better (> 0.80) than a 2-dimensional quantitative pD method [70]. In healthy subjects, MSUS of MCP joints using an 18 MHz transducer yielded an excellent interobserver kappa (0.83) for erosions [71]. A fair to good concordance (kappa 0.36–0.76) of a semiquantitative MCP score for cartilage damage was described in RA patients in 2010 [72].

Subclinical joint changes in asymptomatic feet of RA patients were recently assessed. Concordance between MSUS and radiograms was low (kappa 0.08–0.40). Inter-reader agreement was excellent for bone erosion (kappa = 1), good for quantitative synovitis (0.64) and moderate (0.47) for pD signal [73].In 2011, the interobserver reliability of a synovitis MSUS resulted in moderate concordance (kappa 0.50) for quantification of synovitis in the radiocarpal joint [74].

Szkudlarek et al showed in thirty RA patients with active disease that MSUS agreement was good for erosions (kappa 0.78) and pD (0.72), and excellent for synovitis (0.81) evaluatingfive joints (second and third MCP, second PIP, first and second MTP) that were scanned by two experienced sonographers. [75]

The Swiss Sonography in Arthritis and Rheumatism (SONAR) group had previously developed a consistent MSUS method for assessing RA activity utilizing B-mode and pD scores [76]. The same group evaluated synovitis and erosion in six differentMSUS machines. Overall, agreement was not more than moderate. Considering only high-quality machines, kappa concordance was better for synovitis (0.64) than erosion (0.41) [77].

Yet in 2005, the EULAR promoted the "Train the trainers" course aiming to evaluate MSUS interobserver reliability in RA. Clinically dominant joint regions (shoulder, knee, ankle/toe, wrist/finger) were examined. Concordance was particularly high for bone lesions, bursitis, and tendon tears (kappa = 1). As a whole, interobserver concordance, sensitivities, and specificities were comparable with MRI [78].

The reliability of the Backhaus 7-joint score was evaluated in 2012 and the best interobserver concordance was obtained for bone erosions in second MTP (plantar side), with kappa of 1. Agreement for pD in palmar side of wrist was good (0.79). Intraobserver reliability of the method was moderate to substantial [79].

In our own experience, we have been employing a 10-joint score exclusively of hand/wrist joints (dorsal aspects of wrists and second and third MCP, and volar aspect of second and third PIP joints of both hands). After evaluating 1380 joints of 60 RA patients, kappa agreement for synovitis ranged from fair to good (0.30–0.70); for cartilage changes, also from fair to good (0.28–0.63; for pD signal, from moderate to absolute agreement (0.53–1); and for erosions, from good to excellent (0.70–0.97) [80].

In 2014, the LUMINA European study assessed the reliability of grading MSUS videoclips with hand pathology in RA by employing non-sophisticated internet tools. Intra-reader concordance for GS/pD synovitis was moderate to good (0.52/0.62), while the interobserver agreement for global synovitis (synovitis and tenosynovitis) was not more than moderate (0.45) [81].

Also recently, a short collegiate consensus attempted to improve MSUS interobserver reliability. Concordance was good for B mode synovitis (0.75) and excellent for pD (0.88). Kappa values were excelllent for small hand joints, but poor to fair in wrists, elbows, ankles and MTP. Admittedly, the consensus meeting was useful to improve agreement in synovits scores of still images. Moreover, the consensus strongly emphasized the need for standards of image acquisition and interpretation [82].

The several studies [68–82] evaluating reliability of MSUS scores have revealed some variation. As a whole, MSUS seems very reliable for bone erosions (kappa ranging from good to excellent); in turn, the grade of agreement for synovitis, although generally moderate to good, has shown more fluctuation. Standardized training seems essential to improve all these outcomes.

Ultrasound scores

A high-resolution machine with a linear high-frequency probe (7.5–18 MHz) should be utilized for evaluation of small joints. In the most widely used scoring systems, semiquantitative GS, generated in the B-mode, synovial proliferation is classified as: zero (absent); 1) mild (slight hipoechoic or anechoic image in articular capsule); 2) moderate (presence of elevation of articular capsule); 3) severe or marked (important distension of articular capsule). The semiquantitative scale of pD signal stratifies inflammatory activity and angiogenesis as follows: zero (absent); 1) mild (one pD signal); 2) moderate (two or more pD signal, meaning < 50% of intraarticular flow); 3) severe or marked (> 50% of intraarticular flow) [83]. In addition, Carotti et al. reported that the resistive index (RI), using spectral Doppler, quantified inflammation in microvessels of finger joints and wrists and discriminated RA synovitis (higher values) from normal subjects [84]. Bone erosions, in turn, are defined according to the OMERACT criteria and are classified as present or absent [85]. Figure 1 illustrates MSUS findings in normal and RA hand joints.

There has been no agreement regarding which joints and tendons should be systematically examined in MSUS of RA patients. A number of different methods and scores have been advocated, without wide concordance to date. As a whole, it was proposed to include dorsal and volar exam of the hands in daily practice and clinical trials [33], but volar examination might not be consensual.

Historically, MSUS scores were firstly proposed in 2005 by two groups of authors [83, 86]. Scheel et al. described different MCP and PIP scores for GS and pD [86]. In 2006, Loeuille et al. reported a 7-joint GS/pD score including wrist, MCP and MTP of dominant side [87]. One year later, an 8-joint system evaluating GS/pD of MCP and MTP of dominant side was proposed by Hensch et al. [88]. In 2008, Iagnocco et al. designed a 10-joint method including MCP, PIP, wrist and knee including tenosynovitis, bursitis and erosion in addition to GS/pD [89]. Also in 2008, a 12-joint simplified MSUS including elbow, wrist, MCP, knee and ankle was reported by Naredo [90].

The 7-joint MSUS score proposed by Backaus et al. in 2009 has been the most largely utilized in recent

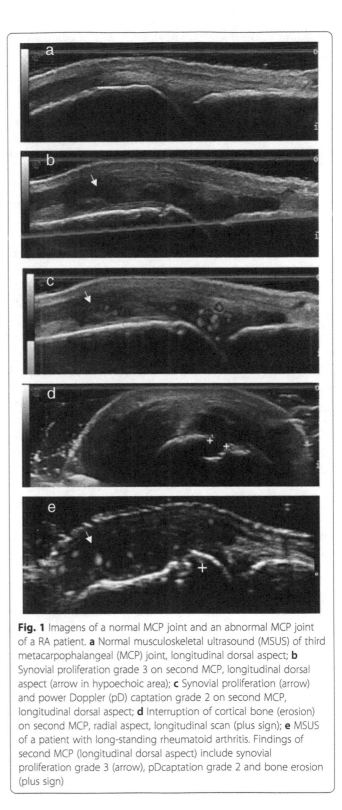

Fig. 1 Imagens of a normal MCP joint and an abnormal MCP joint of a RA patient. **a** Normal musculoskeletal ultrasound (MSUS) of third metacarpophalangeal (MCP) joint, longitudinal dorsal aspect; **b** Synovial proliferation grade 3 on second MCP, longitudinal dorsal aspect (arrow in hypoechoic area); **c** Synovial proliferation (arrow) and power Doppler (pD) captation grade 2 on second MCP, longitudinal dorsal aspect; **d** Interruption of cortical bone (erosion) on second MCP, radial aspect, longitudinal scan (plus sign); **e** MSUS of a patient with long-standing rheumatoid arthritis. Findings of second MCP (longitudinal dorsal aspect) include synovial proliferation grade 3 (arrow), pDcaptation grade 2 and bone erosion (plus sign)

literature and includes five hand and two foot joints of the clinically dominant side: wrist, second and third MCP and proximal interphalangeal (PIP), and second and fifth metatarsophalangeal (MTP) joints. This score also evaluated tenosynovitis and erosive changes [91].

In 2010, Hammer et al. proposed a 78-joint GS/pD score [92]. In 2012, a 6-joint MSUS score of wrists,

MCP and knees utilized synovial effusion in conjunction with the synovial proliferation and pD parameters. This score was practical, trustworthy and sensitive-to-change for evaluating synovial inflammation in RA [93].

Of note, a semi-quantitative 10-joint score of synovial thickness and pD which included only MCP joints was proved a reliable endpoint in a clinical trial [94]. A modified 7-joint score adding dorsal and palmar recesses of the wrists, as well as of small joints of hands and feet, was described in 2014. In a survey of 32 patients with early RA (832 joints examined), GS and pD were sensitive to detect synovitis [95]. A total pD score of 8-joint (bilateral wrist, knee, and the second and third MCP joints), reported in 2015, was found to be a simple and effective tool for monitoring RA activity [96].

Also very recently, a 12-joint score evaluating synovial hypertrophy by B-mode technology and synovitis by pD signal was described. The wrist–hand–ankle–MTP assessments were able to predict unstable remission in RA patients presumably inactive on methotrexate therapy [97].

With such heterogeneity in the previously mentioned scores, it is important to verify if scores with low number of joints correlate well with scores involving more joints, in order to find a set feasible for clinical daily practice. For instance, the 7-joint Backaus score significantly correlated with a 12-joint instrument for monitoring of response to infliximab in RA patients, according to a 2016 study [98].

A novel GS/pD score composed of a bilateral approach of six hand joints (first, second and third MCP joints, second and third PIP joints and radiocarpal joint), two feet joints (second and third MTP) and, in addition, one tendon (extensor carpi ulnaris), performed better than previous scores in a longitudinal analysis [99]. Using a data-driven approach, the same group of authors set out to validate a new MSUS score in a large survey of early or established RA. The set comprising GS/pD scores of seven joints/two tendons (first and second MCP, second MCP, third PIP, radiocarpal, elbow, first and second MTP, tibialis posterior tendon, extensor carpi ulnaris tendon) preserved most of the information when compared to a 9-joint score (which added fifth MCP and fifth MTP) [100].

A systematic review of 14 studies published in 2011 did not yield a consensus as to the minimal number of joints to be included in a global MSUS score [101]. Newer recommendations after critical analysis of the most recent MSUS scores are expected. Table 1 lists, in chronological order, the MSUS scores described so far.

Conclusion

MSUS is an useful instrument to complement the physical examination of RA patients. The method is quick and safe. The GS/pD scales are helpful to detect early synovitis and MSUS is also sensitive in the identification of bone erosions.

The method is of interest to identify subclinical disease activity in patients considered to be in clinical remission and might add relevant information regarding response to therapy. Whether targeted therapy to pD activity would provide superior outcomes compared with treating to clinical targets alone, it is still a matter of open discussion, which was recently highlighted by the Targeted Ultrasound Initiative group [102]. Proper clinical trials are warranted to clarify this point.

Table 1 Musculoskeletal ultrasound scores described in chronological order

Author/reference	Year	Joint characteristic/score elements
Naredo et al. [83]	2005	12-joint (wrists, MCP, PIP, knees); GS/pD
Scheel et al. [86]	2005	Three different MCP/PIP scores; GS/pD
Loeuille et al. [87]	2006	7-joint (wrists, MCP, MTP); GS/pD
Hensch et al. [88]	2007	8-joint (MCP, MTP); GS/pD
Iagnocco et al. [89]	2008	10-joint (MCP, PIP, wrist, knee); GS/pD, tenosynovitis, bursitis, erosion
Naredo et al. [90]	2008	12-joint (elbow, wrist, MCP, knee, ankle); GS/pD, tenosynovitis, bursitis
Backhaus et al. [91]	2009	7-joint (wrist, MCP, PIP, MTP); GS/pD, tenosynovitis, erosion
Hammer et al. [92]	2010	78-joint; GS/pD
Perricone et al. [93]	2012	6-joint (wrists, second MCP and knees); synovial effusion, GS/pD
Seymour et al. [94]	2012	10-joint (MCP); GS/pD
Mendonça et al. [95]	2014	7-joint (wrists, MCP, MTF); GS/pD
Yoshimi et al. [96]	2015	8-joint (wrists, knees, MCP); pD
Aga A et al. [99]	2015	6-joint (MCP, PIP, radiocarpal, MTP, extensor carpi ulnaris); GS/pD
Aga A et al. [100]	2015	7-joint/2 tendon (MCP, PIP, radiocarpal, elbow, MTP, tibialis posterior tendon, extensor carpi ulnaris tendon); GS/pD
Janta I et al. [97]	2016	12-joint (wrist, hand, ankle, MTP); B-mode, pD, tenosynovitis

GS gray scale, *pD* power Doppler, *MCP* metacarpophalangeal joint, *PIP* proximal interphalangeal joint, *MTP* metatarsophalangeal joint

Correlation of MSUS parameters with synovial tissue inflammatory activity and cytokines is also an area to be searched. Exploring this field may disclose new physio-pathological features of synovitis and also better clarify the meaning of MSUS parameters.

Importantly, MSUS is practical, feasible and less expensive than MRI. Quality of MSUS devices is surely an item of major importance. Better training and competency of sonographers, allied to incorporation of modern ultrasound will certainly improve MSUS performance in the following years [103].

For the time being, a number of points regarding employment of MSUS in rheumatological daily practice demand elucidation. Validity and reproducibility of MSUS scores have still to be improved (interobserver concordance is yet variable – just like clinical assessment). Choice of equipment and selection of parameters to be utilized (pD alone, pD plus GS, bone erosions, cartilage changes, synovial effusion, tenosynovitis, spectral Doppler) are also pending issues.

Since a pD signal can be also seen in healthy joints [104], the adding of spectral Doppler and estimate of RI might provide useful information regarding the flow in synovial membrane (low RI are seen in inflamed joints) [105]. New data on reliability of RI as a measure of synovial flow and microvessel inflammation should be available shortly.

Above all, MSUS score standardization, considering the particularities of each affected joint or tendon, is surely a requirement. Solved these questions, MSUS will consolidate its role as a reliable instrument to complement physical examination, appraise disease activity and monitor response to therapy in RA management.

Key messages

1) MSUS can be nowadays considered a complement to physical exam in patients with rheumatoid arthritis (RA).
2) MSUS seems to correlate well with indexes of disease activity in RA patients. Subclinical synovitis seen on MSUS could help the physician in clinical decisions.
3) Standardization of MSUS techniques is necessary to consolidate the method in clinical practice.

Abbreviations
ACR: American College of Rheumatology; DAS: Disease Activity Score; DAS28: Disease Activity Score in 28 joints; EULAR: Europena League Against Rheumatism; GS: gray scale; IL-17: interleukin 17; IL-6: interleukin 6; MCP: metacarpophangeal joint; MRI: magnetic resonance imaging; MSUS: musculoskeletal ultrasound; MTP: metatarsophalangeal joint; OMERACT: Outcome Measures in Rheumatology; pD: power Doppler; RA: rheumatoid arthritis; TNF: tumor necrosis factor; VEGF: vascular endothelial growth factor

Authors' contributions
AP, HS, JPP, IGS, JAM, MCB and JEF carried out literature search and reviewed the articles. AP and HS wrote the manuscript. JPP, IGS, JAM, MCB and JEF reviewed the manuscript and made adjustments to the text and contributed to update the review. All authors read and approved the final manuscript.

Authors' information
JAM is currently the chief of the "Image in Rheumatology" Committee of the Brazilian Society of Rheumatology.
AP and IGS teach rheumatology fellows on the use of ultrasound in Rheumatology.

Author details
[1]Rheumatology Unit, Nossa Senhora da Conceição Hospital, Porto Alegre, RS, Brazil. [2]Rheumatology Department, Sao Lucas Hospital, Faculty of Medicine of Pontifical Catholic University of Rio Grande do Sul (PUCRS), Av Ipiranga, 6690/220, Porto Alegre 90610-000, Brazil. [3]Rheumatology Unit, Pontifical Catholic University of Campinas (PUCCAMP), Campinas, SP, Brazil. [4]Rheumatology Research Unit, Instituto de Medicina Molecular, Faculdade de Medicina, Universidade de Lisboa, Lisbon, Portugal. [5]Rheumatology Department, Hospital de Santa Maria, Lisbon Academic Medical Centre, Lisbon, Portugal.

References
1. Scott D, Wolfe F, Huizinga T. Rheumatoid arthritis. Lancet. 2010;376:1094–108.
2. McInnes I, Schett G. Cytokines in the pathogenesis of rheumatoid arthritis. Nat Rev Immunol. 2007;7:429–42.
3. Ohrndorf S, Backhaus M. Pro musculoskeletal ultrasonography in rheumatoid arthritis. Clin Exp Rheumatol. 2015;33:S50–3.
4. Filippucci E, Iagnocco A, Meenagh G. Ultrasound imaging for the rheumatologist. Clin Exp Rheumatol. 2006;24:1–5.
5. Zayat AS, Ellegaard K, Conaghan PG, Terslev L, EM a H, Freeston JE, et al. The specificity of ultrasound-detected bone erosions for rheumatoid arthritis. Ann Rheum Dis. 2015;74:897–903.
6. Iwamoto T, Ikeda K, Hosokawa J, Yamagata M, Tanaka S, Norimoto A, Sanayama Y, Nakagomi D, et al. Prediction of relapse after discontinuation of biologic agents by ultrasonographic assessment in patients with rheumatoid arthritis in clinical remission: high predictive values of total gray-scale and power Doppler scores that represent residual synovial. Arthritis Care Res. 2014;66:1576–81.
7. Pineda C, Reginato AM, Flores V, Aliste M, Alva M, Aragón-Laínez RA, et al. Pan-American league of associations for rheumatology (PANLAR) recommendations and guidelines for musculoskeletal ultrasound training in the Americas for rheumatologists. J Clin Rheumatol. 2010;16:113–8.
8. Colebatch A, Edwards C, Østergaard M, van der Heijde D, Balint P, D'Agostino M, et al. EULAR recommendations for the use of imaging of the joints in the clinical management of rheumatoid arthritis. Ann Rheum Dis. 2013;72:804–14.
9. Andersen M, Ellegaard K, Hebsgaard JB, Christensen R, Torp-Pedersen S, Kvist PH, et al. Ultrasound colour Doppler is associated with synovial pathology in biopsies from hand joints in rheumatoid arthritis patients: a cross-sectional study. Ann Rheum Dis. 2014;73:678–83.
10. Alivernini S, Peluso G, Fedele AL, Tolusso B, Gremese E, Ferraccioli G. Tapering and discontinuation of TNF-α blockers without disease relapse using ultrasonography as a tool to identify patients with rheumatoid arthritis in clinical and histological remission. Arthritis Res Ther. 2016;18:39.
11. Anandarajah A, Thiele R, Giampoli E, Monu J, Seo GS, Feng C, et al. Patients with rheumatoid arthritis in clinical remission manifest persistent joint inflammation on histology and imaging studies. J Rheumatol. 2014;41:2153–60.
12. Takase K, Ohno S, Takeno M, Hama M, Kirino Y, Ihata A, et al. Simultaneous evaluation of long-lasting knee synovitis in patients undergoing arthroplasty

by power Dopplerultrasonography and contrast-enhanced MRI in comparison with histopathology. Clin Exp Rheumatol. 2012;30:85–92.

13. Koski J. Doppler Imaging and Histology of the Synovium. J Rheumatol. 2012;39:452–3.

14. Paleolog EM. The vasculature in rheumatoid arthritis: cause or consequence? Int J Exp Pathol. 2009;90:249–61.

15. Koski JM, Saarakkala S, Helle M, Hakulinen U, Heikkinen JO, Hermunen H. Power Doppler ultrasonography and synovitis: correlating ultrasound imaging with histopathological findings and evaluating the performance of ultrasound equipments. Ann Rheum Dis. 2006;65:1590–5.

16. Koski JM, Saarakkala S, Helle M, Hakulinen U, Heikkinen JO, Hermunen H, et al. Assessing the intra- and inter-reader reliability of dynamic ultrasound images in power Doppler ultrasonography. Ann Rheum Dis. 2006;65:1658–60.

17. Walther M, Harms H, Krenn V, Radke S, Faehndrich TP, Gohlke F. Correlation of power Doppler sonography with vascularity of the synovial tissue of the knee joint in patients with osteoarthritis and rheumatoid arthritis. Arthritis Rheum. 2001;44:331–8.

18. Kitchen J, Kane D. Greyscale and power Doppler ultrasonographic evaluation of normal synovial joints: correlation with pro- and anti-inflammatory cytokines and angiogenic factors. Rheumatology (Oxford). 2015;54:458–62.

19. Ramirez J, Ruiz-Esquide V, Pomes I, Celis R, Cuervo A, Hernandez M, et al. Patients with rheumatoid arthritis in clinical remission and ultrasound-defined active synovitis exhibit higher disease activity and incresed serum levels of angiogenic biomarkers. Arthritis Res Ther. 2014;16:R5.

20. Strunk J, Heineman E, Neeck G, Schmidt KL, Lange U. A new approach to studying angiogenesis in rheumatoid arthritis by means of power Doppler ultrasonography and measurement of serum vascular endothelial growth factor. Rheumatology. 2004;43:1480–3.

21. Terslev L, Torp-Pedersen S, Bang N, Koenig MJ, Nielsen MB, Bliddal H. Doppler ultrasound findings in healthy wrists and finger joints before and after use of two different contrast agents. Ann Rheum Dis. 2005;64:824–7.

22. Klauser A, Frauscher F, Schirmer M, Halpern E, Pallwein L, Herold M, et al. The value of contrast-enhanced color Doppler ultrasound in the detection of vascularization of finger joints in patients with rheumatoid arthritis. Arthritis Rheum. 2002;46:647–53.

23. Fiocco U, Ferro F, Cozzi L, Vezzù M, Sfriso P, Checchetto C, et al. Contrast medium in power Doppler ultrasound for assessment of synovial vascularity: comparison with arthroscopy. J Rheumatol. 2003;30:2170–6.

24. Szkudlarek M, Court-Payen M, Strandberg C, Klarlund M, Klausen T, Østergaard M. Contrast-enhanced power Doppler ultrasonography of the metacarpophalangeal joints in rheumatoid arthritis. Eur Radiol. 2003;13:163–8.

25. Andersen M, Boesen M, Ellegaard K, Christensen R, Söderström K, Søe N, et al. Synovial explant inflammatory mediator production corresponds to rheumatoid arthritis imaging hallmarks: a cross-sectional study. Arthritis Res Ther. 2014;16:R107.

26. Do Prado AD, Bisi MC, Piovesan DM, Bredemeier M, Batista TS, Petersen L, et al. Ultrasound power Doppler synovitis is associated with plasma IL-6 in established rheumatoid arthritis. Cytokine. 2016;83:27–32.

27. Ball E, Gibson D, Rooney AB. Plasma IL-6 levels correlate with clinical and ultrasound measures of arthritis in patients with systemic lupus erythematosus. Lupus. 2014;23:46–56.

28. Brzustewicz E, Bryl E. The role of cytokines in the pathogenesis of rheumatoid arthritis. Practical and potential application of cytokines as biomarkers and targets of personalized therapy. Cytokine. 2015;76:527–36.

29. Baillet A, Gossec L, Paternotte L, Paternotte S, Etcheto A, Combe B, et al. Evaluation of serum Interleukin-6 level as a surrogate marker of synovial inflammation and as a factor of structural progression in early rheumatoid arthritis: results from a French National Multicenter Cohort. Arthritis Care Res (Hoboken). 2015;67:905–12.

30. Fazaa A, Ben Abdelghani K, Abdeladhim M, Laatar A, Ben Ahmed M, Zakraoui L. The level of interleukin-17 in serum is linked to synovial hypervascularization in rheumatoid arthritis. Jt Bone Spine. 2014;81:550–1.

31. Gullick N, Evans H, Church L, Javaraj D, Filer A. Linking power Doppler ultrasound to the presence of Th17 cells in the rheumatoid. PLoS One. 2010;5:e12516.

32. Van der Heijde D, van 't Hof M, van Riel P, Theunisse L, Lubberts E, van Leeuwen M, et al. Judging disease activity in clinical practice in rheumatoid arthritis: first step in the development of a disease activity score. Ann Rheum Dis. 1990;49:916–20.

33. Vlad V, Berghea F, Libianu S, Balanescu A, Bojinca V, Constantinescu C, Abobului M, Predeteanu D, Ionescu R. Ultrasound in rheumatoid arthritis: volar versus dorsal synovitis evaluation and scoring. BMC Musculoskelet Disord. 2011;12:124.

34. Szkudlarek M, Narvestad E, Klarlund M, Court-Payen M, Thomsen HS, Østergaard M. Ultrasonography of the metatarsophalangeal joints in rheumatoid arthritis: comparison with magnetic resonance imaging, conventional radiography, and clinical examination. Arthritis Rheum. 2004; 50:2103–12.

35. Salaffi F, Filippucci E, Carotti M, Naredo E, Meenagh G, Ciapetti A, et al. Inter-observer agreement of standard joint counts in early rheumatoid arthritis: a comparison with grey scale ultrasonography - a preliminary study. Rheumatology (Oxford). 2008;47:54–8.

36. Ogishima H, Tsuboi H, Umeda N, Horikoshi M, Kondo Y, Sugihara M. Analysis of subclinical synovitis detected by ultrasonography and low-field magnetic resonance imaging in patients with rheumatoid arthritis. Mod Rheumatol. 2014;24:60–8.

37. Mendonca J, Yazbek M, Laurindo I, Bertolo M. Wrist ultrasound analysis of patients with early rheumatoid arthritis. Braz J Med Biol Res. 2011;44:11–5.

38. Rezaei H, Torp-Pedersen S, af Klint E, Backheden M, Kisten Y, Gyori N, et al. Diagnostic utility of musculoskeletal ultrasound in patients with suspected arthritis - a probabilistic approach. Arthritis Res Ther. 2014;16:448–55.

39. Ceponis A, Onishi M, Bluestein H, Kalunian K, Townsend J, Kavanaugh A. Utility of the ultrasound examination of the hand and wrist joints in the management of established rheumatoid arthritis. Arthritis Care Res. 2014;66:236–44.

40. Nakagomi D, Ikeda K, Okubo A, Iwamoto T, Sanayama Y, Takahashi K, et al. Ultrasound can improve the accuracy of the 2010 American College of Rheumatology/European league against rheumatism classification criteria for rheumatoid arthritis to predict the requirement for methotrexate treatment. Arthritis Rheum. 2013;65:890–8.

41. Szkudlarek M, Court-Payen M, Strandberg C, Klarlund M, Klausen T, Ostergaard M. Power Doppler ultrasonography for assessment of synovitis in the metacarpophalangeal joints of patients with rheumatoid arthritis: a comparison with dynamic magnetic resonance imaging. Arthritis Rheum. 2001;44:2018–23.

42. Baillet A, Gaujoux-Viala C, Mouterde G, Pham T, Tebib J, Saraux A, Fautrel B, Cantagrel A, Le Loët X, Gaudin P. Comparison of the efficacy of sonography, magnetic resonance imaging and conventional radiography for the detection of bone erosions in rheumatoid arthritis patients: a systematic review and meta-analysis. Rheumatology (Oxford). 2011;50:1137–47.

43. Ten Cate DF, Luime JJ, Swen N, Gerards AH, De Jager MH, Basoski NM. Role of ultrasonography in diagnosing early rheumatoid arthritis and remission of rheumatoid arthritis - a systematic review of the literature. Arthritis Res Ther. 2013;15:R4.

44. Dougados M, DEvauchelle-Pensec V, Ferlet J, Jousse-Joulin S, D'Agostino M, Backhaus M. The ability of synovitis to predict structural damage in rheumatoid arthritis: a comparative study between clinical examination and ultrasound. Ann Rheum Dis. 2013;72:665–71.

45. Brown A, Conaghan P, Karim Z, Quinn M, Ikeda K, Peterfy C, et al. An explanation for the apparent dissociation between clinical remission and continued structural deterioration in rheumatoid arthritis. Arthritis Rheum. 2008;58:2958–67.

46. Peluso G, Michelutti A, Bosello S, Gremese E, Toluso B, Ferraccioli G. Clinical and ultrasonographic remission determines different changes of relapse in early and long standing rheumatoid arthritis. Ann Rheum Dis. 2011;70:172–5.

47. Do Prado AD, Bisi M, Piovesan D, Bredemeieir M, Silveira I, Mendonça J, et al. Association of clinical examination with gray scale and power Doppler ultrassonography in established rheumatoid arthritis. J Clin Rheumatol. 2016; in press

48. Yoshimi R, Toyota Y, Tsuchida N, Sugiyama Y, Kunishita Y, Kishimoto D, et al. Considerable discrepancy between Patient's assessment and ultrasonography assessment on the most affected joint in rheumatoid arthritis [abstract]. Arthritis Rheumatol. 2015;67:S10.

49. Filer A, de Pablo P, Allen G, Nightingale P, Jordan A, Jobanputra P. Utility of ultrasound joint counts in the prediction of rheumatoid arthritis in patients with very early synovitis. Ann Rheum Dis. 2011;70:500–7.

50. Smolen J, Van Der Heijde D, St Clair E, Emery P, Bathon J, Keystone E, et al. Predictors of joint damage in patients with early rheumatoid arthritis treated with high-dose methotrexate with or without concomitant infliximab: results from the ASPIRE trial. Arthritis Rheum. 2006;54:702–10.

Ultrasound and its clinical use in rheumatoid arthritis: Where do we...

9

51. Damjanov N, Radunovic G, Prodanovic S, Vukovic V, Milic V, SimicPasalic K. Construct validity and reliability of ultrasound disease activity score in assessing joint inflammation in RA: comparison with DAS-28. Rheumatology (Oxford). 2012;51:120–8.

52. Dale J, Purves D, McConnachie A, McInnes I, Porter D. Tightening up? Impact of musculoskeletal ultrasound disease activity assessment on early rheumatoid arthritis patients treated using a treat to target strategy. Arthritis Care Res. 2014;66:19–26.

53. Gärtner M, Mandl P, Radner H, Supp G, Machold K, Aletaha D, et al. Sonographic joint assessment in rheumatoid arthritis: associations with clinical joint assessment during a state of remission. Arthritis Rheum. 2013; 65:2005–14.

54. Backhaus T, Ohrndorf S, Kellner H, Strunk J, Hartung W, Sattler H, et al. The US7 score is sensitive to change in a large cohort of patients with rheumatoid arthritis over 12 months of therapy. Ann Rheum Dis. 2013;72:1163–9.

55. Nguyen H, Ruyssen-Witrand A, Gandjbakhch F, Constantin A, Foltz V, Cantagrel A. Prevalence of ultrasound-detected residual synovitis and risk of relapse and structural progression in rheumatoid arthritis patients in clinical remission: a systematic review and meta-analysis. Rheumatology. 2014;53:2110–8.

56. Saleem B, Brown A, Quinn M, Karim Z, Hensor E, Conaghan P, et al. Can flare be predicted in DMARD treated RA patients in remission, and is it important? A cohort study. Ann Rheum Dis. 2012;71:1316–21.

57. Naredo E, Valor L, De la Torre I, Montoro M, Bello N, Martinez-Barrio J, et al. Predictive value of Doppler ultrasound-detected synovitis in relation to failed tapering of biologic therapy in patients with rheumatoid arthritis. Rheumatology. 2015;54:1408–14.

58. Marks J, Holroyd C, Dimitrov B, Armstrong R, Calogeras A, Cooper C, et al. Does combined clinical and ultrasound assessment allow selection of individuals with rheumatoid arthritis for sustained reduction of anti-tumor necrosis factor therapy? Arthritis Care Res. 2015;67:746–53.

59. Gärtner M, Alasti F, Supp G, Mandl P, Smolen J, Aletaha D. Persistence of subclinical sonographic joint activity in rheumatoid arthritis in sustained clinical remission. Ann Rheum Dis. 2015;74:2050–3.

60. Foltz V, Gandjbakhch F, Etchepare F, Rosenberg C, Tanguy M, Rozenberg S, et al. Power Doppler ultrasound, but not low-field magnetic resonance imaging, predicts relapse and radiographic disease progression in rheumatoid arthritis patients with low levels of disease activity. Arthritis Rheum. 2012;64:67–76.

61. Scirè C, Montecucco C, Codullo V, Epis O, Todoerti M, Caporali R. Ultrasonographic evaluation of joint involvement in early rheumatoid arthritis in clinical remission: power Doppler signal predicts short-term relapse. Rheumatol. 2009;48:1092–7.

62. Zufferey P, Möller B, Brulhart L, Tamborrini G, Scherer A, Finckh A, et al. Persistence of ultrasound synovitis in patients with rheumatoid arthritis fulfilling the DAS28 and/or the new ACR/EULAR RA remission definitions: results of an observational cohort study. Joint Bone Spine. 2014;81:426–32.

63. Yoshimi R, Hama M, Takase K, Ihata A, Kishimoto D, Terauchi K, et al. Ultrasonography is a potent tool for the prediction of progressive joint destruction during clinical remission of rheumatoid arthritis. Mod Rheumatol. 2013;23:456–65.

64. da Silva Chakr RM, Brenol JC, Behar M, Mendonça JA, Kohem CL, Monticielo OA, et al. Is ultrasound a better target than clinical disease activity scores in rheumatoid arthritis with fibromyalgia? A case-control study. PLoS One. 2015;10:e0118620.

65. Iagnocco A, Finucci A, Ceccarelli F, Perricone C, Iorgoveanu V, Valesini G. Power Doppler ultrasound monitoring of response to anti-tumour necrosis factor alpha treatment in patients with rheumatoid arthritis. Rheumatology (Oxford). 2015;54:1890–6.

66. Montoro Alvarez M, Chong OY, Janta I, González C, López-Longo J, Monteagudo I, Valor L, et al. Relation of Doppler ultrasound synovitis versus clinical synovitis with changes in native complement component levels in rheumatoid arthritis patients treated with biologic disease-modifying anti-rheumatic drugs. Clin Exp Rheumatol. 2015;33:141–5.

67. Haavardsholm E, Aga A, Olsen I, Hammer H, Uhlig T, Fremstad H, et al. Aiming for remission in rheumatoid arthritis: clinical and radiographic outcomes from a randomized controlled strategy trial investigating the added value of ultrasonography in a treat-to-target regimen [abstract]. Arthritis Rheumatol. 2015;67:S10.

68. Hart LE, Tugwell P, Buchanan WW, Norman GR, Grace EM, Southwell D. Grading of tenderness as a source of interrater error in the Ritchie articular index. J Rheumatol. 1985;12:716–7.

69. Thompson PW, Hart LE, Goldsmith CH, Spector TD, Bell MJ, Ramsden MF. Comparison of four articular indices for use in clinical trials in rheumatoid arthritis: patient, order and observer variation. J Rheumatol. 1991;18:661–5.

70. Strunk J, Strube K, Rumbaur C, Lange U, Müller-Ladner U. Interobserver agreement in two- and three-dimensional power Doppler sonographic assessment of synovial vascularity during anti-inflammatory treatment in patients with rheumatoid arthritis. Ultraschall Med. 2007;28:409–15.

71. Fodor D, Felea I, Popescu D, Motei A, Ene P, Serban O, Micu M. Ultrasonography of the metacarpophalangeal joints in healthy subjects using an 18 MHz transducer. Med Ultrason. 2015;17:185–91.

72. Filippucci E, da Luz KR, Di Geso L, Salaffi F, Tardella M, Carotti M, et al. Interobserver reliability of ultrasonography in the assessment of cartilage damage in rheumatoid arthritis. Ann Rheum Dis. 2010;69:1845–8.

73. Sant'Ana Petterle G, Natour J, Rodrigues da Luz K, Soares Machado F, dos Santos MF, da Rocha Correa Fernandes A, et al. Usefulness of US to show subclinical joint abnormalities in asymptomatic feet of RA patients compared to healthy controls. Clin Exp Rheumatol. 2013;31:904–12.

74. Luz KR, Furtado R, Mitraud SV, Porglhof J, Nunes C, Fernandes AR, Natour J. Interobserver reliability in ultrasound assessment of rheumatoid wrist joints. ActaReumatol Port. 2011;36:245–50.

75. Szkudlarek M, Court-Payen M, Jacobsen S, Klarlund M, Thomsen HS, Østergaard M. Interobserver agreement in ultrasonography of the finger and toe joints in rheumatoid arthritis. Arthritis Rheum. 2003;48:955–62.

76. Zufferey P, Brulhart L, Tamborrini G, Finckh A, Scherer A, Moller B, et al. Ultrasound evaluation of synovitis in RA: correlation with clinical disease activity and sensitivity to change in an observational cohort study. Jt Bone Spine. 2014;81:222–7.

77. Brulhart L, Ziswiler HR, Tamborrini G, Zufferey P, SONAR/SCQM programmes. The importance of sonographer experience and machine quality with regards to the role of musculoskeletal ultrasound in routine care of rheumatoid arthritis patients. Clin Exp Rheumatol. 2015;33:98–101.

78. Scheel AK, Schmidt WA, Hermann KG, Bruyn GA, D'Agostino MA, Grassi W, et al. Interobserver reliability of rheumatologists performing musculoskeletal ultrasonography: results from a EULAR "train the trainers" course. Ann Rheum Dis. 2005;64:1043–9.

79. Ohrndorf S, Fischer IU, Kellner H, Strunk J, Hartung W, Reiche B, et al. Reliability of the novel 7-joint ultrasound score: results from an inter- and intraobserver study performed by rheumatologists. Arthritis Care Res (Hoboken). 2012;64:1238–43.

80. Bisi M, do Prado A, Rabelo C, Brollo F, da Silveira I, JA M, et al. Articular ultrasonography: interobserver reliability in rheumatoid arthritis. Rev Bras Reumatol. 2014;54:250–4.

81. Vlad V, Berghea F, Iagnocco A, Micu M, Damjanov N, Skakic V, et al. Inter & intra-observer reliability of grading ultrasound videoclips with hand pathology in rheumatoid arthritis by using non- sophisticated internet tools (LUMINA study). Med Ultrason. 2014;16:32–6.

82. Cheung PP, Kong KO, Chew LC, Chia FL, Law WG, Lian TY, Tan YK, Cheng YK. Achieving consensus in ultrasonography synovitis scoring in rheumatoid arthritis. Int J Rheum Dis. 2014;17:776–81.

83. Naredo E, Bonilla G, Gamero F, Uson J, Carmona L, Laffon A. Assessment of inflammatory activity in rheumatoid arthritis: a comparative study of clinical evaluation with grey scale and power Doppler ultrassonography. Ann Rheum Dis. 2005;64:375–81.

84. Carotti M, Salaffi F, Morbiducci J, Ciapetti A, Bartolucci L, Gasparini S, et al. Colour Doppler ultrasonography evaluation of vascularization in the wrist and finger joints in rheumatoid arthritis patients and healthy subjects. Eur J Radiol. 2012;81:1834–8.

85. Wakefield R, Balint P, Szkudlarek M, Fillipucci E, Backhaus M, D'Agostino M. OMERACT 7 Special Interest Group. Musculoskeletal ultrasound including definitions for ultrasonographic pathology. J Rheumatol. 2005;32:2485–7.

86. Scheel AK, Hermann KG, Kahler E, et al. A novel ultrasonografic synovitis scoring system suitable for analyzing finger joint inflammation in rheumatoid arthritis. Arthritis Rheum. 2005;52:733–43.

87. Loeuille D, Sommier JP. ScUSI, an ultrasound inflammatory score, predicts sharp progression at 7 months in RA patients. Arthritis Rheum. 2006;54:S139.

88. Hensch A, Hermann KG. Impact of B mode, power Doppler and contrast enhanced ultrasonography in RA patients on anti-TNF alfa therapy. Arthritis Rheum. 2007;56:S280.

89. Iagnocco A, Filippucci E, Perella C, Ceccarelli F, Cassarà E, Alessandri C, et al. Clinical and ultrasonographic monitoring of response to adalimumabe treatment in rheumatoid arthritis. J Rheumatol. 2008;35:35–40.

90. Naredo E, Rodríguez M, Campos C, Rodríguez-Heredia JM, Medina JA, Giner E, Martínez O, et al. Validity, reproducibility, and responsiveness of a twelve-joint simplified power dopplerultrasonographic assessment of joint inflammation in rheumatoid arthritis. Arthritis Rheum. 2008;59:515–22.

91. Backhaus M, Ohrndorf S, Kellner H, Strunk J, Backhaus T, Hartung W. Evaluation of a novel 7-joint ultrasound score in daily rheumatologic practise: a pilot project. Arthritis Rheum. 2009;61:1194–201.

92. Hammer HB, Sveinsson M, Kongtorp AK, Kvien TK. A 78-joints ultrasonographic assessment is associated with clinical assessments and is highly responsive to improvement in a longitudinal study of patients with rheumatoid arthritis starting adalimumab treatment. Ann Rheum Dis. 2010;69:1349–51.

93. Perricone C, Ceccarelli F, Modesti M, Vavala C, Di Franco M, Valesini G, Iagnocco A. The 6-joint ultrasonographic assessment: a valid, sensitive-to-change and feasible method for evaluating joint inflammation in RA. Rheumatology (Oxford). 2012;51:866–73.

94. Seymour M, Pétavy F, Chiesa F, Perry H, Lukey PT, Binks M, et al. Ultrasonographic measures of synovitis in an early phase clinical trial: a double-blind, randomized, placebo and comparator controlled phase IIa trial of GW274150 (a selective inducible nitric oxide synthase inhibitor in rheumatoid arthritis. Clin Exp Rheumatol. 2012;30:254-61.

95. Mendonça JA, Yazbek MA, Costallat BL, Gutiérrez M, Bértolo MB. The modified US7 score in the assessment of synovitis in early rheumatoid arthritis. Rev Bras Reumatol. 2014;54:287–94.

96. Yoshimi R, Ihata A, Kunishita Y, Kishimoto D, Kamiyama R, Minegishi K, et al. A novel 8-joint ultrasound score is useful in daily practice for rheumatoid arthritis. Mod Rheumatol. 2015;25:379–85.

97. Janta I, Valor L, De la Torre I, MartínezEstupiñán L, Nieto JC, Ovalles-Bonilla JG, et al. Ultrasound-detected activity in rheumatoid arthritis on methotrexate therapy: which joints and tendons should be assessed to predict unstable remission? Rheumatol Int. 2016;36:387–96.

98. Leng X, Xiao W, Xu Z, Zhu X, Liu Y, Zhao D, et al. Ultrasound7 versus ultrasound12 in monitoring the response to infliximab in patients with rheumatoid arthritis. Clin Rheumatol. 2016;35:587–95.

99. Aga A, Lie E, Olsen I, Hammer H, Uhlig T, van der Heijde D, et al. Development of an ultrasound joint inflammation score for rheumatoid arthritis through a data-driven approach. Arthritis Rheumatol. 2015;67:S10.

100. Aga AB, Hammer HB, Olsen IC, Uhlig T, Kvien TK, van der Heijde D, et al. First step in the development of an ultrasound joint inflammation score for rheumatoid arthritis using a data-driven approach. Ann Rheum Dis. 2016;75:1444–51.

101. Mandl P, Naredo E, Wakefield R, Conaghan P, D'Agostino M, OMERACT Ultrasound Task Force, et al. A systematic literature review analysis of ultrasound joint count and scoring systems to assess synovitis in rheumatoid arthritis according to the OMERACT filter. J Rheumatol. 2011;38:2055–62.

102. Wakefield RJ, D'Agostino MA, Naredo E, Buch MH, Iagnocco A, Terslev L, et al. After treat-to-target: can a targeted ultrasound initiative improve RA outcomes? Ann Rheum Dis. 2012;71:799–803.

103. Gutierrez M, Okano T, Reginato AM, Cazenave T, Ventura-Rios L, Bertolazzi C, Pineda C. Pan-American League Against Rheumatisms (PANLAR) Ultrasound Study Group. New Ultrasound Modalities in Rheumatology. J Clin Rheumatol. 2015;21:427–34.

104. Terslev L, Torp-Pedersen E, Qvistgaard E, von der Recke P, Bliddal H. Doppler ultrasound findings in healthy wrists and finger joints. Ann Rheum Dis. 2004;63:644–8.

105. Vlad V, Micu M, Porta F, Radunovic G, Nestorova R, Petranova T, et al. Ultrasound of the hand and wrist in rheumatology. Med Ultrason. 2012;14:42–8.

2

Ultrasound inflammatory parameters and Treg/Th17 cell profiles in established rheumatoid arthritis

Aline Defaveri do Prado[1,2*], Melissa Cláudia Bisi[1], Deise Marcela Piovesan[1], Markus Bredemeier[2], Talita Siara Baptista[3], Laura Petersen[3], Moises Evandro Bauer[3], Inês Guimarães da Silveira[1], José Alexandre Mendonça[4] and Henrique Luiz Staub[1]

Abstract

Background: Imbalance and disfuntion in regulatory T-cells (Tregs) and IL-17 producer lymphocytes (Th17) have been implicated in the pathogenesis of rheumatoid arthritis (RA). Gray scale synovial proliferation (GS), power Doppler signal (pD) and bone erosions seen on high resolution muskuloskeletal ultrasound (MSUS) are hallmarks of destructive articular disease.

Objective: To evaluate the association of peripheral Tregs and Th17 with MSUS findings in RA.

Methods: RA patients (1987 ACR criteria) treated with disease-modifying antirheumatic drugs (DMARDs) were included. Lymphocytes were isolated and immunophenotyped by flow cytometry to investigate regulatory FoxP3+ T cells and IL-17+ cells. MSUS (MyLab 60, Esaote, Genova, Italy, linear probe 6–18 MHz) was performed on hand joints, and a 10-joint US score was calculated for each patient.

Results: Data on lymphocytes subsets were avaiable for 90 patients. The majority of patients were Caucasian women with a median disease duration of 6 years (interquartile range: 2–13 years). Mean DAS28 was 4.28 (SD $\pm$ 1.64) and mean HAQ score was 1.11 (SD $\pm$ 0.83).
There was no significant correlation of 10-joint GS score (rS = 0.122, 95% CI: − 0.124 to 0.336, $P = 0.254$) and 10-joint pD score (rS = 0.056, 95% CI: − 0.180 to 0.273, $P = 0.602$) with the mean percentage of peripheral Treg cells. Also, 10-joint GS score (rS = 0.083, 95% CI: − 0.125 to 0.302, $P = 0.438$) and 10-joint pD score 10 (rS = − 0.060, 95% CI: − 0.271 to 0.150, $P = 0.575$); did not correlate to Th17 profile. No association of bone erosions on MSUS with Treg and Th17 profiles ($P = 0.831$ and $P = 0.632$, respectively) was observed.

Conclusion: In this first study addressing MSUS features and lymphocytes subtypes in established RA, data did not support an association of circulating Tregs and Th17 lymphocytes with inflammatory and structural damage findings on MSUS.

* Correspondence: adprado@gmail.com
[1]Rheumatology Service, Pontifícia Universidade Católica do Rio Grande do Sul (PUCRS), Ipiranga Avenue, 6690 room 220, Porto Alegre, RS CEP 90610-000, Brazil
[2]Rheumatology Service, Hospital Nossa Senhora da Conceição – Grupo Hospitalar Conceição (GHC), Av. Francisco Trein, 596 – 2nd floor, Porto Alegre, RS CEP 91350-200, Brazil
Full list of author information is available at the end of the article

Introduction

Rheumatoid arthritis (RA) is a chronic autoimmune disease characterized by polyarthritis leading to synovial proliferation, pannus formation, bone erosions and joint deformities [1]. Besides the major role of cytokines in the development and progression of the disease, specially TNF-alpha and interleukins (IL) [2], regulatory T cells (Tregs) and lymphocytes producers of IL-17 (Th17) imbalance and disfuntion have also been implicated in the pathogenesis of rheumatoid arthritis (RA) [3].

In recent years, high-resolution musculoskeletal ultrasound (MSUS) has been widely used in clinical rheumatology practice, since it has demonstrated consistent and reproducible results among trained rheumatologists [4]. Synovial proliferation seen on gray scale ultrasound (GS) and synovial power Doppler (pD) signal are characteristics of joint inflammation. The usefulness of MSUS in the setting of RA patient assistance, especially for the detection of subclinical synovitis, RA relapse and structural progression has already been scientifically proved and is included in the current management of rheumatoid arthritis [5, 6].

The linkage between RA inflammatory cells and mediators with articular ultrasonographic abnormalities has been an interesting area of investigation. The association of plasma IL-6, a major inflammatory cytokine, with joint sonographic findings, specially power Doppler, was demonstrated in early RA [7] and established disease [8]. Plasma IL-17 was associated with joint pD and gray scale synovitis in the hands of RA patients [9]. However, the relationship of MSUS findings with circulating suppressive or inflammatory T cell subtypes has not been addressed so far. In the current study, we evaluate the association of MSUS parameters with the T regulatory (Treg) and Th17 cell profiles.

Methods

RA outpatients (classified according to the 1987 American College of Rheumatology criteria) treated exclusively with non-biologic disease-modifying anti-rheumatic drugs (DMARDs) were consecutively included in this prospective cross-sectional study.

MSUS examination was performed using a high resolution machine (MyLab 60, Esaote, Genova, Italy) and a linear high-frequency probe (6–18 MHz) by one of two sonography-trained rheumatologists unware of clinical and laboratory data. Details of MSUS assessment and interobserver agreement is described elsewhere [7]. A single Rheumatologist (DMP) evaluated disease activity using the Disease Activity Score in 28 joints (DAS28) and applied the Health Assessment Questionnaire (HAQ) before MSUS.

A blood sample was taken just before clinical and sonographic evaluation and immediately used for lymphocytes identification. Peripheral lymphocytes were isolated and immunophenotyped by flow cytometry to investigate regulatory FoxP3+ T cells and IL-17+ cells using a commercially available Human Th-17/Treg Phenotyping Kit (BD Biosciences, San Jose, CA, USA), according to manufacturer's instructions.

All blood samples were collected at 8:00 AM and clinical and ultrasound evaluations were performed in the morning, between 8:30 and 11:00 AM.

Statistical analysis

Statistical analyses were performed using SPSS for Windows, version 20.0. Between-group comparisons involving non-normal quantitative variables were performed using the Mann-Whitney or Kruskal-wallis tests, and correlations were assessed using Spearman's rank (r_S). Confidence intervals for correlations were estimated using the Bootstrapping method with 1000 iteractions. Two-tailed P values less than or equal to 0.05 were considered statistically significant.

Results

We evaluated iniatially 101 RA patients, and data on lymphocytes subsets were avaiable for 90 patients (samples from 11 had to be excluded due to technical problems during cytometry) whose clinical and demographic features are described in Table 1. Among them, Caucasian women predominated, with a median disease duration of 6 years (interquartile range: 2–13 years). Mean DAS28 was 4.28 (SD ± 1.64) and mean HAQ score was 1.11 (SD ± 0.83). More than 80% of patients were on methotrexate. Moderate disease activity according to DAS28 was observed in the majority of the sample (67.8%), 32.2% had high and 28.9% had low disease activity (LDA). Only 14.4% of patients were on DAS28 remission.

There was no significant correlation of 10-joint GS score ($r_S = 0.122$, 95% CI: − 0.124 to 0.336, $P = 0.254$) and 10-joint pD score ($r_S = 0.056$, 95% CI: − 0.180 to

Table 1 Clinical and demographic features of the patients ($n = 90$)

	Number of patients (absolute and percent)
Female gender	72 (80.%)
Caucasians	77 (85.6%)
Positive Rheumatoid Factor	64 (63.4%)
Current smoker	12 (13.3%)
Fibromyalgia- associated with RA	4 (4.4%)
Methotrexate[a]	74 (82.2%)
Leflunomide[a]	37 (41.1%)
Hydroxychloroquine[a]	24 (26.7%)
Sulfasalazine[a]	7 (7.8%)

[a]Current use

0.273, $P = 0.602$) with the mean percentage of peripheral Treg cells (Fig. 1). Also, 10-joint GS score ($r_S = 0.083$, 95% CI: -0.125 to 0.302, $P = 0.438$) and 10-joint pD score 10 ($r_S = -0.060$, 95% CI: -0.271 to 0.150, $P = 0.575$; Additional file 1: Figure S1) did not correlate to Th17 profile. There was also no association of MSUS abnormalities in right wrist (one of the most frequently affected joints in RA) with Treg or Th-17 lymphocytes percentage in peripheral blood ($P = 0.459$ and $P = 0.418$, respectively; Additional file 2: Figure S2 and Additional file 3: Figure S3). In addition, no association of bone erosions on MSUS with Treg and Th17 profiles ($P = 0.831$ and $P = 0.632$, respectively) was observed.

In secondary analyses, the mean percentage of peripheral Treg cells was associated with level of disease activity ($p = 0.020$); patients with LDA presented the highest percentage (Additional file 4: Figure S4). There was also a trend for negative association of DAS28 and Treg cells percentage ($r_S = -0.18$, 95% CI: -0.380 to 0.034, $P = 0.088$). Th17 cells tended to be higher in LDA (Additional file 5: Figure S5), but there was no evidence of significant correlation of DAS28 (taken as a continuous variable) with Th17 lymphocytes percentage ($r_S = -0.89$, 95% CI: -0.301 to 0.139, $P = 0.402$).

Discussion

To the best of our knowledge, this is the first study addressing the relation of MSUS features with blood lymphocytes subtypes in RA. Our sample was composed of established RA patients on non-biologic DMARDs. No significant association of MSUS abnormalities with the percentages of circulating Treg and Th-17 cels was observed.

It is well known that RA patients have a higher number of Th-17 lymphocytes and lower number of Treg cells in blood compared to healthy controls [10, 11]. In fact, the imbalance between Th-17 and Treg lymphocytes, where Th-17 lymphocytes seem to be resistant to Treg cells suppression, is a key factor to pathogenic response to autoantibodies [3, 10, 11]. A higher quantity of Treg cells was documented in the inflamed synovium, suggesting once again that Treg are less able to suppress pro inflammatory Th-17 in RA [12]. So, it is possible that joint level MSUS power Doppler may be related to lower activity of synovial (but according to our results, not circulating) Treg lymphocytes. Indeed, synovial Th-17 cells were associated with persistently positive pD signal in the knee of RA patients [13]. It seems that synovial Th17 and Treg lymphocytes subsets are more important than circulating ones in RA pathogenesis.

In a secondary analysis, we observed higher percentages of Treg cells in patients with clinical low disease activity (LDA). These results are similar to those reported by XX et al., which showed levels of Tregs similar to healthy controls in patients with low disease activity or

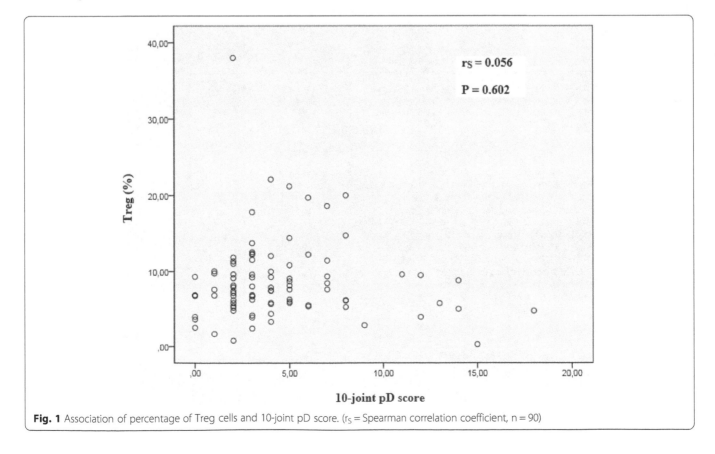

Fig. 1 Association of percentage of Treg cells and 10-joint pD score. (r_S = Spearman correlation coefficient, n = 90)

remission [14]. This may possibly reflect a improved Treg/Th-17 balance in patients whose disease is better controlled.

Conclusion

Our data did not show correlation of inflammatory and structural damage MSUS findings with peripheral blood Treg and Th17 cell profiles in established RA under treatment with non-biologic DMARDs.

Additional files

Additional file 1: Figure S1. Association of percentage of Th-17 lymphocytes and 10-joint pD score.(r_S = Spearman correlation coefficient, n = 90).

Additional file 2: Figure S2. Association of percentage of circulating Treg lymphocytes and grading of power Dopper synovitis (0–3) in the right wrist (Kruskal-Wallis test, n = 90).

Additional file 3: Figure S3. Association of percentage of circulating Th-17 lymphocytes and grading of power Dopper synovitis (0–3) in the right wrist (Kruskal-Wallis test, n = 90).

Additional file 4: Figure S4. Association of percentage of Treg cells and level of disease activity according to DAS28 (Kruskal-Wallis test, n = 90).

Additional file 5: Figure S5. Association of percentage of Th-17 lymphocytes and level of disease activity according to DAS28 (Kruskal-Wallis test, n = 90).

Acknowledgements
Not applicable.

Author's contributions
ADdP and MCB – performed all ultrasound examinations. MB and ADdP – performed the statistical analysis, wrote and revised the manuscript. DMP – performed all clinical evaluations for the study (DAS 28, HAQ, clinical history). TSB and LP – performed all laboratory work (lymphocyte identification). ADdP, MEB, IGdS, JAM, and HLS – design the study, revised the collected data, revised the literature and revised the final manuscript. All authors read and approved the final manuscript.

Author details
[1]Rheumatology Service, Pontifícia Universidade Católica do Rio Grande do Sul (PUCRS), Ipiranga Avenue, 6690 room 220, Porto Alegre, RS CEP 90610-000, Brazil. [2]Rheumatology Service, Hospital Nossa Senhora da Conceição – Grupo Hospitalar Conceição (GHC), Av. Francisco Trein, 596 – 2nd floor, Porto Alegre, RS CEP 91350-200, Brazil. [3]Laboratory of Immunosenescence, Institute of Biomedical Research, Pontificia Universidade Católica do Rio Grande do Sul (PUCRS), Av. Ipiranga, 6690, 2nd floor, Porto Alegre, RS CEP 90610-000, Brazil. [4]Rheumatology Department, Pontifícia Universidade Católica de Campinas (PUCCAMP), Av. John Boyd Dunlop, S/N, Campinas, SP CEP 13034-685, Brazil.

References
1. Firestein G. Etiology and Pathogenis of rheumatoid arthritis. In: Firestein GS, Budd RC, Gabriel SE, McInnes IB, O'Dell JR, editors. Kelley's textbook of rheumatology. Philadelphia: Saunders; 2013. p. 1059–108.
2. McInnes I, Buckley C, Isaacs J. Cytokines in rheumatoid arthritis — shaping the immunological landscape. Nat Rev Rheumatol. 2016;12:63–8.
3. Kima EY, Moudgilb KD. Immunomodulation of autoimmune arthritis by pro-inflammatory cytokines. Cytokine. 2017;98:87–96.
4. Bisi M, do Prado A, Rabelo C, Brollo F, da Silveira I, JA M, et al. Articular ultrasonography: interobserver reliability in rheumatoid arthritis. Rev Bras Reum. 2014;54:250–4.
5. Colebatch A, Edwards C, Østergaard M, van der Heijde D, Balint P, D'Agostino M, et al. EULAR recommendations for the use of imaging of the joints in the clinical management of rheumatoid arthritis. Ann Rheum Dis. 2013;72:804–14.
6. D'Agostino MA, Terslev L, Wakefield R, et al. Novel algorithms for the pragmatic use of ultrasound in the management of patients with rheumatoid arthritis: from diagnosis to remission. Ann Rheum Dis Published Online First: [23 August 2016] doi:https://doi.org/10.1136/annrheumdis2016-209646.
7. Baillet A, Gossec L, Paternotte S, Etcheto A, Combe B, Meyer O, et al. Evaluation of serum Interleukin-6 level as a surrogate marker of synovial inflammation and as a factor of structural progression in early rheumatoid arthritis: results from a French National Multicenter Cohort. Arthritis Care Res (Hoboken). 2015;67:905–12.
8. Do Prado AD, Bisi MC, Piovesan DM, Bredemeier M, Batista TS, Petersen L, et al. Ultrasound power Doppler synovitis is associated with plasma IL-6 in established rheumatoid arthritis. Cytokine. 2016;83:27–32.
9. Fazaa A, Ben Abdelghani K, Abdeladhim M, Laatar A, Ben Ahmed M, Zakraoui L. The level of interleukin-17 in serum is linked to synovial hypervascularization in rheumatoid arthritis. Jt Bone Spine. 2014;81:550–1.
10. Wang W, Shao S, Jiao Z. The Th17/Treg imbalance and cytokine environment in peripheral blood of patients with rheumatoid arthritis. Rheumatolol Int. 2012;32:887–93.
11. Niu W, Cai B, Huang Z. Disturbed Th17/Treg balance in patients with rheumatoid arthritis. Rheumatolol Int. 2012;32:2731–6.
12. Jiao Z, Wang W, Jia R, Li J, You H, Chen I. Accumulation of FoxP3-expressing CD4+CD25+ T cells with distinct chemokine receptors in synovial fluid of patients with active rheumatoid arthritis. Scand J Rheumatol. 2007;36:28–33.
13. Gullick N, Evans H, Church L, Javaraj D, Filer A. Linking power Doppler ultrasound to the presence of Th17 cells in the rheumatoid. PLoS One. 2010;5:e 12516.
14. Chen J, Li J, Gao H, Wang C, Luo J, Lv Z, Li X. Comprehensive evaluation of different T-helper cell differentiation and function in rheumatoid arthritis. J Biomed Biotechnol. 2012. https://doi.org/10.1155/2012/535361.

3

Disease activity is associated with LV dysfunction in rheumatoid arthritis patients without clinical cardiovascular disease

Punchong Hanvivadhanakul[1][*][†] and Adisai Buakhamsri[2][†]

Abstract

Objectives: The cross-sectional study aimed to assess left ventricular systolic function using global longitudinal strain (GLS) by speckle-tracking echocardiography (STE) and arterial stiffness using cardio-ankle vascular index (CAVI) in Thai adults with rheumatoid arthritis (RA) and no clinical evidence of cardiovascular disease (CVD).

Methods: Confirmed RA patients were selected from a list of outpatient attendees if they were 18 years (y) without clinical, ECG and echocardiographic evidence of CVD, diabetes mellitus, chronic kidney disease, and excess alcoholic intake. Controls were matched with age and sex to a list of healthy individuals with normal echocardiograms. All underwent STE and CAVI.

Results: 60 RA patients (females = 55) were analysed. Mean standard deviation of patient and control ages were 50 ± 10.2 and 51 ± 9.9 y, respectively, and mean duration of RA was 9.0 ± 6.8 y. Mean DAS28-CRP and DAS28-ESR were 2.9 ± 0.9 and 3.4 ± 0.9, respectively. There was no between-group differences in left ventricular ejection fraction (LVEF), LV sizes, LVMI, LV diastolic function and CAVI were within normal limits but all GLSs values was significantly lower in patients vs. controls: 17.6 ± 3.4 vs 20.4 ± 2.2 ($p = 0.03$). Multivariate regression analysis demonstrated significant correlations between GLSs and RA duration ($p = 0.02$), and GLSs and DAS28-CRP ($p = 0.041$).

Conclusions: Patients with RA and no clinical CV disease have reduced LV systolic function as shown by lower GLSs. It is common and associated with disease activity and RA disease duration. 2D speckle-tracking GLSs is robust in detecting this subclinical LV systolic dysfunction.

Keywords: Rheumatoid arthritis, Subclinical LV dysfunction, Global longitudinal strain, DAS28-CRP, Disease duration

Introduction

Rheumatoid arthritis (RA) is a systemic autoimmune disease, characterised by chronic joint inflammation and destruction. Extra-articular organ involvement, such as the skin, eyes, heart, lungs, and blood vessels may also cause clinically significant pathology and affect clinical outcomes and quality of life. Compared to the general population, patients with RA have a 8–15 year reduced life expectancy [1] due principally to cardiovascular complications, most commonly atherosclerotic diseases

and congestive heart failure (CHF) [2]. Although the pathophysiologic mechanism is not clearly defined, the chronic inflammatory state of RA itself seems to play a pivotal role in both vascular changes and impaired myocardial function [3, 4]. Previous studies have shown that asymptomatic left ventricular myocardial dysfunction is common, both systolic and diastolic abnormalities at rates of; 45 and 31% respectively [5–10]. Some studies have also shown increased left ventricular mass in RA patients [5, 11, 12]. However, most of the studies were conducted in western and middle eastern countries. There are few studies from Asian populations and the outcomes differ [13, 14]. Thus, the present study was conducted to determine left ventricular structure and function and arterial wall stiffness. Specifically, we used left ventricular deformation (global longitudinal strain or

* Correspondence: phanvivad@gmail.com
†Punchong Hanvivadhanakul and Adisai Buakhamsri contributed equally to the study.
¹Division of Rheumatology, Department of Medicine, Faculty of Medicine, Thammasat University, 99/209 Moo 18, Paholyothin Road, Klong Luang, Pathumthanee 12120, Thailand
Full list of author information is available at the end of the article

GLS) to assess subclinical LV systolic dysfunction [15] and measured the cardio-ankle vascular index (CAVI) to evaluate arterial stiffness (LV afterload). CAVI is a simple bedside tool to estimate the combined stiffness of the aorta, iliac, femoral, and tibial arteries. Arterial stiffness may affect the structure and function of the left ventricle [16]. We hypothesized that GLSs and CAVI may be associated with LV functional and structural change, respectively, in patient with RA and no clinical CV disease.

Patients and methods

Study population
This was a cross-sectional study of patients with proven rheumatoid arthritis who had been followed up at the Rheumatology clinic of Thammasat University Hospital (TUH) between August 2015 and July 2017. All underwent a medical history, thorough physical examination, and medical record review to assess their eligibility for the study. To be included, they had to: (i) be at least 18 years (y) old, (ii) have fulfilled the 1987 American College of Rheumatology (ACR) classification criteria [17] or the 2010 ACR/European League Against Rheumatism (EULAR) classification RA criteria [18], (iii) have been under outpatient follow-up for ≥2 y, and (iv) have given written informed consent. Patients were excluded if they had one of the following: arterial hypertension, coronary heart disease, valvular heart disease, CHF, diabetes mellitus, chronic kidney disease, aortic/peripheral arterial disease, clinically significant arrhythmia or alcoholic intake.

Control subjects
Control subjects were obtained from our echocardiography database of 100 healthy normal subjects, previously enrolled in an unrelated echocardiography study. They were declared healthy if they had normal findings in all following aspects: medical history, physical examination and no current intake of any medication. Additionally, 12-lead electrocardiogram and comprehensive echocardiogram must be normal. They were then age- and sex-matched with the RA patients. Age-matching was limited at +/- 2 years. This study was approved by the Ethics Committee of the Faculty of Medicine, Thammasat University. Informed consent was obtained from all participants included in the study.

Clinical data collection
Patient data were recorded on to standard case report forms and included age, sex, body mass index, smoking status, waist circumference, and pertinent physical signs (e.g. locations of tender and/or swollen joints). Disease activity and functional status were assessed by the Disease Activity Score 28 (DAS28), C-reactive protein (CRP), erythrocyte sedimentation rate (ESR) and a health assessment questionnaire (HAQ). The medical records were also reviewed to determine disease duration, medication use, cumulative dosage of corticosteroids and methotrexate, and radiographic joint erosions.

Patient blood sampling
After 12 h of overnight fasting, blood was drawn to determine the following laboratory investigations: fasting blood glucose, lipid profile (total cholesterol, triglyceride, high-density lipoprotein, and low-density lipoprotein), serum creatinine, calculated glomerular filtration rate (GFR), CRP, ESR, rheumatoid factor (RF), and anti-citrullinated peptide antibody (ACPA). RF was detected by latex agglutination (Plasmatec Laboratory Co, Cambridge, UK) and serum ACPA by immunofluorescence (Thermo Fisher Scientific EliA, Germany); an ACPA level ≥ 5.6 IU/mL was positive, according to the manufacturer's instructions.

Echocardiograms
Transthoracic two-dimensional (2-D) echocardiography was performed in all participants with an iE33 ultrasound machine equipped with an S5 transducer (Philips medical imaging, Andover, MA). Standard echocardiographic apical and short-axis views were obtained in accordance with the American Society of Echocardiography and European Association of Cardiovascular Imaging recommendations [19]. 2-D images were carefully adjusted to avoid over gain, which may affect the distance measurement used for LV mass calculation. Second-harmonic images were acquired for speckle tracking imaging. With high frame rate B-mode scans (40–90 frames/s) Pulsed-wave Doppler imaging were also obtained in the apical four-chamber view for assessment of the septal and lateral mitral annulus (Ea). These images with at least 3 loops of each apical LV view were stored in a digital cine-loop format for off-line analysis.

Left ventricular mass (LVM) was calculated by two different methods, as recommended by the American and European guidelines [19]: (i) M-mode tracing of the LV in the parasternal long-axis and cube formula, and (ii) 2-D method using the LV short-axis view at papillary muscle level, apical four-chamber view and area-length formula. LVM values obtained from these two methods were then indexed with body surface area and reported as LV mass index (LVMI). LV hypertrophy was present if LVMI by either method exceeding a cut-off values according to gender: (i) linear method: 95–115 g/m^2 and (ii) 2-D method: 88–102 g/m^2 for women and men, respectively. All other echocardiographic data were used to determine cardiac dimensions, left ventricular systolic and diastolic functions in compliance with standard criteria [19, 20].

LV longitudinal strain [LS] measurement with speckle-tracking technique was performed in Excelera workstation (QLAB11, Philips) by an experienced cardiologist blinded to subject group. Speckle-tracking echocardiography (STE) utilizes a software specialized for tracking acoustic markers in standard 2-D grey scale images over one cardiac cycle [21, 22]. Strain is a parameter of myocardial deformation expressed as a negative percentage value since the left ventricle shortens along its longitudinal axis during systole. The reduced absolute strain values (less negative strain) reflect diminished contractile function. In brief, LV myocardium (region of interest) was manually traced from medial to lateral mitral annulus in each standard apical view with good 2-D image quality. The software then performed automatic tracking of echocardiographic speckles over a cardiac cycle. The tracking quality was determined visually and the process repeated if the result was poor. If the tracking was still at poor quality, we excluded that segment from calculation of mean GLS. Any patient with more than 1 segment of poor tracking quality was not enrolled to final analysis. Longitudinal-strain (LS) curve over one cardiac cycle was generated-with-measured maximal LS during systole in each view. Global longitudinal strain during systole (GLSs) was the automated average value from 2 different cardiac cycles. In this study, GLS values were reported as absolute number (higher number means more shortening of myocardium).

Cardio-ankle vascular stiffness index (CAVI)

CAVI, an index of arterial stiffness, was determined using a dedicated device (VaSera VS-2000, Fukuda Denshi, Japan). Participants laid in the supine position for at least 20 min before testing. Blood pressure cuffs were then applied to the upper (brachial artery) and lower (just above ankle) extremities on both sides to obtain arterial pressures by oscillometry while echocardiograms and cardiac phonograms were being recorded. Pulse wave velocity (PWV) was measured; PWV = the length from aortic valve to the ankle divided by the combination of two time intervals (time from aortic valve closing to the notch of the brachial pulse wave and time from the rise of the brachial pulse wave to the ankle pulse wave). CAVI was automatically calculated using following equation [16]:

$$CAVI = a \times \left[(2\rho/\varDelta P) \times \ln(Ps/Pd) \times PWV^2 \right] + b$$

where ρ is blood density, $\varDelta P$ is 'Ps−Pd', Ps/Pd are systolic/diastolic pressures and a/b are constants.

　According to the manufacturer's instructions, there are 3 categories of CAVI value; normal (CAVI< 8.0), borderline (CAVI = 8.0 - < 9.0) and abnormal (CAVI ≥9.0). All measurements were performed.

Reproducibility of LVM and GLSs measurements

Echocardiographic data sets of 12 patients (corresponding to 10% of the studied population) were randomly chosen to assess intra- and interobserver variability of LVMI and GLSs. The measurements were performed twice by the same observer separated by 1-week interval and by a second observer blinded to the results of the first observer. Measurement variabilities were assessed using intraclass correlation coefficients. The intraobserver correlation coefficients for LVMI and GLSs were 0.92 and 0.95 respectively and those of LVMI and GLSs were 0.88 and 0.92, respectively. Thus, overall reproducibility was good.

Statistical analysis

Continuous variables were expressed as mean ± standard deviation (SD) and categorical variables as frequencies. Between-group comparisons were performed using Wilcoxon rank sum tests, Chi-square test or Fisher's exact test where appropriate. Multiple regression analysis, adjusted for age, gender, blood pressure, BMI, heart rate and LVMI (where appropriate) were used to examine associations between LVMI or global LV strain (in separate model) and characteristics of RA disease. The correlation of CAVI and GLSs was assessed with Pearson's correlation coefficient. All tests were two-sided and a value of ≤0.05 was considered statistically significant. Data analysis was performed using SPSS software version 14.0 (SPSS Inc., Chicago, Illinois).

Results

Two hundred and eighty patients with RA have been screened and 62 were initially enrolled but two were later excluded from the final analysis because: (i) one male patient had hypertension diagnosed during the study even though prior BP recordings at study enrolment were normal. Hypertension was confirmed by 24-h ambulatory blood pressure monitoring. He had echocardiographic-LVH (LVMI 122 g/m^2 and 110 g/m^2 by M-mode and 2-D, respectively) and borderline CAVI (8.8), and (ii) a female who was lost to follow-up; her echocardiogram and CAVI were within normal limits. General clinical characteristics are presented in Table 1. Features of RA patients are detailed in Table 2. The important echocardiographic findings including LVMI, GLSs and CAVI (in the patient group) are shown in Tables 3 and 4.

Patients with rheumatoid arthritis

The 60 RA patients (female = 55) had a mean age of 51 ± 9.9 y; most were non-smokers (95%). Dyslipidemia and impaired fasting glucose were present in 18 (30%) and 8 (13%) patients, respectively, but all had normal eGFR values. Mean (range) RA duration was 7 (2–32) y.

Table 1 Clinical characteristics of patients with rheumatoid arthritis and age/sex-matched healthy controls

Clinical characteristics	Patients $n = 60$	Controls $n = 60$	P-value
Age (years)	50 ± 10.2	51 ± 9.9	0.8
Women	55 (92%)	55 (92%)	1.0
BMI (kg/m^2)	22 ± 3	21 ± 2.5	0.64
Systolic blood pressure (mmHg)	120 ± 9.7	117 ± 8.8	0.5
Diastolic blood pressure (mmHg)	75 ± 7.7	73 ± 10	0.2
Heart rate (BPM)	74 ± 7	77 ± 9	0.6
Smoking history	3 (5%)	None	< 0.01
Dyslipidemia	17(28%)	None	< 0.01

No patients had rheumatoid nodule. Biological agent was not used in our patient cohort. Rheumatoid factor (RF) was positive in 32 (54%) patients and anti-citrullinated peptide antibody (ACPA) in 43 (72%) patients; both were positive in 31 (52%) patients. The DAS28-CRP, DAS28-ESR and HAQ scores were 2.9 ± 0.9, 3.4 ± 1.0 and 0.5 ± 0.6, respectively.

Cardiac geometry and function

Cardiac chamber sizes including the left ventricle and left atrium were normal in all patients. LVEF and doppler-based diastolic function were also normal by the American Society of Echocariography criteria [23, 24]. Estimated left atrial pressure was normal and there was no echocardiographic evidence of pulmonary hypertension in all patients.

Table 2 Clinical characteristics of 60 patients with rheumatoid arthritis and regression analysis for factors associated with systolic global longitudinal strain

Clinical parameters	Value	Adjusted univariate coefficient[a] (SE)	P-value
Clinical			
Duration of RA (years)	9.0 ± 6.8 (2–40)	1.68 (0.76)	0.02
HAQ disability index	0.55 ± 0.6 (0–2.25)	1.1 (0.49)	0.58
Rheumatoid nodule	0	NA	NA
DAS28-CRP	2.9 ± 0.9 (1.48–5.66)	1.44 (0.72)	0.041
DAS28-ESR	3.4 ± 0.9 (1.05–6.25)	0.67 (0.43)	0.7
Joint erosion	25 (42%)	0.8 (0.62)	0.09
Medications			
Methotrexate	58 (96%)	0.03 (0.01)	0.79
Cumulative dose of methotrexate (g)	2.9 ± 1.4 (0–5.36)	0.26 (0.02)	0.47
Sulfasalazine	30 (50%)	0.72 (0.13)	0.61
Hydroxychloroquine	18 (23%)	0.4 (0.27)	0.53
Leflunomide	20 (30%)	0.74 (0.81)	0.8
Other DMARDs	31 (52%)	0.1 (0.05)	0.72
Corticosteriod	29 (48%)	0.7 (0.49)	0.93
Cumulative dose of corticosteroid (g)	2.8 ± 4.6(0–23)	0.33 (0.09)	0.82
NSAIDs	13 (22%)	0.92 (0.55)	0.44
Laboratory			
CRP[b] (mg/dL)	10.1 ± 15 (0.3–65.2)	0.52 (0.38)	0.56
ESR[b](mm/hr)	30 ± 19 (3–81)	0.81 (0.62)	0.7
Positive RF or ACPA	45 (75%)	0.59 (1.0)	1.0

Continuous data are expressed as mean ± SD (min-max), categorical data as n (%)

ACPA Anti-citrullinated peptide antibodies, *CRP* C-reactive protein, *DAS28* Disease Activity Score 28, *DMARDs* Disease-modifying antirheumatic drugs, *ESR* Erythrocyte sedimentation rate, *HAQ* Health assessment questionnaire, *RA* Rheumatoid arthritis, *RF* Rheumatoid factor, *NA* Not available or not applicable

[a]Adjusted for age, gender, blood pressure, body mass index, heart rate and left ventricular mass index

[b]Log-transformed

Table 3 Disease activity scores in patients with rheumatoid arthritis

Disease activity	DAS28-CRP N (%)	DAS28-ESR N (%)
Remission (< 2.6)	26 (43)	12 (20)
Low (2.6 to < 3.2)	10 (16)	13 (22)
Moderate (3.2 to < 5.1)	23 (38)	33 (55)
Severe (≥ 5.1)	1 (3)	2 (3)

LV mass index (LVMI)

LVMI was slightly higher with M mode than the 2-D method. Men had higher LVMI than women subjects, However, all patients had normal LVMI independent of measurement methods. No correlation was found between LVMI and other variables of RA disease, blood pressure and CAVI.

Systolic global longitudinal strain (GLSs)

GLSs were normal for all patients when using the general cut-off point of normal limit [23, 25, 26] but were significantly lower than the controls: $17.6 \pm 3.4\%$ vs. $20.4 \pm 2.2\%$ ($p = 0.03$). Duration of rheumatoid disease and DAS28-CRP score were significantly associated with lower absolute value of GLSs after adjustment for age, gender, blood pressure, body mass index, heart rate and left ventricular mass index (univariate coefficient (SE); 1.68 (0.76), $p = 0.02$ for duration of disease and 1.44 (0.72), $p = 0.041$ for DAS28-CRP).

Cardio-ankle velocity index (CAVI)

CAVIs (Table 5) were normal in almost all patients (96%) while a few were in borderline category (4%) and

Table 5 Cardio-Ankle vascular stiffness index in patients with rheumatoid arthritis

CAVI category	Value[a]	N (% of total)
Normal (< 8)	6.7 ± 1.5	58 (96)
Borderline (8 to < 9)	8.5 ± 4.2	2 (4)
Abnormal (≥9)	NA	0 (0)

[a]Mean ± SD, categorical data as n (%)ʲ

none had abnormal CAVI. There was no correlation between CAVI and GLSs ($r = -0.13$, $p = 0.6$).

Discussions

We have demonstrated that LV systolic function of patient with RA is worse than those of matched healthy subject. This subclinical LV systolic dysfunction as shown by lower GLSs (although still in normal range) is common in patients with chronic RA and independently associated with disease activity and RA duration. All RA patients in our study underwent prospectively comprehensive echocardiographic examinations. Cardiac geometry (i.e. chamber sizes) and all echocardiographic parameters of systolic/diastolic function (except GLSs) were within normal limits and were not significantly different from those of the control subjects. We did not find LVH (determined by LVMI) in our RA patients even when using two different methods of assessment. This contrasts with other studies which have reported high rates of increased LVM/LVMI in RA patients [12, 27, 28]. In general, significant proportions of RA patients have co-existing cardiovascular risk factors such as hypertension or an increased Framingham Risk Score, which have been reported in up to 40% of RA patients [13].

Table 4 Echocardiographic parameters and systolic global longitudinal strain of patients with rheumatoid arthritis and age and sex-matched control subjects

Parameters	Patients	Controls	P-value
LV end-diastolic volume index[a] (mL/m^2)	52 ± 8	54 ± 7	0.10
LV end-systolic volume index[a] (mL/m^2)	22 ± 5	24 ± 4	0.38
LV ejection fraction[a]	57 ± 4	56 ± 3	0.50
Left atrial volume index (mL/m^2)	26 ± 6	24 ± 5	0.67
LV mass index (gm/m^2) (M-mode)	74 ± 8	76 ± 12	0.40
LV mass index (gm/m^2) (2D-method)	72 ± 7	75 ± 10	0.09
LV hypertrophy[b]	0	0	NS
LV diastolic dysfunction[c]	0	0	NS
Average E' (septal and lateral) (cm/s)	12.4 ± 2.5	13.1 ± 3.2	0.2
E/E'	6.2 ± 1.6	6.8 ± 2.1	0.35
Systolic global longitudinal strain (%)	17.6 ± 3.4	20.4 ± 2.2	0.03

E' Mitral annulus tissue velocity curing early diastole, E Peak mitral inflow velocity during early diastole

NS Not significant

[a]Modified Simpson's method

[b]According to 2015 American Society of Echocardiography: recommendations for cardiac chamber quantification by echocardiography

[c]According to 2016 American Society of Echocardiography: recommendations for the evaluation of left ventricular diastolic function by echocardiography

This study was meticulously designed to avoid confounding factors that affect LV mass, like arterial hypertension, diseases associated with LV pressure/volume loading and hypertrophic/infiltrative cardiomyopathy. These had been ruled out by reviewing medical records, conducting detailed physical examinations, ECGs and echocardiograms prior to enrolment. Importantly, we also performed CAVI in all patients to detect abnormal arterial stiffness which can be present in chronic inflammatory diseases like RA [29–31]. CAVI has been used to assess arterial stiffness in subjects at risk of or with clinically overt cardiovascular disease [32, 33]; increased arterial stiffness is related to changes in LV geometry and LV mass independent of arterial blood pressure [34–36]. However, CAVI results in our study were mostly normal with no patient having an abnormal CAVI. This together with strict study inclusion criteria, may partly explain the absence of LVH in our patients i.e. LVH as defined by LVMI higher than normal limits, is uncommon in RA patients if conditions causing increased LV afterload are absent.

Conventional parameters of LV systolic and diastolic function in our patients were also normal. We also used GLSs to assess subclinical changes of LV systolic function and found that even though our RA patients had significantly lower values vs. controls, all values were within normal limits (higher than 15.9%) [25] and were independent of LV diastolic function. Since GLSs is more sensitive to change in LV systolic function than LVEF, our findings demonstrate subtle LVSD in RA. GLSs, as a marker of LVSD, has previously been shown to be abnormal in early stage heart disease and have prognostic significance in many cardiac disorders such as chemotherapy-related cardiomyopathy [37] and hypertrophic cardiomyopathy [38].

Our results were also in line with a study in patients with RA by Fine et al. [9] who demonstrated a reduction of LV longitudinal strain independent of LVEF and the degree of LV diastolic dysfunction. We identified DAS28-CRP and duration of disease as independent factors affecting subclinical LVSD; both factors are indicative of the severity and duration of inflammation. Using a simplified Disease Activity Index of < 3.3, Midtbø et al. [39] have shown that when RA is in remission, patients have improved LV function (assessed by stress corrected mid-wall shortening and global longitudinal strain) compared to patients with active disease. Proposed mechanisms of LV systolic dysfunction in RA include chronic inflammation, oxidative stress and myocyte dysfunction, interstitial fibrosis and endothelial dysfunction that leads to impaired perfusion [3]. These can reasonably explain our findings that disease activity determined subclinical LV systolic dysfunction in our patient cohort.

Analysis model of current study showed that factors such as age, use of DMARDs or corticosteroids and inflammatory markers were not associated with LVSD. Their effects may have been masked as they were likely incorporated into DAS28-CRP and duration of disease. In addition, the ESR, which may be influenced by many factors and is a less sensitive marker of RA disease activity compared to CRP [40, 41]. Methotrexate and prednisolone were commonly prescribed; thus, the association of these drugs to LVSD may not be able to demonstrate.

As our studied population were Asian, whether ethnic difference plays any role on the final results are yet to be determined. General consideration deserves to be mentioned. First, prevalence of CV risk factors in Asians with RA appears to be lower than that of non-Asian population (US and European population) [42]. These risk factors including hypertension, diabetes, dyslipidemia and central obesity (or, collectively, metabolic syndrome) have direct and indirect insult to myocardial function. Second, geometric changes of the heart due to those underlying disease and/or races may have impact on left ventricular function [43]. Third, genetic susceptibility may increases disease severity and chronicity of systemic inflammation. Although it was not well established in RA, genetic susceptibilities specific to some ethnic groups were demonstrated in other rheumatic diseases such as SLE [44, 45]. Fourth, disparity of ethnic-related socioeconomic level (ability to access proper treatment, timely diagnosis/follow-up) may also account for the different changes of cardiovascular structure. Thus, these ethnic-related factors potentially affect LV systolic function and, inevitably, GLSs.

Study limitations

Circumferential and radial strains were not studied in our patients as these parameters are less reproducible than longitudinal strain [46]. Analysis of GLSs is dependent on quality of two-dimensional image. Poor speckle tracking will directly affect the reliability of GLS value. The power of our study to detect small change in LV geometry and function was limited by the small number of cases and controls (60/group). This, however, was the result of rigorous inclusion criteria to ascertain that the patients had no underlying CVD, which would have been a confounding factor in our study results. A small difference may not be detected if only a universal normal cut-off point was used. We did not take serial measurements, so a temporal relationship between disease activity and left ventricle function could not be demonstrated; this is an avenue of future research to see if we can replicate the results of other long term RA studies [47, 48]. Cardiac biomarkers, like cardiac troponin and NT-proBNP, were not studied in our patients and could have supported (or otherwise) the findings of subclinical LVSD. There were no patients with abnormal CAVIs; thus, we could not explore potential associations with cardiac function parameters. Both DAS28-ESR and DAS28-CRP may have limited power in estimation of disease activity. While DAS28 ESR reflects disease activity in the previous few weeks, DAS28-CRP does so but for a shorter term. Simplified and clinical disease activity indices (SDAI, CDAI) were not associated with LV systolic function (GLSs) in our study. Presence of smoker and dyslipidemia in patient group may possibly affect the its GLS results. We did sensitivity analysis including only those with no smoking history or dyslipidemia and found no effect on main results. However, it was unable to exclude possible effect of this two factors on GLS if studied population was larger.

Conclusions

Patients with RA and no clinical CV disease have reduced LV systolic function when comparing to that of matched healthy subjects. It is demonstrated by the lower GLSs values while conventional echocardiographic parameters of LV systolic function are still unchanged. This subclinical LV systolic dysfunction is common and associated with disease activity and RA disease duration.

Clinical perspective

2D-STE GLS can be easily performed with most echocardiogram machines. This technique provides the opportunities to identify subclinical LV systolic dysfunction in at-risk RA patients, including presence of multiple CV risk factors, high disease activity or long disease duration in particular. Serial GLSs measurement may be an interesting strategy and considered as a long-term follow-up tool in these patients. Further studies are needed to evaluate a proper GLSs cut-off point (or delta change); to understand mechanism(s), consequences and therapeutic implications of subclinical LV systolic dysfunction.

Abbreviations
2-D: Two-dimensional; ACPA: Anti-citrullinated peptide antibody; ACR: American College of Rheumatology; CAVI: Cardio-ankle vascular index; CHF: Congestive heart failure; CRP: C-reactive protein; CVD: Cardiovascular disease; DAS28: Disease Activity Score 28; ESR: Erythrocyte sedimentation rate; EULAR: European League Against Rheumatism; GFR: Glomerular filtration rate; GLS: Global longitudinal strain; GLSs: Global longitudinal strain during systole; HAQ: Health assessment questionnaire; LS: LV longitudinal strain; LV: Left ventricular; LVEF: Left ventricular ejection fraction; LVMI: LV mass index; LVOT: LV outflow tract; PWV: Pulse wave velocity; RA: Rheumatoid arthritis; RF: Rheumatoid factor; STE: Speckle-tracking echocardiography; TUH: Thammasat University Hospital; y: Years

Acknowledgements
We thank the patients and control subjects for agreeing to participate in this study. This study was supported by Thammasat university research grant (TP 2-37-2559).Dr. Bob Taylor kindly reviewed the paper.

Authors' contributions
PH and AB contribute to this study equally. PH collected, analyzed, and interpreted the patient data regarding rheumatoid arthritis. AB performed echocardiogram examination, analyzed, and interpreted data. AB was a major contributor in writing the manuscript. All authors read and approved the final manuscript.

Author details
[1]Division of Rheumatology, Department of Medicine, Faculty of Medicine, Thammasat University, 99/209 Moo 18, Paholyothin Road, Klong Luang, Pathumthanee 12120, Thailand. [2]Division of Cardiology, Department of Medicine, Faculty of Medicine, Thammasat University, 99/209 Moo 18, Paholyothin Road, Klong Luang, Pathumthanee 12120, Thailand.

References
1. Wolfe F, Freundlich B, Straus WL. Increase in cardiovascular and cerebrovascular disease prevalence in rheumatoid arthritis. J Rheumatol. 2003;30(1):36–40.
2. Avina-Zubieta JA, Thomas J, Sadatsafavi M, Lehman AJ, Lacaille D. Risk of incident cardiovascular events in patients with rheumatoid arthritis: a meta-analysis of observational studies. Ann Rheum Dis. 2012;71(9):1524–9.
3. England BR, Thiele GM, Anderson DR, Mikuls TR. Increased cardiovascular risk in rheumatoid arthritis: mechanisms and implications. BMJ. 2018;361: k1036.
4. Targonska-Stepniak B, Biskup M, Biskup W, Majdan M. Diastolic dysfunction in rheumatoid arthritis patients with low disease activity. Clin Rheumatol. 2019;38(4):1131–7.
5. Corrao S, Salli L, Arnone S, Scaglione R, Pinto A, Licata G. Echo-Doppler left ventricular filling abnormalities in patients with rheumatoid arthritis without clinically evident cardiovascular disease. Eur J Clin Investig. 1996;26(4):293–7.
6. Wislowska M, Sypula S, Kowalik I. Echocardiographic findings, 24-hour electrocardiographic Holter monitoring in patients with rheumatoid arthritis according to Steinbrocker's criteria, functional index, value of Waaler-rose titre and duration of disease. Clin Rheumatol. 1998;17(5):369–77.
7. Liang KP, Myasoedova E, Crowson CS, Davis JM, Roger VL, Karon BL, et al. Increased prevalence of diastolic dysfunction in rheumatoid arthritis. Ann Rheum Dis. 2010;69(9):1665–70.
8. Sitia S, Tomasoni L, Cicala S, Atzeni F, Ricci C, Gaeta M, et al. Detection of preclinical impairment of myocardial function in rheumatoid arthritis patients with short disease duration by speckle tracking echocardiography. Int J Cardiol. 2012;160(1):8–14.
9. Fine NM, Crowson CS, Lin G, Oh JK, Villarraga HR, Gabriel SE. Evaluation of myocardial function in patients with rheumatoid arthritis using strain imaging by speckle-tracking echocardiography. Ann Rheum Dis. 2014;73(10):1833–9.
10. Cioffi G, Viapiana O, Ognibeni F, Dalbeni A, Gatti D, Adami S, et al. Prevalence and factors related to left ventricular systolic dysfunction in asymptomatic patients with rheumatoid arthritis. A prospective tissue Doppler echocardiography study. Herz. 2015;40(7):989–96.
11. Wislowska M, Jaszczyk B, Kochmanski M, Sypula S, Sztechman M. Diastolic heart function in RA patients. Rheumatol Int. 2008;28(6):513–9.
12. Cioffi G, Viapiana O, Ognibeni F, Dalbeni A, Giollo A, Adami S, et al. Prevalence and factors related to inappropriately high left ventricular mass in patients with rheumatoid arthritis without overt cardiac disease. J Hypertens. 2015;33(10):2141–9.
13. Dougados M, Soubrier M, Antunez A, Balint P, Balsa A, Buch MH, et al. Prevalence of comorbidities in rheumatoid arthritis and evaluation of their monitoring: results of an international, cross-sectional study (COMORA). Ann Rheum Dis. 2014;73(1):62–8.
14. Jin S, Li M, Fang Y, Li Q, Liu J, Duan X, et al. Chinese Registry of rheumatoid arthritis (CREDIT): II. prevalence and risk factors of major comorbidities in Chinese patients with rheumatoid arthritis. Arthritis Res Ther. 2017;19(1):251.
15. Smiseth OA, Torp H, Opdahl A, Haugaa KH, Urheim S. Myocardial strain imaging: how useful is it in clinical decision making? Eur Heart J. 2016; 37(15):1196–207.

16. Sun CK. Cardio-ankle vascular index (CAVI) as an indicator of arterial stiffness. Integr Blood Press Control. 2013;6:27–38.

17. Arnett FC, Edworthy SM, Bloch DA, McShane DJ, Fries JF, Cooper NS, et al. The American Rheumatism Association 1987 revised criteria for the classification of rheumatoid arthritis. Arthritis Rheum. 1988;31(3):315–24.

18. Aletaha D, Neogi T, Silman AJ, Funovits J, Felson DT, Bingham CO 3rd, et al. 2010 rheumatoid arthritis classification criteria: an American College of Rheumatology/European League Against Rheumatism collaborative initiative. Arthritis Rheum. 2010;62(9):2569–81.

19. Lang RM, Badano LP, Mor-Avi V, Afilalo J, Armstrong A, Ernande L, et al. Recommendations for cardiac chamber quantification by echocardiography in adults: an update from the American Society of Echocardiography and the European Association of Cardiovascular Imaging. Eur Heart J Cardiovasc Imaging. 2015;16(3):233–70.

20. Nagueh SF, Smiseth OA, Appleton CP, Byrd BF 3rd, Dokainish H, Edvardsen T, et al. Recommendations for the evaluation of left ventricular diastolic function by echocardiography: an update from the American Society of Echocardiography and the European Association of Cardiovascular Imaging. J Am Soc Echocardiogr. 2016;29(4):277–314.

21. Reisner SA, Lysyansky P, Agmon Y, Mutlak D, Lessick J, Friedman Z. Global longitudinal strain: a novel index of left ventricular systolic function. J Am Soc Echocardiogr. 2004;17(6):630–3.

22. Langeland S, D'Hooge J, Wouters PF, Leather HA, Claus P, Bijnens B, et al. Experimental validation of a new ultrasound method for the simultaneous assessment of radial and longitudinal myocardial deformation independent of insonation angle. Circulation. 2005;112(14):2157–62.

23. Lang RM, Badano LP, Mor-Avi V, Afilalo J, Armstrong A, Ernande L, et al. Recommendations for cardiac chamber quantification by echocardiography in adults: an update from the American Society of Echocardiography and the European Association of Cardiovascular Imaging. J Am Soc Echocardiogr. 2015;28(1):1–39 e14.

24. Nagueh SF, Smiseth OA, Appleton CP, Byrd BF 3rd, Dokainish H, Edvardsen T, et al. Recommendations for the evaluation of left ventricular diastolic function by echocardiography: an update from the American Society of Echocardiography and the European Association of Cardiovascular Imaging. Eur Heart J Cardiovasc Imaging. 2016;17(12):1321–60.

25. Yingchoncharoen T, Agarwal S, Popovic ZB, Marwick TH. Normal ranges of left ventricular strain: a meta-analysis. J Am Soc Echocardiogr. 2013;26(2):185–91.

26. Voigt JU, Pedrizzetti G, Lysyansky P, Marwick TH, Houle H, Baumann R, et al. Definitions for a common standard for 2D speckle tracking echocardiography: consensus document of the EACVI/ASE/Industry Task Force to standardize deformation imaging. Eur Heart J Cardiovasc Imaging. 2015;16(1):1–11.

27. Myasoedova E, Davis JM 3rd, Crowson CS, Roger VL, Karon BL, Borgeson DD, et al. Brief report: rheumatoid arthritis is associated with left ventricular concentric remodeling: results of a population-based cross-sectional study. Arthritis Rheum. 2013;65(7):1713–8.

28. Corrao S, Argano C, Pistone G, Messina S, Calvo L, Perticone F. Rheumatoid arthritis affects left ventricular mass: systematic review and meta-analysis. Eur J Intern Med. 2015;26(4):259–67.

29. Klocke R, Cockcroft JR, Taylor GJ, Hall IR, Blake DR. Arterial stiffness and central blood pressure, as determined by pulse wave analysis, in rheumatoid arthritis. Ann Rheum Dis. 2003;62(5):414–8.

30. Crilly MA, Kumar V, Clark HJ, Scott NW, Macdonald AG, Williams DJ. Arterial stiffness and cumulative inflammatory burden in rheumatoid arthritis: a dose-response relationship independent of established cardiovascular risk factors. Rheumatology (Oxford). 2009;48(12):1606–12.

31. Rudominer RL, Roman MJ, Devereux RB, Paget SA, Schwartz JE, Lockshin MD, et al. Independent association of rheumatoid arthritis with increased left ventricular mass but not with reduced ejection fraction. Arthritis Rheum. 2009;60(1):22–9.

32. Miyoshi T, Doi M, Hirohata S, Sakane K, Kamikawa S, Kitawaki T, et al. Cardio-ankle vascular index is independently associated with the severity of coronary atherosclerosis and left ventricular function in patients with ischemic heart disease. J Atheroscler Thromb. 2010;17(3):249–58.

33. Sato Y, Nagayama D, Saiki A, Watanabe R, Watanabe Y, Imamura H, et al. Cardio-ankle vascular index is independently associated with future cardiovascular events in outpatients with metabolic disorders. J Atheroscler Thromb. 2016;23(5):596–605.

34. Urbina EM, Dolan LM, McCoy CE, Khoury PR, Daniels SR, Kimball TR. Relationship between elevated arterial stiffness and increased left ventricular mass in adolescents and young adults. J Pediatr. 2011;158(5):715–21.

35. Chung CM, Lin YS, Chu CM, Chang ST, Cheng HW, Yang TY, et al. Arterial stiffness is the independent factor of left ventricular hypertrophy determined by electrocardiogram. Am J Med Sci. 2012;344(3):190–3.

36. Totaro S, Khoury PR, Kimball TR, Dolan LM, Urbina EM. Arterial stiffness is increased in young normotensive subjects with high central blood pressure. J Am Soc Hypertens. 2015;9(4):285–92.

37. Thavendiranathan P, Poulin F, Lim KD, Plana JC, Woo A, Marwick TH. Use of myocardial strain imaging by echocardiography for the early detection of cardiotoxicity in patients during and after cancer chemotherapy: a systematic review. J Am Coll Cardiol. 2014;63(25 Pt A):2751–68.

38. Afonso LC, Bernal J, Bax JJ, Abraham TP. Echocardiography in hypertrophic cardiomyopathy: the role of conventional and emerging technologies. JACC Cardiovasc Imaging. 2008;1(6):787–800.

39. Midtbo H, Semb AG, Matre K, Kvien TK, Gerdts E. Disease activity is associated with reduced left ventricular systolic myocardial function in patients with rheumatoid arthritis. Ann Rheum Dis. 2017;76(2):371–6.

40. Castrejon I, Ortiz AM, Garcia-Vicuna R, Lopez-Bote JP, Humbria A, Carmona L, et al. Are the C-reactive protein values and erythrocyte sedimentation rate equivalent when estimating the 28-joint disease activity score in rheumatoid arthritis? Clin Exp Rheumatol. 2008;26(5):769–75.

41. Fleischmann RM, van der Heijde D, Gardiner PV, Szumski A, Marshall L, Bananis E. DAS28-CRP and DAS28-ESR cut-offs for high disease activity in rheumatoid arthritis are not interchangeable. RMD Open. 2017;3(1):e000382.

42. Yiu KH, Tse HF, Mok MY, Lau CS. Ethnic differences in cardiovascular risk in rheumatic disease: focus on Asians. Nat Rev Rheumatol. 2011;7(10):609–18.

43. Buakhamsri A, Popovic ZB, Lin J, Lim P, Greenberg NL, Borowski AG, et al. Impact of left ventricular volume/mass ratio on diastolic function. Eur Heart J. 2009;30(10):1213–21.

44. Manzi S, Meilahn EN, Rairie JE, Conte CG, Medsger TA Jr, Jansen-McWilliams L, et al. Age-specific incidence rates of myocardial infarction and angina in women with systemic lupus erythematosus: comparison with the Framingham study. Am J Epidemiol. 1997;145(5):408–15.

45. Mok CC, Kwok CL, Ho LY, Chan PT, Yip SF. Life expectancy, standardized mortality ratios, and causes of death in six rheumatic diseases in Hong Kong, China. Arthritis Rheum. 2011;63(5):1182–9.

46. Mor-Avi V, Lang RM, Badano LP, Belohlavek M, Cardim NM, Derumeaux G, et al. Current and evolving echocardiographic techniques for the quantitative evaluation of cardiac mechanics: ASE/EAE consensus statement on methodology and indications endorsed by the Japanese Society of Echocardiography. J Am Soc Echocardiogr. 2011;24(3):277–313.

47. Ikonomidis I, Tzortzis S, Lekakis J, Paraskevaidis I, Andreadou I, Nikolaou M, et al. Lowering interleukin-1 activity with anakinra improves myocardial deformation in rheumatoid arthritis. Heart. 2009;95(18):1502–7.

48. Spethmann S, Rieper K, Riemekasten G, Borges AC, Schattke S, Burmester GR, et al. Echocardiographic follow-up of patients with systemic sclerosis by 2D speckle tracking echocardiography of the left ventricle. Cardiovasc Ultrasound. 2014;12:13.

4

Quadriceps muscle properties in rheumatoid arthritis: Insights about muscle morphology, activation and functional capacity

Denise Blum[1], Rodrigo Rodrigues[2,3]* ⓘ, Jeam Marcel Geremia[2], Claiton Viegas Brenol[1], Marco Aurélio Vaz[2] and Ricardo Machado Xavier[1]

Abstract

Background: Rheumatoid arthritis (RA) is an inflammatory and chronic autoimmune disease that leads to muscle mass loss and functional capacity impairment, potentiated by physical inactivity. Despite evidences demonstrate neuromuscular impairments in RA patients, aging effects may have masked the results of similar previous studies. The aim of study was to verify (i) the effects of RA on functional capacity and muscle properties in middle-aged patients and (ii) the association between age, clinical characteristics, quadriceps muscle properties and functional capacity.

Methods: Thirty-five RA women and 35 healthy age-matched women were compared with the following outcomes: (i) physical activity level through the International Physical Activity Questionnaire (IPAQ); (ii) timed-up and go (TUG) test; (iii) isometric knee extensor muscular strength; and (iv) vastus lateralis muscle activation and muscle architecture (muscle thickness, pennation angle and fascicle length) during an isometric test. An independent Student t-test and partial correlation (controlled by physical activity levels) were performed, with $p < 0.05$.

Results: Compared with healthy women, RA presented (i) lower physical activity level (-29.4%; $p < 0.001$); (ii) lower isometric knee extensor strength (-20.5%; $p < 0.001$); (iii) lower TUG performance (-21.7%; $p < 0.001$); (iv) smaller muscle thickness (-23.3%; $p < 0.001$) and pennation angle (-14.1%; $p = 0.011$). No differences were observed in muscle activation and fascicle length. Finally, the correlation demonstrated that, with exception of TUG, muscle strength and muscle morphology were not associated with age in RA, differently from healthy participants.

Conclusion: Middle-aged RA patients' impairments occurred due to the disease independently of the aging process, except for functional capacity. Physical inactivity may have potentiated these losses.

Keywords: Arthritis, rheumatoid, Quadriceps muscle, Electromyography, Muscular atrophy, Muscle strength

Introduction

Rheumatoid arthritis (RA) is a chronic autoimmune disease that causes joint inflammation and progressive joint destruction [1]. Its main symptoms are joint pain, morning stiffness and fatigue [2]. In industrialized countries,

RA affects 0.5–1% of adults, with 5–50 per 100,000 new cases annually. Fifty percent for RA's development risk has been attributed to genetic factors [2]. Moreover, RA patients usually avoid physical activities due to their fear of exacerbating the disease symptoms [3], which contributes to an enhanced pro-inflammatory burden and high level of disease activity [4]. However, regular muscle contraction may suppress pro-inflammatory activity [5], and, consequently, attenuate the disease's activity level.

* Correspondence: rodrigo.esef@gmail.com
[2]Laboratório de Pesquisa do Exercício, Universidade Federal do Rio Grande do Sul, Porto Alegre, Brazil
[3]Centro Universitário da Serra Gaúcha, Caxias do Sul, Brazil
Full list of author information is available at the end of the article

One of RA's structural manifestations is rheumatoid cachexia that consists of a muscle mass reduction due to an increased muscle protein catabolism induced by inflammatory cytokines [6, 7]. This muscle mass loss generates an impairment in RA patients physical function and functional capacity [8].

Previous studies observed a smaller vastus lateralis (VL) pennation angle, cross-sectional area (CSA) and volume in RA patients compared to healthy subjects [1, 6]. However, functional capacity impairment [1, 9], without changes in knee extensor muscle activity and strength, has been observed [1, 6, 9]. Despite RA's mechanisms are not completely clear, the identification of neuromuscular changes induced by RA is critical in order to create adequate rehabilitation programs able to improve the patients' functional capacity [1, 6, 7]. Previous clinical studies demonstrated a relationship between knee extensor morphological parameters, muscular strength, and functional capacity in knee osteoarthritis [10], cancer [11] and chronic obstructive pulmonary disease (COPD) patients [12].

Although changes in quadriceps morphological parameters were observed in RA patients [1, 6, 9], it is important to note that the contribution of muscle activation parameters to the observed knee extensor muscle strength impairment in RA patients is uncertain [1, 6, 13]. Despite the losses in muscle mass, muscle strength, and functional capacity observed in RA patients in previous studies [1, 6, 13], their neuromuscular parameters results were probably masked due to aging effects. Similar results to those in RA were observed for strength [14, 15], functional capacity [16], VL muscle thickness [17, 18], pennation angle [18] and activation [19] with aging, which are also augmented by physical inactivity [20].

Thus, despite functional and neuromuscular changes were observed in RA patients [1, 6, 13], the aging effects might have masked the true neuromuscular adaptations due to RA. Based in these observed limitations, the first aim of the present study was to verify the RA impact on quadriceps muscle properties, muscular strength and functional capacity in middle-aged RA women compared with healthy controls, matched by sex and age. In addition, we wanted to verify if there is an association between age, clinical characteristics, muscle parameters and functional capacity in both groups.

Material and methods

Subjects

RA's patients that presented functional classes I (able to perform usual activities of daily living, including self-care, vocational and avocational activities) and II (able to perform usual self-care and vocational activities, but limited in avocational activities), according to the American Rheumatism Association's 1992 revised criteria [21] and at least 3 years of confirmed diagnosis were recruited from the rheumatology service of Hospital de Clínicas de Porto Alegre. Exclusion criteria included the presence of any cardiovascular, neuromuscular and metabolic diseases, inability to walk or flex the knee and knee replacement, pain or swelling in the knee joint. Additionally, juvenile RA patients were also excluded. The recruited RA patients were compared with age and sex matched healthy controls (GC), which were recruited from the local community. A written informed consent was obtained from all participants before starting the experiment. The study was approved by the Hospital Ethical Research Committee (number 09–634) and was conducted respecting the ethical standards of the Declaration of Helsinki General Assembly Meeting (October 2008).

At the lab, participants performed the following evaluations: (i) questionnaires and scales; (ii) body composition measurements; (iii), knee extensor muscle architecture, muscle activation, muscular strength, and (iv) the Timed-Up and Go (TUG) test. All neuromuscular parameters were measured on the participants' right limb, based on a previous study [1].

RA disease activity, pain score, physical activity and function

Disease activity in RA patients was estimated using the composite score of the Disease Activity Score-28 with Erythrocyte Sedimentation Rate (DAS28-ESR). Scores below 2.6 indicated remission, from 2.6 to 3.1 low, from 3.2 to 5.1 moderate, and higher than 5.1 indicated high disease activity [22].

Physical activity level was determined through the International Physical Activity Questionnaire (IPAQ), which captures the activities' intensity performed during leisure time, at work, during domestic tasks and active transport. The sum of all these activities is defined as the total physical activity and was presented in met.min.-week [17].

Additionally, the self-assessed physical function was obtained through the Health Assessment Questionnaire (HAQ), which includes questions about the performance on activities of daily living [23]. Also, before any physical test, the pain level was evaluated with a 0–100 mm visual analogue scale (VAS), where 0 and 100 mm corresponded to no pain and intolerable pain, respectively.

Functional capacity and knee extensor muscular strength

The TUG test measures the time for an individual to rise from a chair, walk 3 m to touch a marker on a wall, turn 180°, return to the chair and sit down [16]. Time was recorded by a stopwatch, and participants were instructed not to use their hands when rising from or sitting back down on the chair.

Maximal knee-extensor muscle strength was measured with a Biodex System 3 dynamometer (Biodex Medical

Systems, Shirley, NY, USA). Volunteers were positioned on the dynamometer according to the manufacturer's recommendations for knee evaluations, with the hip angle fixed at 85°, knee flexed at 90° and the trunk, hips and thighs firmly strapped to the apparatus. Subjects performed a warm-up protocol consisting of 10 submaximal knee extension/flexion repetitions at an angular velocity of $90°.s^{-1}$. Next, subjects were instructed to execute the test with the highest possible effort to develop maximal knee extension, and verbal encouragement was provided throughout the test. Three knee extensor isometric tests at 90° of knee flexion (0° = full knee extension) were executed, with a 2-min resting period between contractions [24, 25]. The peak torque obtained from these three contractions was normalized to body mass (Nm/Kg) and used for analysis.

Muscle architecture measurements

A B-mode ultrasonography system (SSD-4000; Aloka Inc., Tokyo, Japan) with a linear-array probe (60 mm, 7.5 MHz) was used to determine VL muscle thickness, pennation angle and fascicle length. The same investigator, with extensive experience in ultrasonography, performed all ultrasound measurements, and high reliability values were obtained in the study [24]. Muscle architecture measurements were obtained with the volunteer seated in the dynamometer, during maximal isometric contraction at 90° of knee flexion. The images were recorded during all data collection through a DVD and synchronized (Horita Video Stop Watch VS – 50; Horita Co., Inc., California, USA) to the isokinetic dynamometer using a single pulse generator. During synchronization, the button was pressed before the isometric test, sending the pulse sampled on a separate channel of the data collection system, which allowed the identification of the exact time of the isometric peak torque and the corresponding ultrasound images used for data analysis during contraction [26].

Scans were taken at the midpoint between the great trochanter and the femur lateral condyle. The ultrasonography probe was covered with water-soluble transmission gel and oriented parallel to the VL muscle fascicles and perpendicular to the skin. The transducer orientation relative to the longitudinal axis of the thigh was different between subjects due to their individual anatomical characteristics. Probe alignment was considered appropriate when several muscle fascicles could be easily delineated without interruption across the image. Ultrasonography images were digitized and analyzed with Image J software (National Institutes of Health, Bethesda, Maryland).

Muscle thickness was considered the distance between deep and superficial aponeuroses, and was calculated through the mean value of five parallel lines drawn at right angles between the superficial and deep aponeuroses along each ultrasonography image. The best fascicle in each image was used for pennation angle and fascicle length analysis. Pennation angle was calculated as the angle between the muscle fascicle and the deep aponeurosis, whereas fascicle length was measured as the length of the fascicular path between the two aponeuroses. When fascicle length was greater than the probe surface, the fascicle line was extrapolated and calculated through a trigonometric function. This mathematical procedure has been used in several studies involving VL fascicle length evaluations [17, 24] (Fig. 1). After that, fascicle length measurement was normalized and expressed as percent of thigh length (distance between the femur lateral condyle and the great trochanter) [27].

Muscle activation

An 8-channel EMG system (AMT-8, Bortec Biomedical Ltd., Calgary, Canada) was synchronized with the dynamometer through a Windaq data acquisition system (Dataq Instruments Inc., Ohio, USA), and used to evaluate the VL electrical activity during the isometric knee-extensor test. Skin preparation and electrode positioning for EMG evaluation followed standard procedures [28]. Passive electrodes (Meditrace 100, Kendall, Boca Raton, USA) were positioned in bipolar configuration (inter-electrode distance: 2.2 cm) on the VL muscle (2/3 on the line from the anterior superior iliac spine to the patella's lateral side). A reference electrode was fixed on the tibia's medial surface.

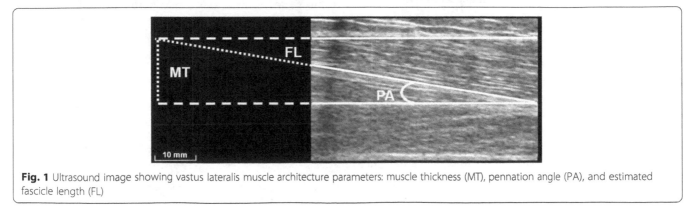

Fig. 1 Ultrasound image showing vastus lateralis muscle architecture parameters: muscle thickness (MT), pennation angle (PA), and estimated fascicle length (FL)

Raw EMG signals were digitized with a sampling frequency of 2000 Hz per channel with a DI-720 16 bits analogue-to-digital board (Dataq Instruments Inc., Ohio, USA), and stored for subsequent analysis. Data were exported to MATLAB® software (MathWorks Inc., Natick, USA), where they were filtered using a Butterworth band-pass filter, with cut-off frequencies of 20 and 500 Hz. Root mean square (RMS) values were calculated from 1-s segments of the EMG signals obtained from the plateau of the knee-extensor isometric torque. Participants performed an additional knee extensor isometric test at 75° of knee flexion (optimal angle for maximal knee extensor strength production) [17] to normalize EMG data obtained during the isometric test at 90° (expressed in percent of maximum).

Table 1 Subjects' characteristics

	CG ($n = 35$)	RA ($n = 35$)	p-value
Age (years)	45.33 ± 12.50	47.92 ± 14.37	0.438
Body mass (Kg)	64.39 ± 9.84	66.53 ± 14.97	0.754
Height (m)	1.62 ± 0.05	1.60 ± 0.07	0.634
Body Mass Index (kg.m^{-2})	24.53 ± 4.23	25.81 ± 5.08	0.249
Pain (VAS)	0.65 ± 1.68	3.00 ± 2.87*	**< 0.001**
IPAQ (met.min.week)	1351.47 ± 425.12	956.19 ± 291.09*	**< 0.001**
HAQ (pts)	N.A	0.43 ± 0.07	N.A
DAS 28-ESR (pts)	N.A	3.81 ± 0.72	N.A
Disease Duration (years)	N.A	12.31 ± 4.32	N.A

CG Control Group, *RA* Rheumatoid Arthritis, *IPAQ* International Physical Activity Questionnaire, *VAS* Visual Analogue Scale, *DAS 28-ESR* Disease Activity Scores, *HAQ* Health Assessment Questionnaire, *NA* Not Applicable; *difference between-group

Statistical analysis

Sample size was determined from the data obtained in a previous study similar to ours [1] for the variables knee extensor isometric torque, vastus lateralis pennation angle and fascicle length obtained during contraction. Effect size (ES) (Cohen's *d*) was calculated for each group (RA patients and healthy subjects) based on mean and SD values. Assuming the ES obtained in each outcome, $\alpha = 0.05$ and $\beta = 0.95$ in an independent Student t-test, a minimum of 30 participants (15 in each group) were needed for knee isometric torque, 70 participants (35 in each group) for vastus lateralis pennation angle and 28 participants (14 in each group) for vastus lateralis fascicle length. Thus, we adopted the number of 70 participants as the minimum necessary to observe significant differences at the main muscular outcomes used in our study.

Data normality was tested through the Shapiro-Wilk test. Data sphericity was tested by Mauchly test, and Greenhouse-Geisser correction factor was used when the sphericity was violated. An independent Student t-test was used to compare all between-groups outcomes. Effect size was calculated for each paired comparison (*d*). Cohen's *d* was interpreted based in the following classification (< 0.2: trivial; > 0.2: small; > 0.50: moderate; > 0.80: large) [29].

Moreover, a partial correlation analysis using the physical activity levels as covariant was performed between all neuromuscular outcomes [VL structure and activation, TUG and knee-extensor isometric torque] and age for both groups. Finally, in the RA patients, additional association analysis between neuromuscular outcomes and clinical characteristics (HAQ, DAS28-ESR, disease duration, accumulated and current dose of glucocorticoids and level of pain) were performed. A significance level of 5% was adopted for all analyses and all statistical procedures were performed in SPSS 20.0.

Results

Thirty-five RA women and 35 healthy women (CG) were recruited to participate in the study. RA patients had lower level of physical activity compared to the CG. The Health Assessment Questionnaire (HAQ) score was 0.43 ± 0.07 points and the disease activity score (DAS 28-ESR) was 3.81 ± 0.72 points, indicating that most patients displayed a moderate disease activity (27/35, 77%). The RA patients' average disease duration was 12.3 ± 4.3 years (Table 1).

All RA patients were under treatment with specific drugs for the disease. Thirty-four patients were taking prednisolone (range 5–30 mg/day, average dose 10.9 mg/day). Thirty-one of them combined this drug with methotrexate (range 10–25 mg/wk., average dose 18.5 mg/wk), and five of them combined prednisolone with other drugs (three using leflunomide, average dose of 20 mg/wk., and two using hydroxychloroquine, average dose of 240 mg/wk). RA patients also displayed higher VAS pain levels compared to controls (Table 1).

Regarding functional capacity, knee-extensor muscular strength and neuromuscular outcomes, RA patients

Table 2 Functional capacity, muscular strength and neuromuscular outcomes data of RA patients and healthy controls

Outcome	CG ($n = 35$)	RA ($n = 35$)	p-value	ES
TUG (sec)	8.42 ± 1.37	10.80 ± 2.72*	**< 0.001**	1.10
Torque (Nm/Kg)	1.94 ± 0.59	1.40 ± 0.46*	**< 0.001**	−1.02
VL RMS (%MIVC)	92.81 ± 21.96	99.25 ± 41.32	0.412	0.20
Muscle thickness (cm)	1.72 ± 0.31	1.37 ± 0.34*	**< 0.001**	−1.08
Pennation angle (°)	9.95 ± 1.81	8.65 ± 2.36*	**0.011**	− 0.62
Fascicle length (%)	25.61 ± 3.83	25.25 ± 5.56	0.749	− 0.07

CG Control Group, *RA* Rheumatoid Arthritis Group, *ES* Effect size, *TUG* Time-up-and go test, *VL* Vastus lateralis muscle; *difference between-group

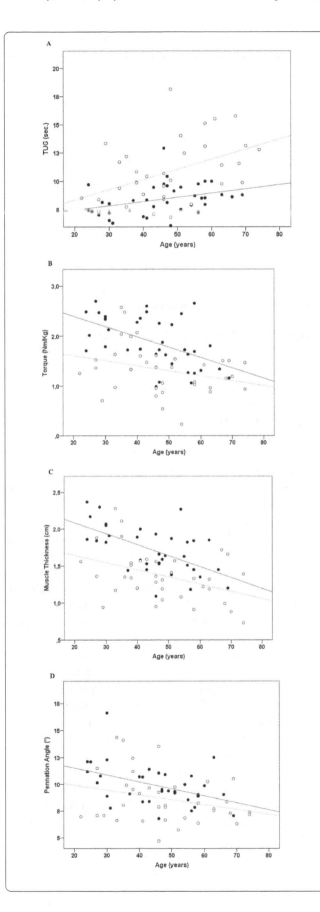

Fig. 2 Partial correlation analysis (controlling by physical activity levels) was significant between TUG and Age in both RA ($r = 0.438$; $p = 0.010$) and CG ($r = 0.336$; $p = 0.048$) **a**, Torque and Age in the CG ($r = -0.498$; $p = 0.002$), but not in RA ($r = -0.317$; $p = 0.089$) (**b**), Muscle Thickness and Age in the CG ($r = -0.576$; $p < 0.001$), but not in RA ($r = -0.310$; $p = 0.092$) (**c**) and Pennation Angle and Age in the CG ($r = -0.462$; $p = 0.005$), but not in RA ($r = -0.260$; $p = 0.137$) (**d**). Black dots = CG; White dots = RA. Solid line = CG; Dashed line = RA

showed lower TUG performance (– 21.7%, i.e. longer duration) and knee-extensor isometric torque (– 20.5%) compared to the CG. RA patients showed smaller VL muscle thickness (– 23.3%) and pennation angle (– 14.1%). No between-group differences were observed in the normalized VL fascicle length and activation (Table 2).

The partial correlations (part r) using physical activity levels as a covariant, demonstrated a significant association between: (i) TUG and age in both RA ($r = 0.438$; $p = 0.010$) and CG ($r = 0.336$; $p = 0.048$); (ii) knee extensor isometric torque and age in the CG ($r = -0.498$; $p = 0.002$), but not in RA ($r = -0.317$; $p = 0.089$); (iii) muscle thickness and age in the CG ($r = -0.576$; $p < 0.001$), but not in RA ($r = -0.310$; $p = 0.092$) and (iv) pennation angle and age in the CG ($r = -0.462$; $p = 0.005$), but not in RA ($r = -0.260$; $p = 0.137$) (Fig. 2 A-D). No association was observed between age and normalized VL fascicle length and activation in both groups ($p > 0.05$). Additionally, in the RA, no association was observed between clinical characteristics [HAQ, DAS28-ESR, current and accumulated dose of glucocorticoids, disease duration and pain] and functional and neuromuscular outcomes [TUG, torque, VL muscle thickness, pennation angle, fascicle length and activation] ($p > 0.05$) (Table 3).

Discussion

Our results demonstrated impairment in functional capacity, muscular strength and muscle morphology in RA patients compared to healthy subjects. Except for the TUG, muscle strength and muscle properties were not associated with age in RA, as opposed to healthy participants in which there was an association. These results suggest that the differences observed between RA and CG, except for functional capacity, occurred due to the disease, not to the aging process. The losses in functionality and muscular strength have been commonly explained by changes in neuromuscular outcomes (muscle activity and muscle architecture properties) [11, 30, 31], although muscle activity did not play a role in our case.

Impairment in muscle activation is a possible explanation for muscle strength and functional capacity losses. A previous study [13] observed a significant quadriceps inhibition (8%) in RA compared to healthy participants, which helped to explain the knee extensor muscular strength impairment. Muscle inhibition mechanisms in

Table 3 RA patients association between neuromuscular outcomes and clinical characteristics controlled by physical activity level

	TUG	Torque	VL RMS	Muscle thickness	Pennation Angle	Fascicle Length
Disease duration	$r = -0.030$	$r = 0.180$	$r = 0.224$	$r = -0.003$	$r = -0.310$	$r = 0.318$
	$p = 0.879$	$p = 0.328$	$p = 0.244$	$p = 0.988$	$p = 0.102$	$p = 0.093$
DAS28-ESR	$r = -0.248$	$r = 0.161$	$r = -0.202$	$r = 0.036$	$r = -0.126$	$r = 0.161$
	$p = 0.194$	$p = 0.404$	$p = 0.294$	$p = 0.851$	$p = 0.515$	$p = 0.404$
HAQ	$r = -0.119$	$r = -0.017$	$r = -0.161$	$r = -0.013$	$r = -0.081$	$r = -0.057$
	$p = 0.539$	$p = 0.929$	$p = 0.403$	$p = 0.948$	$p = 0.676$	$p = 0.770$
Current dose of GC	$r = -0.201$	$r = 0.069$	$r = -0.104$	$r = 0.131$	$r = 0.092$	$r = 0.018$
	$p = 0.296$	$p = 0.721$	$p = 0.592$	$p = 0.498$	$p = 0.634$	$p = 0.927$
Accumulated dose of GC	$r = -0.172$	$r = 0.125$	$r = -0.030$	$r = 0.084$	$r = -0.121$	$r = 0.164$
	$p = 0.373$	$p = 0.518$	$p = 0.877$	$p = 0.663$	$p = 0.531$	$p = 0.395$
Pain	$r = -0.088$	$r = 0.076$	$r = -0.002$	$r = 0.232$	$r = 0.128$	$r = 0.111$
	$p = 0.649$	$p = 0.697$	$p = 0.993$	$p = 0.225$	$p = 0.509$	$p = 0.566$

DAS28-ESR Disease Activity Score-28 with Erythrocyte Sedimentation Rate, *HAQ* Health Assessment Questionnaire, *GC* Glucocorticoids

RA are unknown, but abnormal afferent information from articular mechanoreceptors, due to joint damage, effusion and pain, have been proposed to explain the voluntary activation impairment and decreased muscular strength [32]. Our study did not demonstrate an impairment in VL muscle activation during maximal tests, similar to what has been observed in previous studies [1, 6]. The absence of pain or swelling in the knee joint of our patients might explain the lack of impairment in VL muscle activation.

RA patients presented lower muscle thickness and pennation angle during the knee-extensor maximal isometric test compared to the CG. Previous studies observed a decrease in VL physiological cross-sectional area (PCSA) [1] and muscle volume [6] caused by RA, which probably led to a reduction in muscle thickness [30, 31] and a smaller force generating capacity [33]. No between-groups differences were observed in fascicle length, agreeing with a previous study [1]. A previous study [34] pointed that an increase in muscle thickness due to training may occur by an increase in pennation angle (addition of in-parallel sarcomeres) or fascicle length (addition of sarcomeres in-series). Thus, the observed smaller muscle thickness in our study was explained by the reduction in pennation angle and not by the fascicle length [35], indicating a parallel loss of sarcomeres due to the rheumatic disease.

Neuromuscular losses observed in our study were also observed in previous studies in patients with chronic disease [10–12, 36]. In RA patients, quadriceps weakness is usually associated with muscle atrophy resulting from the inflammatory process induced by the disease [37], causing proteolytic events, and resulting in cell breakdown and death [38]. In our study, most of the patients displayed a moderate disease activity (77%), which was not associated with neuromuscular parameters. In addition, pain and

disability induced by disease limit the patient's daily living activities [13]. It is interesting to observe that physical inactivity contributes to an enhanced pro-inflammatory condition, and regular muscle contraction may suppress pro-inflammatory activity [5]. Additionally, a higher physical activity level was associated with higher muscle mass [20]. As the disease [39] and physical activity levels [40] are related to poorer muscle performance, and physical inactivity contributes to enhancing pro-inflammatory processes, we believe that our findings are in line with these reports, as the RA group showed lower physical activity levels compared to CG.

Besides physical activity, the use of glucocorticoids is a common strategy to fight the disease and to substantially reduce the rate of erosion progression in RA when used with other anti-rheumatoid drugs [41]. Although the chronic use of glucocorticoids induces muscle atrophy due to increased protein breakdown and decreased protein synthesis [42], this consequence particularly occurs if high doses are used for prolonged periods [43]. We observed that our patients showed an average dose of 10.9 mg/day, being classified as a medium dose (between 7.5–30 mg/day) [44]. The occurrence of myopathy in patients receiving glucocorticoids is rare at low doses [45]. Additionally, the accumulated and current dose of glucocorticoids reported by our patients were not associated with neuromuscular outcomes. Therefore, it is unlikely that our results were related with the use of glucocorticoids. Future research should be directed towards studying the long-term effects of glucocorticoid treatment in RA and its influence on body composition, muscle mass and functional capacity.

To the best of our knowledge, this is the first study to demonstrate a muscle morphology impairment solely related to the rheumatic disease and not to the aging process. The RA patients and healthy subjects age in previous studies [1, 6] was quite high (average 59–60 years), indicating a possible aging effect that might have masked the true neuromuscular adaptations due to RA. VL muscle thickness is reduced in the elderly [17, 18], and a muscle mass reduction is considered the major cause for the strength loss [14]. An age-related decline in pennation angle has also been previously reported [18], and is thought to be due to reductions in fiber number and/or fiber diameter that accompany sarcopenia [33]. Our results demonstrated that the neuromuscular adaptations induced by RA occurred independently from the aging process, since, when controlling the physical activity levels, age was not associated with strength and muscle properties, with exception of TUG, differently from what was observed in healthy participants. TUG is a simple test embedding several tasks (stand up from a chair, walk forward, turn around an obstacle, walk back to the chair, and sit down) represented by total time. It is possible that the TUG single components may have presented a different behavior across the aging process [46] and combined with RA. This hypothesis should be further explored.

Decrease in functional capacity and muscular strength could be partially explained by changes in tendon stiffness [47], also observed in RA patients' patellar tendon [9]. The reduction in tendon stiffness is likely due to local and systemic effects of cytokines on the tendon structural characteristics [48]. In addition, the reduction in mechanical overload due to a decrease in physical activity level could potentiate tendon stiffness impairment [9, 47]. Although we did not measure this outcome, the reduced muscular strength and functional capacity might also be explained by changes in patellar tendon stiffness, since a reduction in tendon stiffness impairs the rate of force development [49] and, consequently, daily living activity (i.e. TUG).

One of the main study limitations was the absence of other tests to evaluate functional capacity, which might have helped us to understand different aspects of functional impairment. Tests such as the 30-s sit-to-stand test and descending stairs might have helped us to identify other functional responses. The lack of dynamic maximal strength measurements are also a limitation, as a low knee extensor muscle shortening velocity decreases the RA patients ability to perform basic activities [50]. Finally, the absence of other quadriceps portions (i.e. vastus medialis and rectus femoris) analysis is also a limitation, since quadriceps muscle neuromuscular parameters have been found as the best dynamic strength predictors [51].

Conclusion

Middle-aged RA patients presented impairment in functional capacity, quadriceps muscle strength and muscle morphology due to the rheumatic disease, not to the aging process, except for functional capacity. We believe that the combination between physical inactivity and chronic inflammation caused by the disease in RA patients might explain the observed changes. Thus, an increase in the physical activity level may be a safe and effective strategy to minimize the functional losses due to this rheumatic disease.

Abbreviations
%MIVC: Maximal isometric voluntary contraction; CG: Control group; COPD: Chronic obstructive pulmonary disease; CSA: Cross-sectional area; DAS28: Disease activity score; EMG: Electromyography; ES: Effect size; FL: Fascicle length; GC: Glucocorticoids; HAQ: Health Assessment Questionnaire; IPAQ: International physical activity questionnaire; MT: Muscle thickness; PA: Pennation angle; PCSA: Physiological cross-sectional area; RA: Rheumatoid arthritis; RMS: Root mean square; TUG: Timed up and go; VAS: Visual analogic scale; VL: Vastus lateralis

Acknowledgements
This work was conducted during a scholarship supported by the International Cooperation Program CAPES/COFECUB at the Federal University of Rio Grande do Sul. Financed by CAPES – Brazilian Federal Agency for Support and Evaluation of Graduate Education within the Ministry of Education of Brazil.

Authors' contributions
DB: the conception, acquisition of data, analysis and interpretation of data, draft of the article revising it critically for important intellectual content and final approval of the version to be submitted; RR: acquisition of data, analysis and interpretation of data, draft of the article revising it critically for important intellectual content, final approval of the version to be submitted and correspondent author; JMG: acquisition of data, data analysis, critical revision of the article, final approval of the version to be submitted; CVB: critical revision of the article, final approval of the version to be submitted; MAV: interpretation of data, draft of the article revising it critically for important intellectual content, final approval of the version to be submitted; RMX: conception, interpretation of data, draft of the article revising it critically for important intellectual content, final approval of the version to be submitted

Author details
[1]Serviço de Reumatologia, Hospital de Clínicas de Porto Alegre, Universidade Federal do Rio Grande do Sul, Porto Alegre, Brazil. [2]Laboratório de Pesquisa do Exercício, Universidade Federal do Rio Grande do Sul, Porto Alegre, Brazil. [3]Centro Universitário da Serra Gaúcha, Caxias do Sul, Brazil.

References
1. Matschke V, Murphy P, Lemmey AB, Maddison P, Thom JM. Skeletal muscle properties in rheumatoid arthritis patients. Med Sci Sports Exerc. 2010; 42(12):2149–55. https://doi.org/10.1249/MSS.0b013e3181e304c3.
2. Scott DL, Wolfe F, Huizinga TW. Rheumatoid arthritis. Lancet. 2010; 376(9746):1094–108. https://doi.org/10.1016/S0140-6736(10)60826-4.
3. Geuskens GA, Burdorf A, Hazes JM. Consequences of rheumatoid arthritis for performance of social roles--a literature review. J Rheumatol. 2007;34(6): 1248–60.
4. Li Y, Yao L, Liu S, Wu J, Xia L, Shen H, et al. Elevated serum IL-35 levels in rheumatoid arthritis are associated with disease activity. J Investig Med. 2019;67(3):707–10. https://doi.org/10.1136/jim-2018-000814.
5. Bruunsgaard H. Physical activity and modulation of systemic low-level inflammation. J Leukoc Biol. 2005;78(4):819–35. https://doi.org/10.1189/jlb.0505247.
6. Matschke V, Murphy P, Lemmey AB, Maddison PJ, Thom JM. Muscle quality, architecture, and activation in cachectic patients with rheumatoid arthritis. J Rheumatol. 2010;37(2):282–4. https://doi.org/10.3899/jrheum.090584.

7. Huffman KM, Jessee R, Andonian B, Davis BN, Narowski R, Huebner JL, et al. Molecular alterations in skeletal muscle in rheumatoid arthritis are related to disease activity, physical inactivity, and disability. Arthritis Res Ther. 2017; 19(1):12. https://doi.org/10.1186/s13075-016-1215-7.

8. de Santana FS, Nascimento Dda C, de Freitas JP, Miranda RF, Muniz LF, Santos Neto L, et al. Assessment of functional capacity in patients with rheumatoid arthritis: implications for recommending exercise. Rev Bras Reumatol. 2014;54(5):378–85. https://doi.org/10.1016/j.rbr.2014.03.021.

9. Matschke V, Jones JG, Lemmey AB, Maddison PJ, Thom JM. Patellar tendon properties and lower limb function in rheumatoid arthritis and ankylosing spondylitis versus healthy controls: a cross-sectional study. ScientificWorldJournal. 2013;2013:514743. https://doi.org/10.1155/2013/ 514743.

10. Gur H, Cakin N. Muscle mass, isokinetic torque, and functional capacity in women with osteoarthritis of the knee. Arch Phys Med Rehabil. 2003;84(10): 1534–41. https://doi.org/10.1016/s0003-9993(03)00288-0.

11. Williams GR, Deal AM, Muss HB, Weinberg MS, Sanoff HK, Nyrop KA, et al. Skeletal muscle measures and physical function in older adults with cancer: sarcopenia or myopenia? Oncotarget. 2017;8(20):33658–65. https://doi.org/ 10.18632/oncotarget.16866.

12. Butcher SJ, Pikaluk BJ, Chura RL, Walkner MJ, Farthing JP, Marciniuk DD. Associations between isokinetic muscle strength, high-level functional performance, and physiological parameters in patients with chronic obstructive pulmonary disease. Int J Chron Obstruct Pulmon Dis. 2012;7: 537–42. https://doi.org/10.2147/COPD.S34170.

13. Bearne LM, Scott DL, Hurley MV. Exercise can reverse quadriceps sensorimotor dysfunction that is associated with rheumatoid arthritis without exacerbating disease activity. Rheumatology (Oxford). 2002;41(2): 157–66. https://doi.org/10.1093/rheumatology/41.2.157.

14. Reeves ND, Narici MV, Maganaris CN. In vivo human muscle structure and function: adaptations to resistance training in old age. Exp Physiol. 2004; 89(6):675–89. https://doi.org/10.1113/expphysiol.2004.027797.

15. Suzuki T, Bean JF, Fielding RA. Muscle power of the ankle flexors predicts functional performance in community-dwelling older women. J Am Geriatr Soc. 2001;49(9):1161–7. https://doi.org/10.1046/j.1532-5415.2001.49232.x.

16. Selva Raj I, Bird SR, Shield AJ. Ultrasound measurements of skeletal muscle architecture are associated with strength and functional capacity in older adults. Ultrasound Med Biol. 2017;43(3):586–94. https://doi.org/10.1016/j. ultrasmedbio.2016.11.013.

17. Baroni BM, Geremia JM, Rodrigues R, Borges MK, Jinha A, Herzog W, et al. Functional and morphological adaptations to aging in knee extensor muscles of physically active men. J Appl Biomech. 2013;29(5):535–42. https://doi.org/10.1123/jab.29.5.535.

18. Kubo K, Kanehisa H, Azuma K, Ishizu M, Kuno SY, Okada M, et al. Muscle architectural characteristics in women aged 20-79 years. Med Sci Sports Exerc. 2003;35(1):39–44. https://doi.org/10.1097/00005768-200301000-00007.

19. Piasecki M, Ireland A, Stashuk D, Hamilton-Wright A, Jones DA, McPhee JS. Age-related neuromuscular changes affecting human vastus lateralis. J Physiol. 2016;594(16):4525–36. https://doi.org/10.1113/JP271087.

20. Raguso CA, Kyle U, Kossovsky MP, Roynette C, Paoloni-Giacobino A, Hans D, et al. A 3-year longitudinal study on body composition changes in the elderly: role of physical exercise. Clin Nutr. 2006;25(4):573–80. https://doi. org/10.1016/j.clnu.2005.10.013.

21. Hochberg MC, Chang RW, Dwosh I, Lindsey S, Pincus T, Wolfe F. The American College of Rheumatology 1991 revised criteria for the classification of global functional status in rheumatoid arthritis. Arthritis Rheum. 1992;35(5):498–502. https://doi.org/10.1002/art.1780350502.

22. Prevoo ML. Van 't Hof MA, Kuper HH, van Leeuwen MA, van de Putte LB, van riel PL. modified disease activity scores that include twenty-eight-joint counts. Development and validation in a prospective longitudinal study of patients with rheumatoid arthritis. Arthritis Rheum. 1995;38(1):44–8. https:// doi.org/10.1002/art.1780380107.

23. Fries JF, Spitz PW, Young DY. The dimensions of health outcomes: the health assessment questionnaire, disability and pain scales. J Rheumatol. 1982;9(5):789–93.

24. Baroni BM, Rodrigues R, Franke RA, Geremia JM, Rassier DE, Vaz MA. Time course of neuromuscular adaptations to knee extensor eccentric training. Int J Sports Med. 2013;34(10):904–11. https://doi.org/10.1055/s-0032-1333263.

25. Rodrigues R, Baroni BM, Pompermayer MG, de Oliveira LR, Geremia JM, Meyer F, et al. Effects of acute dehydration on neuromuscular responses of

26. Geremia JM, Baroni BM, Bobbert MF, Bini RR, Lanferdini FJ, Vaz MA. Effects of high loading by eccentric triceps surae training on Achilles tendon properties in humans. Eur J Appl Physiol. 2018;118(8):1725–36. https://doi. org/10.1007/s00421-018-3904-1.

27. Kumagai K, Abe T, Brechue WF, Ryushi T, Takano S, Mizuno M. Sprint performance is related to muscle fascicle length in male 100-m sprinters. J Appl Physiol (1985). 2000;88(3):811–6. https://doi.org/10.1152/ jappl.2000.88.3.811.

28. SENIAM. Surface ElectroMyoGraphy for the Non-Invasive Assessment of Muscles. Available in < http://www.seniam.org/2017> [Accessed in April 2012].

29. Cohen, J. Statistical Power Analysis for the Behavioral Sciences (2nd ed.). Hillsdale: Lawrence Erlbaum Associates, Publishers;1988.

30. de Boer MD, Seynnes OR, di Prampero PE, Pisot R, Mekjavic IB, Biolo G, et al. Effect of 5 weeks horizontal bed rest on human muscle thickness and architecture of weight bearing and non-weight bearing muscles. Eur J Appl Physiol. 2008;104(2):401–7. https://doi.org/10.1007/s00421-008-0703-0.

31. Fitts RH, Riley DR, Widrick JJ. Functional and structural adaptations of skeletal muscle to microgravity. J Exp Biol. 2001;204(Pt 18):3201–8.

32. Palmieri-Smith RM, Villwock M, Downie B, Hecht G, Zernicke R. Pain and effusion and quadriceps activation and strength. J Athl Train. 2013;48(2): 186–91. https://doi.org/10.4085/1062-6050-48.2.10.

33. Narici MV, Maganaris CN, Reeves ND, Capodaglio P. Effect of aging on human muscle architecture. J Appl Physiol (1985). 2003;95(6):2229–34. https://doi.org/10.1152/japplphysiol.00433.2003.

34. Franchi MV, Reeves ND, Narici MV. Skeletal Muscle Remodeling in Response to Eccentric vs. Concentric Loading: Morphological, Molecular, and Metabolic Adaptations. Front Physiol. 2017;8:447. https://doi.org/10.3389/ fphys.2017.00447.

35. Narici M, Cerretelli P. Changes in human muscle architecture in disuse-atrophy evaluated by ultrasound imaging. J Gravit Physiol. 1998;5(1):P73–4.

36. Mesquita R, Wilke S, Smid DE, Janssen DJ, Franssen FM, Probst VS, et al. Measurement properties of the timed up & go test in patients with COPD. Chron Respir Dis. 2016;13(4):344–52. https://doi.org/10.1177/ 1479972316647178.

37. Roth SM, Metter EJ, Ling S, Ferrucci L. Inflammatory factors in age-related muscle wasting. Curr Opin Rheumatol. 2006;18(6):625–30. https://doi.org/10. 1097/01.bor.0000245722.10136.6d.

38. Narici MV, Maganaris CN. Adaptability of elderly human muscles and tendons to increased loading. J Anat. 2006;208(4):433–43. https://doi.org/10. 1111/j.1469-7580.2006.00548.x.

39. Uutela TI, Kautiainen HJ, Hakkinen AH. Decreasing muscle performance associated with increasing disease activity in patients with rheumatoid arthritis. PLoS One. 2018;13(4):e0194917. https://doi.org/10.1371/journal. pone.0194917.

40. Vardar-Yagli N, Sener G, Saglam M, Calik-Kutukcu E, Arikan H, Inal-Ince D, et al. Associations among physical activity, comorbidity, functional capacity, peripheral muscle strength and depression in breast cancer survivors. Asian Pac J Cancer Prev. 2015;16(2):585–9. https://doi.org/10.7314/apjcp. 2015.16.2.585.

41. Kirwan JR, Bijlsma JW, Boers M, Shea BJ. Effects of glucocorticoids on radiological progression in rheumatoid arthritis. Cochrane Database Syst Rev. 2007;1:CD006356. https://doi.org/10.1002/14651858.CD006356.

42. Schakman O, Kalista S, Barbe C, Loumaye A, Thissen JP. Glucocorticoid-induced skeletal muscle atrophy. Int J Biochem Cell Biol. 2013;45(10):2163–72. https://doi.org/10.1016/j.biocel.2013.05.036.

43. McKay LIC, J.A. Physiologic and pharmacologic effects of corticosteroids. In: Kufe DWPR, Weichselbaum RR, editors. Holland-Frei Cancer Medicine, 6th edition, Hamilton (ON): BC Decker 2003.

44. Buttgereit F, da Silva JA, Boers M, Burmester GR, Cutolo M, Jacobs J, et al. Standardised nomenclature for glucocorticoid dosages and glucocorticoid treatment regimens: current questions and tentative answers in rheumatology. Ann Rheum Dis. 2002;61(8):718–22. https://doi.org/10.1136/ ard.61.8.718.

45. McDonough AK, Curtis JR, Saag KG. The epidemiology of glucocorticoid-associated adverse events. Curr Opin Rheumatol. 2008;20(2):131–7. https:// doi.org/10.1097/BOR.0b013e3282f51031.

46. Mangano GRA, Valle MS, Casabona A, Vagnini A, Cioni M. Age-Related Changes in Mobility Evaluated by the Timed Up and Go Test Instrumented

through a Single Sensor. Sensors (Basel). 2020;20(3):E719. https://doi.org/10.3390/s20030719.

47. Geremia JM, Bobbert MF, Casa Nova M, Ott RD, Lemos Fde A, Lupion Rde O, et al. The structural and mechanical properties of the Achilles tendon 2 years after surgical repair. Clin Biomech (Bristol, Avon). 2015;30(5):485–92. https://doi.org/10.1016/j.clinbiomech.2015.03.005.

48. Jain A, Nanchahal J, Troeberg L, Green P, Brennan F. Production of cytokines, vascular endothelial growth factor, matrix metalloproteinases, and tissue inhibitor of metalloproteinases 1 by tenosynovium demonstrates its potential for tendon destruction in rheumatoid arthritis. Arthritis Rheum. 2001;44(8):1754–60. https://doi.org/10.1002/1529-0131(200108)44:8<1754:: AID-ART310>3.0.CO;2-8.

49. Bojsen-Moller J, Magnusson SP, Rasmussen LR, Kjaer M, Aagaard P. Muscle performance during maximal isometric and dynamic contractions is influenced by the stiffness of the tendinous structures. J Appl Physiol (1985). 2005;99(3):986–94. https://doi.org/10.1152/japplphysiol.01305.2004.

50. Sayers SP, Guralnik JM, Thombs LA, Fielding RA. Effect of leg muscle contraction velocity on functional performance in older men and women. J Am Geriatr Soc. 2005;53(3):467–71. https://doi.org/10.1111/j.1532-5415.2005.53166.x.

51. Trezise J, Blazevich AJ. Anatomical and neuromuscular determinants of strength change in previously untrained men following heavy strength training. Front Physiol. 2019;10:1001. https://doi.org/10.3389/fphys.2019.01001.

5

Fears and beliefs of people living with rheumatoid arthritis

Penélope Esther Palominos[1,2]*, Andrese Aline Gasparin[1], Nicole Pamplona Bueno de Andrade[1], Ricardo Machado Xavier[1,2], Rafael Mendonça da Silva Chakr[1,2], Fernanda Igansi[1] and Laure Gossec[3]

Abstract

Objective: To assess the main fears and beliefs of people with rheumatoid arthritis (RA) and their effect on treatment outcomes;

Methods: A systematic literature review was conducted in Pubmed/Medline; original articles published up to May 2017, reporting fears and/or beliefs of adult patients with RA were analyzed. Fears and beliefs were collected by two independent researchers and grouped into categories.

Results: Among 474 references identified, 84 were analyzed, corresponding to 24,336 RA patients. Fears were reported in 38.4% of the articles ($N = 32/84$): most studies described fears related to pharmacological therapy (50.0%, $N = 16/32$) and fear of disability (28.1%, $N = 9/32$). Beliefs were reported in 88.0% of articles ($N = 74/84$) and were found to moderate the patient-perceived impact of RA in 44.6% ($N = 33/74$), mainly the emotional impact (18.9%, $N = 14/74$); measures of function, quality of life, fatigue and pain were also found to be affected by patients' beliefs in 8.1% ($N = 6/74$), 6.8% ($N = 5/74$), 2.7% ($N = 2/74$) and 2.7% ($N = 2/74$) of the articles, respectively. Beliefs about therapy were linked to adherence in 17.6% of articles ($N = 13/74$) and beliefs about cause of RA predicted coping patterns in 12.2% of publications ($N = 9/74$). Only 9.5% ($N = 8/84$) of articles reported fears and/or beliefs of patients living outside Europe and North America: there was only one work which recruited patients in Latin America and no article included patients from Africa.

Conclusion: In RA, patients' beliefs are linked to impact of disease and non-adherence. Further research is needed on fears/beliefs of patients living outside Europe and North America.

Keywords: Fears, Beliefs, Rheumatoid arthritis

Background

Despite the growing interest of rheumatologists into the patients' perspective in the last decade and the wide use of patient-reported outcomes in the assessment of Rheumatoid Arthritis (RA), the main fears and beliefs of this group of patients and their consequences on treatment outcomes are unclear [1, 2]. This theme has been explored through qualitative and quantitative methodology in different populations with a large amount of fears and beliefs being reported and even conflicting data being published about the consequences of patients' perceptions [3–5]. While some authors, for example, found an association between higher concern scores about drugs with non-adherence, other found no association between patients' beliefs and maintenance of disease-modifying antirheumatic drugs (DMARDs) [3–5].

The subjectivity of fear and beliefs, the small patient samples in some studies and the limited knowledge about the consequences of patients' fears and beliefs on treatment outcomes may lead some rheumatologists to be unconvinced about the importance of the theme.

A systematic literature review would help to obtain an overview. Furthermore, cultural background may play a role in fears and beliefs [6, 7].

* Correspondence: penelopepalominos@gmail.com
[1]Universidade Federal do Rio Grande do Sul (UFRGS), Programa de Pós Graduação em Ciências Médicas (PPGCM), Rua Ramiro Barcelos 2400, segundo andar, Porto Alegre 90035-903, Brazil
[2]Department of Rheumatology, Hospital de Clinicas de Porto Alegre, Rua Ramiro Barcelos 2350, sexto andar, Porto Alegre 90035-903, Brazil
Full list of author information is available at the end of the article

This systematic literature review aimed to obtain an overview on fears and beliefs of patients living with RA reported in the medical literature, as well as assess the consequences of fears and beliefs on impact of disease and treatment outcomes. It also investigated if published studies reporting fears and beliefs are representative of all continents.

Methods

A systematic literature review was conducted in PubMed Medline up to 25 May 2017, using the Preferred Reporting Items for Systematic Reviews and Meta-Analyses statement as a guideline in the development of the study protocol and reporting of the results [8].

Search and selection process

Publications were identified through the following research strategy:

("interviews as topic"[MeSH Terms] OR "narration"[MeSH Terms] OR "surveys and questionnaires"[MeSH Terms] OR "qualitative research"[MeSH Terms]) AND ("arthritis/psychology"[MeSH Terms] OR "arthritis, rheumatoid"[MeSH Terms]) AND ("fears"[All Fields] OR "beliefs"[All Fields] OR "attitude to health/psychology"[MeSH Terms] OR "behavior and behavior mechanisms/psychology"[MeSH Terms] OR "affective symptoms/psychology"[MeSH Terms])

Inclusion criteria

All original articles reporting fears and/or beliefs of adult patients diagnosed with RA were included in the analysis; fears and beliefs were defined according to the Cambridge English Dictionary respectively as "a strong emotion caused by great worry about something dangerous, painful or unknown that is happening or might happen" and "the feeling of being certain that something exist or is true". These concepts were useful for making the distinction between articles reporting fears/beliefs and articles reporting coping patterns and psychological status. Articles written in English, Spanish, French, Italian and Portuguese and published up to 25 May 2017 were considered.

Both qualitative studies (data obtained through individual interview and/or focus groups), quantitative studies (information obtained through questionnaires) and mixed designs (articles including qualitative and quantitative methods) were included.

When RA and other clinical conditions (i.e. systemic lupus erythematosus, osteoarthritis, chronic pain etc) were included in the same study, the article was included in the analysis only if fears and/or beliefs of patients with RA were described separately from the other clinical condition.

Exclusion criteria

articles not reporting fears and/or beliefs, articles reporting fears and/or beliefs of patients with other rheumatic and non-rheumatic diseases, articles assessing children's fears and/or beliefs, studies assessing fears and/or beliefs of patients' spouses, partners and caregivers as well as reviews, letters and editorials were excluded.

Data collection

The selection process was performed by two authors (PEP and AAG) based on the titles and abstracts of the articles, and then on full texts. The articles included were then reviewed by two authors (PEP and NPD) and disagreements were solved by consensus.

General data extraction

Data were obtained on year of publication, study design (qualitative, quantitative or mixed design), number of patients, sampling method (convenience, consecutive, purposeful, systematic random sample), number of centers recruiting patients, the method used for data collection (individual interview, focus groups, questionnaire or mixed methods). When qualitative methodology was employed, the method used for qualitative analysis and for sample size definition was obtained. Demographic data of participants such as gender, mean age, mean disease duration was recorded for each report.

Collection of fear and beliefs

Fears were grouped in categories by PEP and LG (e.g. fears related to pharmacological therapy, fear of falling, fear of exercise relating injury, etc.). Beliefs were grouped in categories according to their consequences (e.g. beliefs about cause of disease predicting coping patterns, beliefs about pharmacological therapy affecting adherence, beliefs affecting impact of disease etc.).

Statistical analysis

Analysis was mainly descriptive; characteristic of articles and patients included were expressed as mean and standard deviation as estimates of central tendency and dispersion, respectively.

Categories of fears and beliefs were presented as number of articles which were included in that category and percentage of articles reporting that specific category among the total number of publication assessing fears or beliefs, respectively. The recruitment of patients worldwide was described as percentage, with the number of articles recruiting patients in each region as numerator and total number of studies reporting that category of fears/beliefs in the denominator.

Results
Description of publications and participants

Of the 474 publications identified by the literature search, 84 were included in the analysis. The list of all articles included in the analysis is provided as Additional file 1.

The main reasons for exclusion were articles assessing fears and/or beliefs from patients with other clinical conditions (52.3%, $N = 204$) and articles not assessing fears and/or beliefs (45.6%, $N = 178$) (Fig. 1).

The 84 articles considered in the analysis included 24,336 subjects with RA; mean age of participants was 54.9 ± 5.0 years old, mean disease duration was 10.7 ± 6.0 years and 74.0% ($N = 18,032$) were females (Table 1).

The sample was recruited by convenience in the majority of analyzed articles (57.1%, $N = 48$), followed by the recruitment of consecutive patients ($N = 14$; 16.7%). Systematic random sampling was described in only 4.8% of articles ($N = 4$).

The majority of trials employed exclusively quantitative methodology (69.0% of the 84 articles analyzed, $N = 58$) with the cross sectional design being the most commonly found (77.6% of the publications reporting only quantitative methods, $N = 45$). Thirty-one percent ($N = 26$) of the 84 articles employed some method of qualitative analysis (both solely or associated with quantitative methods). Among these 26 articles, the majority described the methodology used for analysis of qualitative data (55.5%, $N = 15$) and the inductive thematic analysis/grounded theory was the most cited ($N = 12$, 80.0% of those articles describing the methodology used for qualitative analysis) (Table 1). Six articles (23.0% of the 26 articles employing qualitative methodology) described that the saturation method was used to define the sample size [9].

Fears and/or beliefs were assessed through questionnaires, individual interviews and focus groups in 75.0% ($N = 63$), 20.2% ($N = 17$) and 6.0% ($N = 5$) of articles, respectively (Table 1).

All articles employing quantitative methodology ($N = 58$) assessed beliefs trough questionnaires and more than 50 different tools assessing fears and/or beliefs were described; the most frequently used were the original, and brief versions of the "Illness Perception Questionnaire" (IPQ) [10, 11] (22.4%, $N = 13$) and the "Beliefs about Medicines Questionnaire" (BMQ) (18.9%, $N = 11$) [12].

Disagreements between the two authors collecting the characteristics of publications, demographic data

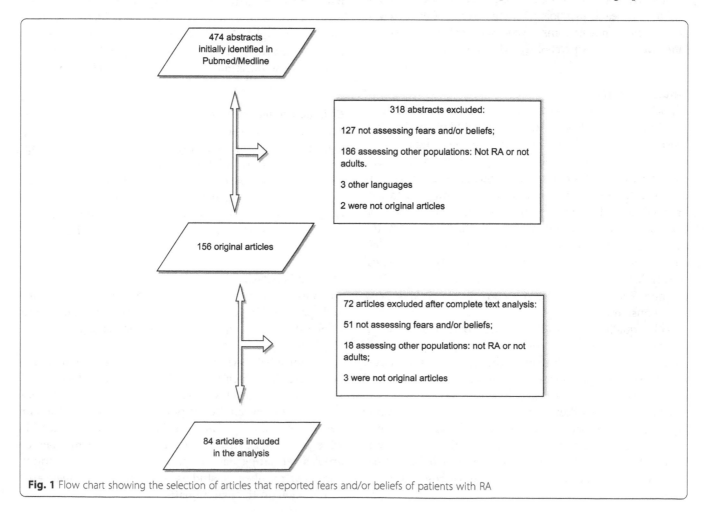

Fig. 1 Flow chart showing the selection of articles that reported fears and/or beliefs of patients with RA

Table 1 Characteristics of the publications and patients included in the analysis

	All articles (N = 84)	Studies employing only qualitative methodology N = 18	Studies employing only quantitative methodology N = 58	Studies with mixed (qualitative and quantitative) methodology N = 8
Total number of patients	24,336	334	23,539	463
Female sex N [a]	18,032	201	17,577	254
Age of participants (mean ± SD)[a]	54.9 ± 5.0	56.4 ± 7.2	54.5 ± 4.8	56.3 ± 2.1
Disease duration in years (mean ± SD) [a]	10.7 ± 6.0	13.9 ± 7.2	10.1 ± 5.9	11.2 ± 4.2
Method used for assessment of fears and/or beliefs N (%) of articles using the method [b]				
Individual interviews	17 (20.2)	13 (72.2)	NA	4 (50.0)
Focus groups	5 (6.0)	4 (22.2)	NA	1 (12.5)
Individual interviews and focus groups	1 (1.2)	1 (5.6)	NA	0 (0.0)
Questionnaire	63 (75.0)	NA	58 (100.0)	5(62.5)

SD standard deviation, N number, NA non applicable
[a]Numbers calculated on available data
[b]The final result can be greater than 100% since some articles employed more than one method to assess fear and/or beliefs

of participants and fears/beliefs occurred in 7.1% of articles when describing study design and in 5.7% of publication when demographic data of patients were analyzed. All disagreements were solved by consensus. There were no disagreements about fears and beliefs presented in the publications.

Fears

Thirty two articles (38.0% of the 84 analyzed publications) reported fears experienced by AR patients (Table 2). Articles reporting patient's concerns about pharmacological therapy and/or reporting factors that influenced these fears about drugs were the most

Table 2 Fears of people living with RA reported in the analyzed articles

Fears	Articles N (% of the 32 articles reporting fears) [a]	Total number of patients	N (%) of studies recruiting participants in Europe in each category/ Number of patients recruited in Europe	N (%) of studies recruiting participants in North America / Number of patients recruited in North America	N (%) of studies recruiting participants outside Europe and North America / Number of patients recruited outside Europe and North America
Fears related to pharmacological therapy	16 (50.0)	1085	13 (81.3) / 867 (760 in UK, 101 in Netherlands, 6 in Sweden)	2 (12.5) /78 (60 in Canada, 18 USA)	1(6.2)/140 (140 in Egypt)
Fear of consequences of disease in the future and disability	9 (28.1)	1049	6 (66.7) / 707 (460 in UK, 199 in Greece, 48 in Sweden)	1 (11.1)/ 30 (30 in USA)	2 (22.2) /312 (101 in United Arab Emirates, 211 in Australia)
Fears related to pregnancy and parenting role	3 (9.4)	211	3 (100.0) / 211 (102 in UK, 25 in France, 84 in Netherlands)	–	–
Fear of falling	3 (9.4)	5172	1(33.3)/48 (48 in Sweden)	1 (33.3) / 128 (128 in USA)	1 (33.3) / 4996 (4996 in Japan)
Fear of exercise related injury/ fear of exercise increasing RA symptoms	3 (9.4)	4289	3 (100.0) / 4289 (4283 in Sweden, 6 in UK)	–	–
Fear to disturb other people	2 (6.3)	38	1 (50.0)/ 8 (8 in UK)	1 (50.0) / 30 (30 in USA)	–
Fear of infections	2 (6.3)	54	2(100.0)/ 54 (48 in Sweden, 6 in UK)	–	–
Fear of negative evaluation from other people due to appearance	1 (3.1)	89	1 (100.0)/89 (89 in UK)	–	–

[a]Some articles reported more than one category of fears
N number; UK United Kingdom, USA United States of America

reported (50.0% of the 32 articles reporting fears, $N = 16$). Fears about pharmacological therapy were related to both synthetic and biological DMARDs (Table 3). Beliefs about drugs seemed to change with the course of disease and personal experiences with the drug [4, 13–15]; according to Ostlund et al., for example, initial beliefs and expectations about methotrexate were challenged as patients initiated treatment and began experiencing varying degrees of effectiveness and side effects [13]. Demographic factors, such as age and educational level were also found to influence fear about drugs, with older patients and subjects with lower educational level experiencing higher concern about DMARDs [5, 6, 14]. People with RA and different ethnicities may have different views about DMARDS even when they are living in the same country: Kumar et al. described higher concern about drugs among RA patients with an Asiatic origin living in United Kingdom when compared with White British patients who lived in the same country [6, 16].

Fear of disease progression and disability was the second most described category ($N = 9/32$ articles reporting fears, 28.1%) (Table 2);

Fears related to pregnancy and parenting roles were reported in three articles (9.4% of the 32 articles reporting fears) (Table 2). Patients who participated in these articles were recruited in Europe and reported the fear of drugs causing birth defects, fear of genetic transfer, fear of being unable to fulfill parenting roles, fear of not being able to prevent accidents and fear of dropping a small baby or toddler [17–19].

Other reported concerns were: the fear of falling ($N = 3/32$ articles, 9.4%), the fear of exercise related injury/ fear of having symptoms increased by exercise ($N = 3/32$ articles, 9.4%) and fear of negative evaluation from other people due to appearance ($N = 1/32$ articles, 3.1%).

Some examples of the fear to disturb other people ($N = 2/32$ articles, 6.3%) included: the fear to disturb family members and partners at home due to night pain, fear to disturb other patients and nurses in the hospital due to night pain, the fear of taking the spouses' time and giving them too much responsibilities [20, 21].

Patients with RA also reported fear of infections such as catching colds; these fears were reported in 6.3% ($N = 2$) of those articles reporting fears. Some patients were afraid of taking exercise in public places such as swimming pools because they thought that having RA made them more susceptible to infections [22, 23].

Only four articles (12.5% of those reporting fears) included patients living outside Europe and North America. No articles reported fears of patients from Latin America or Africa.

Beliefs

Seventy-four articles, corresponding to 88.0% of the total 84 analyzed articles, reported at least one belief. Main categories of beliefs and their consequences were described in Table 4.

Patient's beliefs about RA influenced impact of disease and assessment of health domains

Patients' beliefs were reported to influence the impact of RA ($N = 33$, 44.6% of the 74 articles assessing beliefs), mediated by their consequences in 8 health domains (Table 4).

Beliefs affecting the emotional domain were reported in 14/74 articles (18.9%). Perceptions of greater symptomatology and greater stress, beliefs on serious consequences of RA, beliefs on lower ability to handle or cope with disease and beliefs on its owns responsibility in the development of RA were reported to amplify the negative emotional impact of disease and contribute to depressive mood and anxiety [24–29].

Patients' beliefs affecting measures of function were reported in 6 publications (8.1% of articles reporting beliefs). Among RA patients, helplessness (patients'

Table 3 Fears related to synthetic and biological DMARDs

Fears	Author and year of publication
Fear of treatment failure	Sanderson 2009 [60]
Fear of being taken of a drug	Sanderson 2009 [60]
Fear of side effects of treatment (mainly long- term side effects)	Goodacre 2004 [4] Popa-Lisseanu 2005 [61] Wong 2007 [5] Sanderson 2009 [60] Fitzcharles 2009 [62] Kumar 2011 [43] Van den Bent 2011 [63] Hayden 2015 [14] Gadallah 2015 [42] Pasma 2015 [15] Nota 2015 [64]
Fear of "too many pills/too many drugs", fear of over-prescription	Popa-Lisseanu 2005 [61] Wong 2007 [5] Fitzcharles 2009 [62]
Fear of drug interaction	Fitzcharles 2009 [62]
Fear of addiction	Goodacre 2004 [4] Wong 2007 [5] Sanderson 2009 [60] Fitzcharles 2009 [62] Kumar 2011 [43] Van den Bent 2011 [63] Nota 2015 [64]
Fear of masking disease	Fitzcharles 2009 [62]
Fear of drugs causing reduced life expectancy	Goodacre 2004 [4]
Fear of being disappointed with a new treatment	Nyman 1999 [46]
Fear of too many changes in therapy	Kumar 2011 [43]

beliefs that they were not able to control pain and the course of disease) has a lower but statistically significant correlation with disability [30]. People who attributed more symptoms to RA, believe in a long illness duration, and held stronger beliefs that it would have negative consequences also presented greater disability on disease-specific measures of functioning; on the other side, stronger beliefs of personal control were associated with lower levels of disability, as were stronger beliefs in the ability of treatment to control RA [6, 26, 31–33].

Health-related quality of life (HRQOL) was found to be influenced by patients' beliefs in 5 articles (6.8% of the 72 publications assessing beliefs). Fears about the consequences of the RA were independently correlated to physical HRQOL, i.e., patients who believe in worse consequences of RA had worse scores in the physical component of quality of life measures; patient global assessment of disease activity was also a significant predictor of poor mental and physical HRQOL [6, 33–36].

Other health domains affected by patients' beliefs were: fatigue (2.7% of the publications assessing beliefs, N = 2 articles), pain (2.7%, N = 2), well-being (2.7%, N = 2), disease activity (1.4%, N = 1) and sexual life (1.4%, N = 1).

Among the 33 articles reporting consequences of patients' beliefs on health domains, only one manuscript recruited RA patients living outside Europe and North America.

Beliefs about pharmacological and non-pharmacological therapy affected patients' adherence

Beliefs about pharmacological and non-pharmacological therapy, including exercise and devices, were sometimes found to affect adherence to therapy (17.6% of articles reporting beliefs, N = 13). Among the 13 articles in this category, four publication (30.8%) studied the influence of patients' beliefs on adherence to physical activity. These references concluded that patient's beliefs about the usefulness of exercise for managing disease and their perceptions of positive social support for participation in exercise were highly correlated with physical activity participation [37–40]. Other eight articles in the same category (61.5%) analyzed the consequences of patients' beliefs about drugs on adherence. Although most patients with RA believed their synthetic and biological DMARDS were necessary to preserve joint structures, reduce pain and increase quality of life, levels of concern about side effects were high and related to non-adherence [3, 5, 15, 16, 41–44].

Table 4 Beliefs of people living with rheumatoid arthritis reported in the analyzed articles

Beliefs and their consequences	Articles N (% of the 74 articles reporting beliefs)[a]	Total number of patients	Studies recruiting participants in Europe N (%) / Number of patients recruited in Europe	Studies recruiting participants in North America N (%) / Number of patients recruited in North America	Studies recruiting participants outside Europe and North America N (%) / Number of patients recruited outside Europe and North America
Beliefs about the RA affecting impact of disease	33 (44.6)	9146			
Emotional impact	14 (18.9)	6404	6 (42.9) / 901	7 (50.0) / 945	1 (7.1)/ 4558
Function	6 (8.1)	715	4 (66.7)/ 370	2 (33.3) / 345	–
Quality of life	5 (6.8)	1034	4 (80.0) / 623	1 (20.0) / 411	–
Fatigue	2 (2.7)	186	1 (50.0) / 64	1 (50.0) / 122	–
Pain	2 (2.7)	299	–	2 (100.0) / 299	–
Well being	2 (2.7)	123	–	2 (100.0) / 123	–
Disease activity	1 (1.4)	322	1 (100.0) / 322	–	–
Sexual life	1 (1.4)	63	1 (100.0) / 63	–	–
Beliefs about pharmacological and non-pharmacological therapy affecting adherence	13 (17.6)	2464	10 (77.0) / 1999	2 (15.4) / 325	1 (7.6) / 140
Beliefs about cause of disease affecting coping strategies and adherence	9 (12.1)	961	8 (88.9) / 750	–	1 (11.1)/ 211
Beliefs affecting decision on therapy	1 (1.4)	142	–	1 (100.0) / 142	–
Beliefs affecting detection, tolerance and reporting of side effects	1 (1.4)	29	1 (100.0) / 29	–	–

N number; RA rheumatoid arthritis, [a]Some articles reported more than one category of beliefs

Beliefs about cause of disease predicted copping patterns and adherence

Beliefs about cause of disease expressed by RA patients in 9 studies (12.1% of articles reporting beliefs) included: hereditarity, stress, unexpressed grief, diet, occupational factors/overwork, lack of exercise, God's will, weather conditions, biological reasons/immune system failure/autoimmunity, accident/chance and karmic explanation (disease caused by past "bad" actions) [18, 36, 43, 45–50]. Beliefs about cause of disease predicted copping patterns: Salminem et al., for example, observed that 40.0% of RA patients believe diet contributed to their disease, more so if longer disease duration and higher education and 51% changed their diet after diagnosis, usually reducing consumption of animal fat and red meat [45].

Nyman et al. also showed that psychological factors, such as stress, overwork, anxiety or a distressing life event, for example bereavement or divorce were cited by 59.7% of AR patients as triggers factors leading to disease [46]. Other authors also demonstrated that most part of RA patients believe the cause of their disease was psychological in nature and that RA patients more readily admitted that psychological factors contributed to their illness compared to osteoarthritis patients [36, 50]. The psychological attribution as cause of RA seemed to have negative consequences: it was positively correlated with patient-related delay between beginning of symptoms and the first visit with general practitioner as well as with the tendency to use dysfunctional coping strategies [47, 49].

The analyzed work also described that patients who believed that the cause of RA was a biological one, viewed medicines less negatively than those who held the view that stress, God or fate were important causative factors [43].

Patients' beliefs influenced decision making during clinical visits

One article (1.4% of the 74 articles reporting beliefs) concluded that patient's beliefs about consequences of RA and high level of concern about disease were more likely to have their treatment escalated, independently of disease activity [51]. In this work, high disease activity was not associated with future escalation of treatment in patients reporting low levels of perceived consequences, concern, and emotional impact; the combination of disease activity and illness beliefs better predicted future escalation of treatment in RA patients than either factor in isolation [51].

Beliefs about DMARDs affected detection, tolerance and reporting of side effects

One qualitative study (1.4% of the 74 articles reporting beliefs) reported a relation between patients' beliefs about DMARDs and the reporting of side effects, with people more prepared to tolerate and do not report side effects when medication was perceived as beneficial or the number of alternatives perceived as limited. When DMARDs were not perceived as beneficial, concerns about side effects were voiced more frequently and the rationale for continued use was questioned [4].

Among the 74 articles reporting beliefs, only three (4.0%) described perceptions of patients with RA living outside Europe and North America (Table 4).

When all the 84 articles were analyzed, only 9.5% ($N = 8$) of them reported fears and/or beliefs of patients living outside Europe and North America: there was only one work which recruited patients in Latin America and no article included patients from Africa.

Discussion

This systematic literature review demonstrated that patients with RA have several beliefs about disease and its treatment and these beliefs influenced global impact of disease, adherence to therapy and copping patterns. Fears regarding the use of DMARDs and the fear of functional disability due to disease progression were the most reported in literature. It also highlighted areas where further original research is required: studies assessing patients' fears and beliefs were conducted mainly in Europe and North America and there is limited knowledge on fears and beliefs of patients living with RA in Asia, Africa, Latin America and Oceania.

Beliefs were shown to influence the patient-perceived impact of RA and, specially, the emotional / psychological impact of disease. This fact seems to be relevant since the prevalence of depression and anxiety is significant among people with RA [52]. Health professionals responsible for the management of RA patients should try to identify unjustified fears and erroneous beliefs that could amplify the psychological impact of disease. To minimize the patients' feeling of culpability by clarifying wrong beliefs about cause of disease, as well as to reinforce patients' ability to cope with consequences of RA are some strategies that can be adopted by health professionals. Since patients who attribute more symptoms to the rheumatic disease have higher psychological impact, it seems appropriate to help patients to recognize symptoms that are really attributed to RA and to differentiate them from those caused by comorbidities such as depression, anxiety and fibromyalgia [24, 28].

Although the emotional domain was the most cited, outcome measures evaluating other health domains as function, quality of life, pain and fatigue were also influenced by patients' perceptions. Since beliefs in more severe consequences of rheumatic disease and feelings of helplessness were associated with worse outcome measures of functioning it is convenient to consider beliefs when facing to patients with poor function not otherwise explained by disease activity [26, 30, 32, 33].

Moreover, this systematic literature review provides rheumatologists new evidence to consider patient's fears and beliefs when facing people with RA who are non-adherent to therapy. Recent work, which used pharmacy dispensing data to calculate medication possession ratios (MPR) and determine patients' adherence (MPR ≥ 0.80), demonstrated that patients with RA have low adherence to conventional and biological DMARDs [53, 54]. Mena-Vázquez et al. found that 88.8% of RA patients showed good adherence to biological drugs but only 61.2% also correctly took concomitant conventional synthetic DMARDs [54]. Another work from Calip et al. found lower rates of adherence to biological therapy: only 37.0% of RA patients were adherent, and the lower rates of adherence (17.0%) were found among young patients in their third year of treatment [53]. Fears related to pharmacological therapy were the most reported in our literature review and almost 20.0% of articles reported that patients' beliefs about therapy were found to affect adherence to treatment, reinforcing the idea that fears and beliefs may have an important role in explaining non-adherence. Since the fear of functional disability was the second most described patients' concern, it could be a strategy to increase adherence to DMARDS to instruct the patients about the ability of these drugs to avoid future structural damage and loss of function.

Although it seems plausible that to offer better knowledge on RA treatment could be a good strategy to improve non-adherence, some authors found that motivational-interviewing-guided group sessions about DMARDs use were not effective to change patients' beliefs about necessity of these drugs and concerns about therapy; this intervention did not improved rates of non-adherence [55]. Van den Bent et al. tested another intervention aiming to change patients' beliefs about medicines and improve non-adherence: a written report informing the physician about the medicine use and the adherence rate was sent to the rheumatologist by the researcher [56]. Adherence did not change after the intervention, compared to adherence assessment prior to the intervention and beliefs about medication were not significantly altered [56]. Further research is necessary to ensure effective strategies aiming to reduce erroneous fears and beliefs that could negatively affect the adherence to therapy in RA patients.

This work brings to light the paucity of published articles reporting fears and/or beliefs of RA patients living in Latin America, Africa, Oceania and Asia. Since nationality was found to influence, among RA patients, the perceptions about trust in physicians and the choice of the RA priority domains, it is convenient to rheumatologists working outside Europe and North America to gain more insight on fear and beliefs of their patients [7, 57].

In addition to differences among nationalities, the diversity of opinions among distinct ethnical groups living in the same country also exists; in United Kingdom, for example, Kumar et al. demonstrated that non-English-speaking RA patients (patients of South Asian origin) usually believe that RA is caused by a God's will and that they do not have an active role in therapy, while English-speaking patients usually believe that the cause of disease is a biological one and view DMARDs less negatively [43]. Salminem et al. also interviewed Punjabi women living in United Kingdom and remarked that this group made sense of the development of RA as a consequence of past "bad" actions. This "karmic explanation" to the development of disease lead patients to hide symptoms from others in order to avoid a moral judgement and stigmatization [48]. Further research comparing fear and beliefs among people of different ethnic and cultural backgrounds would be interesting.

Other gap in publications was remarked: most articles included only patients with long disease duration, and the perception of patients with early RA was rarely described [58]. Further studies allowing comparison of fear and beliefs of patients in different stages of RA is necessary since it has been shown that beliefs about the consequences of disease and expectations of patients varied according to the stage of RA and familiarity with other people with the same clinical condition [13, 18].

This study has some weaknesses. It is not exhaustive since the one database assessed was PubMed/Medline; however this is the most important database of biomedical research articles covering more than 5600 journals published in more than 80 countries; articles in five languages were included in the analysis and there was no limit of date for the search.

This work included all studies reporting fear and/or beliefs of patients with RA found with our search strategy regardless of their quality level to optimize the number of reported fear and beliefs. The appraisal of qualitative research, for example, is still a challenge since there is no consensus on a tool for quality evaluation in this type of studies. According to Dixon-Woods et al., there are over 100 tolls described to evaluate quality in qualitative research, some adopting non-reconcilable positions on a number of issues [59].

It is possible that among the studies employing some method of qualitative analysis, some work were probably not exhaustive since less than a quarter of those articles reported that the principle of saturation was used to define the sample size [9].

Despite its limitations, this work highlights several fears and beliefs of patients with RA, allowing rheumatologists and other health professionals to create strategies to minimize fears and beliefs that could affect negatively the management of disease.

Conclusion

In RA, patients' beliefs influenced global impact of disease, adherence to therapy and copping patterns. The most common fears of RA patients were related to the consequences of RA and the use of DMARDs. Further research is needed on fears and beliefs of patients living outside Europe and North America.

Additional file

Additional file 1: List of the 84 articles included in the analysis

Abbreviations
BMQ: Beliefs about medicines questionnaire; DMARDs: Disease- modifying antirheumatic drugs; HRQOL: Health-related quality of life; IPQ: Illness perception questionnaire; MPR: Medication possession ratios; RA: Rheumatoid arthritis

Authors' contributions
All authors meet the authorship criteria, giving substantial contribution to the conception of the work, data acquisition and analysis, drafting or reviewing the work for intellectual content and giving final approval of the version to be published. The authors agree to be accountable for all aspects of the work in ensuring that questions related to the accuracy or integrity of any part of the work are appropriately investigated and resolved.

Author details
[1]Universidade Federal do Rio Grande do Sul (UFRGS), Programa de Pós Graduação em Ciências Médicas (PPGCM), Rua Ramiro Barcelos 2400, segundo andar, Porto Alegre 90035-903, Brazil. [2]Department of Rheumatology, Hospital de Clinicas de Porto Alegre, Rua Ramiro Barcelos 2350, sexto andar, Porto Alegre 90035-903, Brazil. [3]Sorbonne Universités, UPMC Univ Paris 06, Institut Pierre Louis d'Epidémiologie et de Santé Publique, GRC-UPMC 08 (EEMOIS); Department of Rheumatology, Pitié Salpêtrière Hospital, AP-HP, 47-83 Boulevard de l'Hôpital, 75013 Paris, France.

References
1. Gossec L, Dougados M, Dixon W. Patient-reported outcomes as end points in clinical trials in rheumatoid arthritis. RMD Open. 2015;1(1):e000019.
2. Kalyoncu U, Dougados M, Daurès J-P, Gossec L. Reporting of patient-reported outcomes in recent trials in rheumatoid arthritis: a systematic literature review. Ann Rheum Dis. 2009;68(2):183–90.
3. Neame R, Hammond A. Beliefs about medications: a questionnaire survey of people with rheumatoid arthritis. Rheumatology. 2005;44(6):762–7.
4. Goodacre LJ, Goodacre JA. Factors influencing the beliefs of patients with rheumatoid arthritis regarding disease-modifying medication. Rheumatology. 2004;43(5):583–6.
5. Wong M, Mulherin D. The influence of medication beliefs and other psychosocial factors on early discontinuation of disease-modifying anti-rheumatic drugs. Musculoskeletal Care. 2007;5(3):148–59.
6. Kumar K, Gordon C, Toescu V, Buckley CD, Horne R, Nightingale PG, et al. Beliefs about medicines in patients with rheumatoid arthritis and systemic lupus erythematosus: a comparison between patients of south Asian and white British origin. Rheumatology. 2008;47(5):690–7.
7. Berrios-Rivera J, Street R Jr, Popa-Lisseanu M, Kallen M, Richardson M, Janssen N. Trust in physicians and elements of the medical interaction in patients with rheumatoid arthritis and systemic lupus erythematosus. Arthritis Rheum. 2006;55(3):385–93.
8. PRISMA: transparent report of systematic reviews and metanalysis. Acessed 1 May 2017.
9. Depoy E, Gitlin L. Introduction to research: understanding and applying multiple strategies. Fourth Edi. St. Louis: Elsevier, Mosby; 1998.
10. Weinman J, Petrie K, Moss-Morris R, Horne R. The illness perception questionnaire: a new method for assessing illness perceptions. Psychology and Health Psychol Heal. 1996;11:431–46.
11. Broadbent E, Petrie KJ, Main J, Weinman J. The brief illness perception questionnaire. J Psychosom Res. 2006;60(6):631–7.
12. Horne R, Weinman J, Hankins M. The beliefs about medicines questionnaire: the development and evaluation of a new method for assessing the cognitive representation of medication. Psychol Health. 1999;14(1):1–24.
13. Östlund G, Björk M, Valtersson E, Sverker A. Lived experiences of sex life difficulties in men and women with early RA – the Swedish TIRA project. Musculoskeletal Care. 2015;13(4):248–57.
14. Hayden C, Neame R, Tarrant C. Patients' adherence-related beliefs about methotrexate: a qualitative study of the role of written patient information. BMJ Open. 2015;5(5):e006918.
15. Pasma A, Van't Spijker A, Luime JJ, Walter MJM, Busschbach JJV, Hazes JMW. Facilitators and barriers to adherence in the initiation phase of disease-modifying antirheumatic drug (DMARD) use in patients with arthritis who recently started their first DMARD treatment. J Rheumatol. 2015;42(3):379–85.
16. Kumar K, Raza K, Nightingale P, Horne R, Chapman S, Greenfield S, et al. Determinants of adherence to disease modifying anti-rheumatic drugs in white British and south Asian patients with rheumatoid arthritis: a cross sectional study. BMC Musculoskelet Disord. 2015;16(1):396.
17. Barlow JH, Cullen LA, Rowe IF. Comparison of knowledge and psychological well-being between patients with a short disease duration (≤1 year) and patients with more established rheumatoid arthritis (≥10 years duration). Patient Educ Couns. 1999;38(3):195–203.
18. Berenbaum F, Chauvin P, Hudry C, Mathoret-Philibert F, Poussiere M, De Chalus T, et al. Fears and beliefs in rheumatoid arthritis and spondyloarthritis: a qualitative study. PLoS One. 2014;9(12):e114350.
19. Clowse MEB, Chakravarty E, Costenbader KH, Chambers C, Michaud K. Effects of infertility, pregnancy loss, and patient concerns on family size of women with rheumatoid arthritis and systemic lupus erythematosus. Arthritis Care Res (Hoboken). 2012;64(5):668–74.
20. Coady DA, Armitage C, Wright D. Rheumatoid arthritis patients' experiences of night pain. J Clin Rheumatol. 2007;13(2):66–9.
21. Foxall MJ, Kollasch C, McDermott S. Family stress and coping in rheumatoid arthritis. Arthritis Care Res (Hoboken). 1989;2(4):114–21.
22. Wang M, Donovan-Hall M, Hayward H, Adams J. People's perceptions and beliefs about their ability to exercise with rheumatoid arthritis: a qualitative study. Musculoskeletal Care. 2015;13(2):112–5.
23. Östlund G, Björk M, Thyberg I, Thyberg M, Valtersson E, Stenström B, et al. Emotions related to participation restrictions as experienced by patients with early rheumatoid arthritis: a qualitative interview study (the Swedish TIRA project). Clin Rheumatol. 2014;33(10):1403–13.
24. Van Os S, Norton S, Hughes LD, Chilcot J. Illness perceptions account for variation in positive outlook as well as psychological distress in rheumatoid arthritis. Psychol Health Med. 2012;17(4):427–39.
25. Strahl C, Kleinknecht RA, Dinnel DL. The role of pain anxiety, coping, and pain self-efficacy in rheumatoid arthritis patient functioning. Behav Res Ther. 2000;38(9):863–73.
26. Smith C. A, Wallston K a. Adaptation in patients with chronic rheumatoid arthritis: application of a general model. Health Psychol. 1992;11(3):151–62.
27. Lowe R, Cockshott Z, Greenwood R, Kirwan JR, Almeida C, Richards P, et al. Self-efficacy as an appraisal that moderates the coping-emotion relationship: associations among people with rheumatoid arthritis. Psychol Health. 2008;23(2):155–74.
28. Devins GM, Gupta A, Cameron J, Woodend K, Mah K, Gladman D. Cultural syndromes and age moderate the emotional impact of illness intrusiveness in rheumatoid arthritis. Rehabil Psychol. 2009;54:33–44. 12p
29. Nakajima A, Kamitsuji S, Saito A, Tanaka E, Nishimura K, Horikawa N, et al. Disability and patient's appraisal of general health contribute to depressed mood in rheumatoid arthritis in a large clinical study in Japan. Mod Rheumatol. 2006;16(3):151–7.
30. Nicassio PM, Kay MA, Custodio MK, Irwin MR, Olmstead R, Weisman MH. An evaluation of a biopsychosocial framework for health-related quality of life and disability in rheumatoid arthritis. J Psychosom Res. 2011;71(2):79–85.

31. Scharloo M, Kaptein AA, Weinman J, Hazes JM, Willems LNA, Bergman W, et al. Illness perceptions, coping and functioning in patients with rheumatoid arthritis, chronic obstructive pulmonary disease and psoriasis. J Psychosom Res. 1998;44(5):573–85.

32. Serbo B, Jajic I. Relationship of the functional status, duration of the disease and pain intensity and some psychological variables in patients with rheumatoid arthritis. Clin Rheumatol. 1991;10(4):419–22.

33. Graves H, Scott DL, Lempp H, Weinman J. Illness beliefs predict disability in rheumatoid arthritis. J Psychosom Res. 2009;67(5):417–23.

34. Kotsis K, Voulgari PV, Tsifetaki N, Machado MO, Carvalho AF, Creed F, et al. Anxiety and depressive symptoms and illness perceptions in psoriatic arthritis and associations with physical health-related quality of life. Arthritis Care Res (Hoboken). 2012;64(10):1593–601.

35. Alishiri GH, Bayat N, Fathi Ashtiani A, Tavallaii SA, Assari S, Moharamzad Y. Logistic regression models for predicting physical and mental health-related quality of life in rheumatoid arthritis patients. Mod Rheumatol. 2008;18(6):601–8.

36. Kotsis K, Voulgari PV, Tsifetaki N, Drosos AA, Carvalho AF, Hyphantis T. Illness perceptions and psychological distress associated with physical health-related quality of life in primary Sjögren's syndrome compared to systemic lupus erythematosus and rheumatoid arthritis. Rheumatol Int. 2014;34(12):1671–81.

37. Ehrlich-Jones L, Lee J, Semanik P, Cox C, Dunlop D, Chang RW. Relationship between beliefs, motivation, and worries about physical activity and physical activity participation in persons with rheumatoid arthritis. Arthritis Care Res. 2011;63(12):1700–5.

38. Swardh E, Biguet G, Opava CH. Views on exercise maintenance: variations among patients with rheumatoid arthritis. Phys Ther. 2008;88(9):1049–60.

39. Sperber NR, Allen KD, DeVellis BM, DeVellis RF, Lewis MA, Callahan LF. Differences in effectiveness of the active living every day program for older adults with arthritis. J Aging Phys Act. 2013;21(4):387–401.

40. Iversen MD, Fossel AH, Daltroy LH. Rheumatologist-patient communication about exercise and physical therapy in the management of rheumatoid arthritis. Arthritis Care Res. 1999;12(3):180–92.

41. Morgan C, McBeth J, Cordingley L, Watson K, Hyrich KL, Symmons DPM, et al. The influence of behavioural and psychological factors on medication adherence over time in rheumatoid arthritis patients: a study in the biologics era. Rheumatol (United Kingdom). 2015;54(10):1780–91.

42. Gadallah MA, Boulos DNK, Gebrel A, Dewedar S, Morisky DE. Assessment of rheumatoid arthritis patients' adherence to treatment. Am J Med Sci. 2015; 349(2):151–6.

43. Kumar K, Gordon C, Barry R, Shaw K, Horne R, Raza K. "It's like taking poison to kill poison but I have to get better": a qualitative study of beliefs about medicines in rheumatoid arthritis and systemic lupus erythematosus patients of south Asian origin. Lupus. 2011;20(8):837–44.

44. Lendrem D, Mitchell S, McMeekin P, Bowman S, Price E, Pease CT, et al. Health-related utility values of patients with primary Sjögren's syndrome and its predictors. Ann Rheum Dis. 2014;73(7):1362–8.

45. Salminen E, Heikkilä S, Poussa T, Lagström H, Saario R, Salminen S. Female patients tend to alter their diet following the diagnosis of rheumatoid arthritis and breast cancer. Prev Med (Baltim). 2002;34(5):529–35.

46. Nyman CS, Lutzen K. Caring needs of patients with rheumatoid arthritis. Nurs Sci Q. 1999;12(2):164–9.

47. Van Der Elst K, De Cock D, Vecoven E, Arat S, Meyfroidt S, Joly J, et al. Are illness perception and coping style associated with the delay between symptom onset and the first general practitioner consultation in early rheumatoid arthritis management? An exploratory study within the CareRA trial. Scand J Rheumatol. 2016;45(3):171–8.

48. Sanderson T, Calnan M, Kumar K. The moral experience of illness and its impact on normalisation: examples from narratives with Punjabi women living with rheumatoid arthritis in the UK. Sociol Health Illn. 2015;37(8): 1218–35.

49. Ziarko M, Mojs E, Piasecki B, Samborski W. The mediating role of dysfunctional coping in the relationship between beliefs about the disease and the level of depression in patients with rheumatoid arthritis. Sci World J. 2014;2014:585063.

50. Ahern MJ, McFarlane AC, Leslie A, Eden J, Roberts-Thomson PJ. Illness behaviour in patients with arthritis. Ann Rheum Dis. 1995;54:245–50.

51. Fraenkel L, Cunningham M. High disease activity may not be sufficient to escalate care. Arthritis Care Res. 2014;66(2):197–203.

52. Isik A, Koca SS, Ozturk A, Mermi O. Anxiety and depression in patients with rheumatoid arthritis. Clin Rheumatol. 2007;26(6):872–8.

53. Calip GS, Adimadhyam S, Xing S, Rincon JC, Lee WJ, Anguiano RH. Medication adherence and persistence over time with self-administered TNF-alpha inhibitors among young adult, middle-aged, and older patients with rheumatologic conditions. Semin Arthritis Rheum. 2017 Oct;47(2):157–64.

54. Mena-Vazquez N, Manrique-Arija S, Yunquera-Romero L, Ureña-Garnica I, Rojas-Gimenez M, Domic C, et al. Adherence of rheumatoid arthritis patients to biologic disease-modifying antirheumatic drugs: a cross-sectional study. Rheumatol Int. 2017 Oct;37(10):1709–18.

55. Zwikker HE, Van den Ende CH, Van Lankveld WG, Den Broeder AA, Van den Hoogen FH, Van de Mosselaar B, et al. Effectiveness of a group-based intervention to change medication beliefs and improve medication adherence in patients with rheumatoid arthritis: a randomized controlled trial. Patient Educ Couns. 2014;94(3):356–61.

56. Van den Bemt BJF, den Broeder AA, van den Hoogen FHJ, Benraad B, Hekster YA, van Riel PLCM, et al. Making the rheumatologist aware of patients' non-adherence does not improve medication adherence in patients with rheumatoid arthritis. Scand J Rheumatol. 2011;40(3):192–6.

57. Wen H, Ralph Schumacher H, Li X, Gu J, Ma L, Wei H, et al. Comparison of expectations of physicians and patients with rheumatoid arthritis for rheumatology clinic visits: a pilot, multicenter, international study. Int J Rheum Dis. 2012;15(4):380–9.

58. Townsend A, Adam P, Cox SM, Li LC. Everyday ethics and help-seeking in early rheumatoid arthritis. Chronic Illn. 2010;6(3):171–82.

59. Dixon-Woods M, Sutton A, Shaw R, Miller T, Smith J, Young B, et al. Appraising qualitative research for inclusion in systematic reviews: a quantitative and qualitative comparison of three methods. J Health Serv Res Policy. 2007;12(1):42–7.

60. Sanderson T, Calnan M, Morris M, Richards P, Hewlett S. The impact of patient-perceived restricted access to anti-TNF therapy for rheumatoid arthritis: a qualitative study. Musculoskeletal Care. 2009;7(3):194–209.

61. Popa-Lisseanu MGG, Greisinger A, Richardson M, O'Malley KJ, Janssen NM, Marcus DM, et al. Determinants of treatment adherence in ethnically diverse, economically disadvantaged patients with rheumatic disease. J Rheumatol. 2005;32(5):913–9.

62. Fitzcharles MA, DaCosta D, Ware MA, Shir Y. Patient barriers to pain management may contribute to poor pain control in rheumatoid arthritis. J Pain. 2009;10(3):300–5.

63. Van Den Bemt BJF, Den Broeder AA, Van Den Hoogen FHJ, Benraad B, Hekster YA, Van Riel PLCM, et al. Making the rheumatologist aware of patients' non-adherence does not improve medication adherence in patients with rheumatoid arthritis. Scand J Rheumatol. 2011;40(3):192–6.

64. Nota I, Drossaert CHC, Taal E, Van De Laar MAFJ. Patients' considerations in the decision-making process of initiating disease-modifying antirheumatic drugs. Arthritis Care Res. 2015;67(7):956–64.

6

The REAL study: A nationwide prospective study of rheumatoid arthritis in Brazil

Geraldo da Rocha Castelar-Pinheiro[1*], Ana Beatriz Vargas-Santos[2], Cleandro Pires de Albuquerque[3], Manoel Barros Bértolo[4], Paulo Louzada Júnior[5], Rina Dalva Neubarth Giorgi[6], Sebastião Cezar Radominski[7], Maria Fernanda B. Resende Guimarães[8], Karina Rossi Bonfiglioli[9], Maria de Fátima Lobato da Cunha Sauma[10], Ivânio Alves Pereira[11], Claiton Viegas Brenol[12], Evandro Silva Freire Coutinho[13] and Licia Maria Henrique da Mota[3]

Abstract

Background: There are few data on the epidemiology, clinical manifestations and management of RA in Brazil, even with the recognition of the high direct, indirect and societal costs of this disease. Herein, we report the formation of the REAL - Rheumatoid Arthritis in Real Life, the first nationally representative multicenter prospective observational study in Brazil.

Methods: The REAL study was designed to include a total of 1300 evaluable patients from 13 tertiary care public health centers specialized in RA management and representative of 5 regions of Brazil. Each center was expected to enroll ~ 100 consecutively seen patients and follow them prospectively in a systematic protocol-driven fashion with scheduled visits at baseline, 6 and 12 months. Core clinical, laboratory and patient-reported outcomes measures were required to be collected at each visit.

Results: A total of 1115 patients (89.4% female, mean age of 56.7 years and median disease duration of 12.7 years) were enrolled from 11 participating centers. Almost 80% of patients were of middle-low or low socioeconomic classes. The median educational time was 8 years, with 3.23% being below literacy level. The interval between symptoms and diagnosis varied from 1 to 457 months (median 12 months). Almost half of the patients were on glucocorticoids, 96.5% on DMARDs, with 35.7% on biologics. Median HAQ-DI was 0.875, ranging from 0 to 3. Median DAS28-ESR was 3.5, with 58.7% of patients presenting moderate or high disease activity.

Conclusions: The first large cohort of Brazilian patients with RA in a real-life setting shows several striking differences from previously published cohorts from other countries. The long delay for diagnosis and start of DMARDs may partly explain the high frequency of erosive disease. An elevated percentage of patients on moderate or high disease activity was seen, despite of the high frequency of corticosteroid and biologics utilization. Data from this cohort may enable public health managers of developing countries better allocate the limited resources available for the care of RA patients.

Keywords: Rheumatoid arthritis, Brazilian cohort, Observational study

* Correspondence: castelar@uerj.br
[1]Departamento de Medicina Interna, Disciplina de Reumatologia, Universidade do Estado do Rio de Janeiro, Avenida Nossa Senhora de Copacabana, 978, sala 508, Copacabana, Rio de Janeiro, RJ 22060-002, Brazil
Full list of author information is available at the end of the article

Background

Rheumatoid arthritis (RA) is a systemic, chronic and progressive disease, characterized by synovial inflammation of peripheral joints. Inadequate treatment often results in reduced health-related quality of life and excess mortality [1]. The current concept of RA management relies on early diagnosis, immediate initiation of a disease-modifying antirheumatic drug (DMARD) and effective suppression of inflammation [2]. Advances in diagnostic tools, the availability of new therapeutic options, mainly the biologic agents, and the adoption of a treat-to-target strategy have been of utmost importance for improving patient outcomes [3]. Despite all this progress, in many areas of the world, the diagnosis of RA is delayed and patients remain undertreated, resulting in great negative humanistic and socioeconomic impact [4, 5].

Brazil is the largest country in Latin America, with a multiethnic population of around 200 million inhabitants [6]. There are few data on the epidemiology and management of RA in Brazil, even with the recognition of the high direct, indirect and societal costs of this disease [7]. A better understanding of the profile of RA patients seen in public health care centers in Brazil can underpin public health policy, enabling a rational allocation of resources and the setting of priorities in this sector.

The REAL – Rheumatoid Arthritis in Real Life – is a multicenter prospective observational cohort study, with twelve-month follow-up period. The aims of this study were to describe the demographic, clinical and therapeutic features of Brazilian patients with RA, and to evaluate adherence to treatment, safety of pharmacologic treatment, and impact on quality of life, physical function and work capacity of these patients. In this first report of REAL study, we describe the methodology and the baseline characteristics of this cohort.

Methods

Setting

Thirteen tertiary care public healthcare centers (Appendix 1) specialized in RA management were selected to represent the five geographic regions in Brazil. Eventually, 11 centers from 4 regions enrolled in the program. The recruitment period started on August 12th, 2015 and ended on April 15th, 2016. Patients were followed for ~ 12 months, with systematic data collection at the initial visit (baseline), at the intermediate visit (6 months ±1 month) and at the final visit (12 months ±1 month), with additional descriptive report of any other unscheduled visit.

Participants

The inclusion criteria were 1) fulfillment of the 1987 American Rheumatism Association (ARA) or the 2010 American College of Rheumatology (ACR) / European League Against Rheumatism (EULAR) classification criteria for rheumatoid arthritis [8, 9]; 2) age 18 years or older; and 3) documented medical record data of at least 6 months of follow up in their healthcare center prior to study enrollment.

Each center was expected to enroll ~ 100 patients consecutively. Since all centers were tertiary-care academic rheumatology practices, they were requested to limit the enrollment of biologic-treated patients to roughly the proportion of these patients being treated in their center.

Variables, data sources and data collection

Table 1 shows the study visit protocol, with all the items systematically evaluated and respective time of assessment. Most data were collected during the medical appointments, with previous medical records used as secondary sources. All data were collected on an electronic medical chart and gathered in a centralized dataset.

Initial visit

At the initial visit the study physician formally assessed the RA classification criteria fulfillment and collected demographic and contact data, socioeconomic profile, family history of RA, other autoimmune diseases or associated conditions, personal history of comorbidities and lifestyle habits (smoking, alcohol consumption and physical activity). For the socioeconomic classification we used the Brazilian Economic Classification Criterion (BECC), a score system updated in 2015 that includes variables such as the number of household electrical appliances, level of education of the householder and access to public services [10]. The score range is stratified from A to D-E, with each stratum corresponding to an estimated household income (Table 2).

The study physician also assessed the following RA aspects: disease duration, time between symptoms onset and diagnosis, time to first DMARD prescription, health facility and physician specialty at first contact with healthcare due to RA symptoms, presence of extra-articular manifestations, positive rheumatoid factor (RF) and anti-citrullinated protein antibody (ACPA), and presence of bone erosions on radiographic study on both hands and feet. Erosive disease was defined when an erosion (defined as a cortical break) was seen in at least three separate joints at any of the following sites: the proximal interphalangeal, the metacarpophalangeal, the wrist (counted as one joint) and the metatarsophalangeal joints. In addition, prior pharmacologic treatments for RA were described (with respective reasons for discontinuation), history of orthopedic surgery and history of intra-articular or periarticular steroid injections.

Table 1 Variables assessed in study visits

Variables		Initial visit	Intermediate visit (6 ± 1 months)	Final visit (12 ± 1 months)
Study entry	Invitation	x		
	Informed consent	x		
Medical history with chart review	Evaluation of inclusion and exclusion criteria	x		
	Demographic data	x		
	Socioeconomic data	x		
	Disease duration	x		
	Time from symptoms onset to diagnosis	x		
	Time from symptoms onset to the 1st DMARD	x		
	Local and medical specialty of the physician on the 1st appointment related with the onset of symptoms	x		
	Previous medications/ injections	x		
	History of joint surgeries	x		x
	Comorbidities	x		x
	Extra-articular manifestations	x		x
	Alcohol consumption	x		x
	Smoking	x		x
	Physical exercise frequency	x		x
	Employment situation	x	x	x
	Medications in use/injections	x	x	x
Physical Exam	Blood pressure	x	x	x
	Heart rate	x	x	x
	Body mass index	x	x	x
	Joint count	x	x	x
Patient reported outcomes	Functional capacity (HAQ-DI)	x	x	x
	Pain (VAS)	x	x	x
	General health (VAS)	x	x	x
	Disease activity within in the previous 6 months VAS	x	x	x
	Current disease activity VAS	x	x	x
	Fatigue (VAS)	x	x	x
	Morning stiffness (VAS)	x	x	x
	Quality of life (SF-12 / SF-6D)	x	x	x
	DMARD use and adherence	x	x	x
	Articular index assessment	x	x	x
Laboratory	Erythrocyte sedimentation rate (mm)	x	x	x
	C-reactive protein (mg/dL)	x	x	x
	Rheumatoid factor	x		
	Anti-citrullinated protein antibody	x		
X-ray	Bone erosions of hands and feet	x		
Physician assessment	Assessment of disease activity by a rheumatologist	x	x	x
Disease activity index	DAS28-ESR	x	x	x
	DAS28-CRP	x	x	x
	CDAI	x	x	x
	SDAI	x	x	x

Table 1 Variables assessed in study visits (Continued)

Variables	Initial visit	Intermediate visit (6 ± 1 months)	Final visit (12 ± 1 months)
RADAI	x	x	x

DMARD disease-modifying antirheumatic drug, HAQ-DI Health Assessment Questionnaire-Disability Index, VAS visual analogue scale, SF-12 12-Item Short-Form Health Survey, SF-6D Short-Form 6 dimensions, DAS28 Disease Activity Score 28-joint count, CDAI Clinical Disease Activity Index, SDAI Simplified Disease Activity Index, RADAI Rheumatoid Arthritis Disease Activity Index

Clinical evaluation included vital signs, anthropometric measures, tender and swollen joint counts, and physician score on the visual analogue scale (VAS) of disease activity. Patient reported outcomes included pain (VAS), global health (VAS), current and previous 6 months disease activity (VAS), fatigue (VAS), morning stiffness (VAS) and articular index, in which the patient evaluates the presence of pain and respective intensity in 16 joints. All laboratory tests, including erythrocyte sedimentation rate (ESR) and C-reactive protein (CRP) were recorded. Compliance to prescribed medications as well as scheduled medical appointments and laboratory tests were also recorded.

The disease activity score-28 joints (DAS28), clinical disease activity index (CDAI), simplified disease activity index (SDAI) and the rheumatoid arthritis disease activity index (RADAI) were also calculated for each appointment [11–13].

The translated and validated versions of the Health Assessment Questionnaire-Disability Index (HAQ-DI), Short Form-12 (SF-12) and SF-6D evaluated, respectively, physical function, functional capacity and wellbeing, and health status from the patient's perspective [14–16].

In this report, we summarize important demographic and clinical data at the baseline visit of all enrolled patients.

Intermediate and final visits

At the intermediate and the final visits, some variables from the medical history, such as change in the marital and employment status, onset of new extra-articular manifestations or comorbidities and medical intercurrences were reassessed. All the items within the physical exam domain, the patient reported outcomes, the lab tests ESR and CRP along with the disease activity indexes, were evaluated at the three scheduled visits (Table 1). Additionally, at the final visit, physicians were requested to describe their therapeutic plan.

Ethical aspects

This study was approved by the National Commission of Ethics in Research (CONEP - Comissão Nacional de Ética em Pesquisa) – Ministry of Health. The coordinating center was the Rio de Janeiro State University, and the approval number was 45781015.8.1001.5259. Each of the centers also obtained approval from the respective Institutional Review Boards. All patients signed the informed consent form.

Results

A total of 1115 patients were enrolled in the study. The general demographic and clinical data of the population at the time of the initial evaluation are presented in Tables 3 and 4. Approximately 90% were female, with a mean age of 56.7 years and median disease duration of 12.7 years. The majority of subjects were white, with minorities from Asian and Brazilian-Indian origins making up 1% of the sample. Almost 80% of patients were classified as pertaining to middle-low or low socioeconomic classes. Median BMI was 27 kg/m^2, with 64% of the patients classified as overweight or obese. The median educational time was 8 years, with 3.23% being below literacy level. About 40% were either current or former smokers.

The interval between symptoms and diagnosis varied from 1 to 457 months (median 12 months). The gap between symptoms onset and first DMARD initiation was wider, ranging from 1 to 624 months, but the same median value of 12 months.

The seropositivity rate was similar between RF (78%) and ACPA (77%), but it is important to highlight that the latter was assessed in less than half of the patients.

Interestingly, similar numbers of patients fulfilled the ARA 1987 and the 2010 ACR-EULAR classification criteria for RA, with 80.8% of subjects meeting both criteria. All patients met at least one criteria.

Table 2 Brazilian Economic Classification Criterion (BECC): relation between socioeconomic strata and estimated household income

Socioeconomic Strata	Household income (US dollar[a])
A	5921.00
B1	2623.00
B2	1357.00
C1	766.81
C2	460.65
D-E	217.71

[a]Conversion of Brazilian reais into US dollars made in accordance with the exchange rate of April 16, 2016- US$1,00: R$ 3,5276

Table 3 Baseline demographic data of patients enrolled in the REAL study

Demographic data	Absolute value or %	N
Age, years, median (range)	56.7 (22.1–88.8)	1115
Female gender, %	89.4	1115
Ethnicity/race/color, %		1115
White	56.8	
Pardo[a]	31.3	
Black	10.9	
Others	1.0	
Smoking, %		1115
Smoker	10.9	
Former smoker	28.6	
Never smoked	60.5	
BMI categories, %		1046
Low weight	5.0	
Normal	31.5	
Overweight	35.3	
Obesity	28.2	
Total formal education time, years, median (range)	8 (0–20)	1075
Brazilian Economic Classification Criterion: Socioeconomic Strata: Gross family income in the month in US dollar[b], %		1101
A (5,921.00)	1.4	
B1 (2623.00)	3.5	
B2 (1357.00)	18.4	
C1 (766.81)	27.4	
C2 (460.65)	31.3	
D-E (217.71)	18.0	

[a]Mixed white and black ethnicities. *BMI* Body mass index. [b]Conversion of Brazilian reais into US dollars made in accordance with the exchange rate of April 16, 2016 - US$1,00: R$ 3,5276

Almost half of the patients were on glucocorticoids, 96.5% on DMARDs, with 35.7% on biologics. Of those on biologics ($n = 398$), 15.6% were on monotherapy.

Median HAQ-DI was 0.875, ranging from 0 to 3. Median DAS28-ESR was 3.5, with 58.7% of patients presenting moderate or high disease activity. When assessed by CDAI, the median score represented low disease activity (CDAI = 9), with 46.7% of subjects classified as presenting moderate to high disease activity.

Discussion

We describe the formation of the first large cohort of Brazilian patients with RA in a real-life setting, with consecutive enrollment of subjects and systematic data collection. The demographic, clinical, serological and radiographic characteristics of the patients being followed have several similar but some divergent characteristics from previously published North American, European and Latin American cohorts [17–21]. Particularly notable are the long delay for diagnosis, the high frequency of corticosteroid use and

of erosive disease, as well as, the elevated percentage of patients on moderate or high disease activity. The high frequency of biologic DMARD use, considering the economic limitations in Brazil, is also remarkable. The fact that most patients were either RF or ACPA positive and had a delay in the initiation of DMARD may explain the observed high frequency (almost 60%) of moderate or high disease activity and erosive disease. The ethnic and socioeconomic class distribution reflects the Brazilian population in general, and is considerably different from other international cohorts [17–22]. It is important to note that the socioeconomic class distribution likely reflects the patients seen at the participating centers, which provide free health care within the Brazilian Public Health System -Sistema Único de Saúde (SUS). In Brazil, three quarters of the population is served by this public and free system, with the others using various private and paid health plans [23] and the latter were likely not represented to a significant degree in this study. About 11% of REAL patients were currently smokers, a number lower than

Table 4 Baseline clinical data of patients enrolled in the REAL study

Clinical Data	Absolute value or %	n
Disease duration, years, median (range)	12.7 (0.7–56.9)	1114
Time from symptoms to diagnosis, months, median (range)	12 (1–457)	1078
Time from symptoms to 1st DMARD, months, median (range)	12 (1–624)	994
Patients with ≥1 extra-articular manifestation, %	23.3	1115
Positive rheumatoid factor, %	78.2	1105
Positive anti-citrullinated peptide antibody, %	77.2	477
Erosive disease, %	54.9	1095
Patients fulfilling classification criteria, %:		
ARA 1987	90.0	1115
ACR/EULAR 2010	90.9	1115
Both	80.8	1115
Drugs in use, %:		
Glucocorticoids	47.4	1115
Nonsteroidal anti-inflammatory drugs	9.1	1115
Synthetic DMARD	90.9	1115
Methotrexate	66.5	1115
Biologic DMARD	35.7	1115
Biologic DMARD in monotherapy	5,6	1115
ESR, median (range)	21 (1–140)	923
CRP median (range)	0.7 (0–76.1)	944
Pain (VAS 0–100), median (range)	40 (0–100)	1115
Fatigue (VAS 0–100), median (range)	40 (0–100)	1115
Global health assessment (VAS 0–100), median (range)	38 (0–100)	1115
DAS28-ESR, median (range)	3.5 (0.3–8.2)	923
Remission	26.2	
Low disease activity	15.1	
Moderate disease activity	41.8	
High disease activity	16.9	
CDAI, median (range)	9 (0–70)	1113
Remission	20.1	
Low disease activity	33.2	
Moderate disease activity	27.5	
High disease activity	19.2	
HAQ-DI, median (range)	0.875 (0–3)	1111
SF-12 physical, median (range)	36.1 (17.5–55.9)	1079
SF-12 mental, median (range)	47.1 (14.3–72.0)	1079

ARA American Rheumatism Association, *ACR* American College of Rheumatology, *EULAR* European League Against Rheumatism, *DMARD* disease-modifying antirheumatic drug, *VAS* visual analogue scale, *ESR* erythrocyte sedimentation rate (mm/first hour), *CRP* C-reactive protein (mg/dL), *DAS28* Disease Activity Score 28-joint count, *CDAI*: Clinical Disease Activity Index, *HAQ* Health Assessment Questionnaire-Disability Index, *SF-12* 12-Item Short-Form Health Survey

that published in previous RA studies from other parts of the world (25–33%), but consistent with the relatively low rates of smoking in the Brazilian population (females: 8.2% and males: 12.6%) [24–27]. Subsequent publications will explore the relationship of these differences with clinical and outcome variables.

We recognize several limitations of the REAL study. All the sites enrolled in the study are "reference centers", and thus are unlikely to represent the broader management of RA across the country. It is probable that these patients present more severe disease, with a less favorable prognosis. REAL study was designed to be representative of the entire Brazilian population, but one center in the Northeast (representing 27.9% of population) could not participate because of delays in the Ethics Committee approval. Also, our cohort does not include patients from among the 25% of Brazilian population receiving their healthcare outside of the public health system. On the other hand, the REAL study data reflects perhaps a more optimal standard of care possibly resulting in better outcomes in comparison with those treated in less prepared facilities. Further publications will study multiple management strategies and their effects on patient outcomes.

Conclusions

The first large cohort of Brazilian patients with RA in a real-life setting shows several striking differences from previously published cohorts from other countries. The long delay for diagnosis and start of DMARDs may partly explain the high frequency erosive disease. An elevated percentage of patients on moderate or high disease activity was seen, despite of the high frequency of corticosteroid and biologics utilization. Data from this cohort may enable public health managers of developing countries better allocate the limited resources available for the care of RA patients.

Appendix 1

Table 5 Thirteen tertiary care public healthcare centers specialized in RA management representing the five geographic regions in Brazil

Centers	Number of patients included	Geographic region
Universidade Estadual de Campinas	111	Southeast
Universidade de Brasília	107	Midwest
Universidade Federal do Pará	102	North
Universidade do Estado do Rio de Janeiro	100	Southeast
Universidade Federal do Paraná	100	South
Universidade Federal do Rio Grande do Sul	102	South
Universidade Federal de Santa Catarina	100	South
Universidade de São Paulo - Ribeirão Preto	99	Southeast
Universidade Federal de Minas Gerais	99	Southeast
Hospital do Servidor Público Estadual de São Paulo	99	Southeast
Universidade de São Paulo – São Paulo	98	Southeast
Universidade Federal do Ceará	0	Northeast
Universidade Federal de São Paulo	0	Southeast
TOTAL	1115	

Acknowledgements

Gurkirpal Singh, MD and Leticia Rocha provided technical and writing assistance.

Authors' contributions

All authors made substantial contributions to the acquisition of data, have been involved in drafting the manuscript or revising it critically for important intellectual content, gave final approval of the version to be published and have participated sufficiently in the work to take public responsibility for appropriate portions of the content; and agreed to be accountable for all aspects of the work in ensuring that questions related to the accuracy or integrity of any part of the work are appropriately investigated and resolved. In addition, GRCP, ABVS and LMHM also made substantial contributions to conception and design of the study.

Competing interests

GRCP: Has received consulting fees from AbbVie, Bristol-Myers Squibb, Eli Lilly, Glaxosmithkline, Janssen, Pfizer, Sanofi Genzyme and Roche; ABVS: Has received supporting for international medical events from AbbVie and Janssen; CPA: Has received personal fees and/or non-financial support from Pfizer, AbbVie, AstraZeneca, Janssen, Bristol-Myers Squibb, Roche, Novartis and UCB, outside the submitted work; MBB: Has participated in clinical and/or experimental studies related to this work and sponsored by Roche; has delivered speeches at events related to this work and sponsored by AbbVie and Pfizer; PLJ: Has received supporting for internationals congresses from Bristol-Myers Squibb, UCB and consulting fees from Pfizer; RDNG: Has received consulting fees, speaking fees and supporting for internationals congresses from Roche, Pfizer, Bristol-Myers Squibb, UCB, Eli-Lilly, AbbVie, Abbott and EMS; SCR: Has received consulting and speaking fees from Abbvie, Janssen, Pfizer, Roche and UCB; MFBRG: Has received speaking fees and supporting for congresses from AbbVie, Bristol-Myers Squibb, Janssen, Novartis, Pfizer, Roche and UCB; KRB: Has received speaking fees and supporting for international congresses from Roche, Pfizer, Bristol-Myers Squibb, Abbvie and Janssen; MFLCS: No financial disclosures; CVB: Has participated in clinical and/or experimental studies related to this work and sponsored by AbbVie, BMS, Janssen, Pfizer and Roche; has received personal or institutional support from AbbVie, BMS, Janssen, Pfizer and Roche; has delivered speeches at events related to this work and sponsored by AbbVie, Janssen, Pfizer and Roche; IAP: Has received consulting fees, speaking fees and supporting for internationals congresses from Roche, Pfizer, UCB Pharma, Eli-Lilly, Abbvie and Janssen; ESFC: No financial disclosures; LMHM: Has received personal or institutional support from AbbVie, Janssen, Pfizer and Roche; has delivered speeches at events related to this work and sponsored by AbbVie, Janssen, Pfizer, Roche and UCB.

Author details

[1]Departamento de Medicina Interna, Disciplina de Reumatologia, Universidade do Estado do Rio de Janeiro, Avenida Nossa Senhora de Copacabana, 978, sala 508, Copacabana, Rio de Janeiro, RJ 22060-002, Brazil. [2]Serviço de Reumatologia, Hospital Universitário Pedro Ernesto - Universidade do Estado do Rio de Janeiro, Rio de Janeiro, Brazil. [3]Serviço de Reumatologia, Hospital Universitário de Brasília - Universidade de Brasília, Brasília, Brazil. [4]Disciplina de Reumatologia, Faculdade de Ciências Médicas, Universidade Estadual de Campinas, Campinas, Brazil. [5]Disciplina de Reumatologia, Faculdade de Medicina da Universidade de Ribeirao Preto, Universidade de Sao Paulo, Ribeirão Preto, Brazil. [6]Serviço de Reumatologia, Instituto de Assistência Médica ao Servidor Público Estadual, Hospital do Servidor Público Estadual de São Paulo, São Paulo, Brazil. [7]Disciplina de Reumatologia, Faculdade de Medicina da Universidade Federal do Paraná, Universidade Federal do Paraná, Curitiba, Brazil. [8]Serviço de Reumatologia, Hospital das Clínicas, Universidade Federal de Minas Gerais, Belo Horizonte, Brazil. [9]Disciplina de Reumatologia, Faculdade de Medicina, Universidade de São Paulo, São Paulo, Brazil. [10]Disciplina de Reumatologia, Faculdade de Medicina, Universidade Federal do Pará, Belém, Brazil. [11]Serviço de Reumatologia, Hospital Universitário, Universidade Federal de Santa Catarina, Florianópolis, Brazil. [12]Serviço de Reumatologia, Departamento de Medicina Interna, Universidade Federal do Rio Grande do Sul, Porto Alegre, Brazil. [13]Departamento de Epidemiologia e Métodos Quantitativos em Saúde, Fundação Osvaldo Cruz, Rio de Janeiro, Brazil.

References

1. van der Linden MP, Knevel R, Huizinga TW, et al. Classification of rheumatoid arthritis: comparison of the 1987 American College of Rheumatology criteria and the 2010 American College of Rheumatology/European league against rheumatism criteria. Arthritis Rheum. 2011;63:37–42.
2. Singh JA, Saag KG, Bridges SL Jr, et al. 2015 American College of Rheumatology Guideline for the treatment of rheumatoid arthritis. Arthritis Rheumatol. 2016;68:1–26.
3. Smolen JS, Aletaha D, Barton A, et al. Rheumatoid arthritis. Nat Rev Dis Primers. 2018;4:18001.
4. Sokka T, Kautiainen H, Pincus T, et al. Disparities in rheumatoid arthritis disease activity according to gross domestic product in 25 countries in the QUEST–RA database. Ann Rheum Dis. 2009;68:1666–72.
5. Burgos Vargas R, Cardiel MH. Rheumatoid arthritis in Latin America. Important challenges to be solved Clin Rheumatol. 2015;34(Suppl 1):S1–3.
6. "World Population Prospects: The 2017 Revision" ESA.UN.org (custom data acquired via website). United Nations Department of Economic and Social Affairs, Population Division. https://www.un.org/development/desa/publications/world-population-prospects-the-2017-revision.html. Accessed 10 Feb 2018.
7. Azevedo AB, Ferraz MB, Ciconelli RM. Indirect costs of rheumatoid arthritis in Brazil. Value Health. 2008;11:869–77.
8. Arnett FC, Edworthy SM, Bloch DA, et al. The American rheumatism association 1987 revised criteria for the classification of rheumatoid arthritis. Arthritis Rheum. 1988;31:315–24.
9. Aletaha D, Neogi T, Silman AJ, et al. 2010 rheumatoid arthritis classification criteria: an American College of Rheumatology/European league against rheumatism collaborative initiative. Ann Rheum Dis. 2010;69:1580–8.
10. ABEP. Brazilian Criteria 2015 and social class distribution update for 2016, ABEP - Associação Brasileira de Empresas de Pesquisa/Brazilian Market Research Association – 2016 – http://www.abep.org/criterio-brasil – Accessed 10 Feb 2018.
11. van der Heidjde DMFM, van't Hof MA, PLCM v R, de Putte LBA v. Development of a disease activity score based on judgment in clinical practice by rheumatologists. J Rheumatol. 1993;20:579–81.
12. Aletaha D, Smolen J. The simplified disease activity index (SDAI) and the clinical disease activity index (CDAI): a review of their usefulness and validity in rheumatoid arthritis. Clin Exp Rheumatol. 2005;23(Suppl 39):S100–8.
13. Stucki G, Liang MH, Stucki S, et al. A self-administered rheumatoid arthritis disease activity index (RADAI) for epidemiologic research. Psychometric properties and correlation with parameters of disease activity. Arthritis Rheum. 1995;38:795–8.
14. Ferraz MB, Oliveira LM, Araujo PM, et al. Crosscultural reliability of the physical ability dimension of the health assessment questionnaire. J Rheumatol. 1990;17:813–7.
15. Silveira MF, Almeida JC, Freire RS, et al. Psychometric properties of the quality of life assessment instrument: 12-item health survey (SF-12). Cien Saude Colect. 2013;18:1923–31.
16. Campolina AG, Bortoluzzo AB, Ferraz MB, et al. Validation of the Brazilian version of the generic six-dimensional short form quality of life questionnaire (SF-6D Brazil). Cien Saude Colet. 2011;16:3103–10.
17. Curtis JR, Jain A, Askling J, et al. A comparison of patient characteristics and outcomes in selected European and U.S. rheumatoid arthritis registries. Semin Arthritis Rheum. 2010;40:2–14.
18. Sokka T, Toloza S, Cutolo M, et al. Women, men, and rheumatoid arthritis: analyses of disease activity, disease characteristics, and treatments in the QUEST-RA study. Arthritis Res Ther. 2009;11:R7.
19. van der Zee-Neuen A, Putrik P, Ramiro S, et al. Large country differences in work outcomes in patients with RA – an analysis in the multinational study COMORA. Arthritis Res Ther. 2017;19:216.
20. Estel BAP, Massardo L, Wojdyla D, et al. Is there something we can learn from rheumatoid arthritis in Latin America? A descriptive report on an inception cohort of 1093 patients [abstract]. Ann Rheum Dis. 2008;67:336.
21. Cardiel MH, Pons-Estel BA, Sacnun MP, et al. Treatment of early rheumatoid arthritis in a multinational inception cohort of Latin American patients: the GLADAR experience. J Clin Rheumatol. 2012;18:327–35.
22. https://ww2.ibge.gov.br/english/estatistica/populacao/caracteristicas_raciais/default_raciais.shtm. Accessed 10 Feb 2018.
23. Lewis M, Penteado E, Malik AM. Brazil's mixed public and private hospital system. World Hosp Health Serv. 2015;51:22–6.
24. Balsa A, Lojo-Oliveira L, Alperi-López M, et al. Prevalence of Comorbidities in Rheumatoid Arthritis and Evaluation of Their Monitoring in Clinical Practice: The Spanish Cohort of the COMORA Study. Reumatol Clin. 2017. https://doi.org/10.1016/j.reuma.2017.06.002. [Epub ahead of print]
25. Meissner Y, Richter A, Manger B, et al. Serious adverse events and the risk of stroke in patients with rheumatoid arthritis: results from the German RABBIT cohort. Ann Rheum Dis. 2017;76:1583–90.
26. GBD 2015 Tobacco Collaborators. Smoking prevalence and attributable disease burden in 195 countries and territories, 1990–2015: a systematic analysis from the Global Burden of Disease Study 2015. Lancet. 2017;389:1885–906.
27. Lotufo PA. Smoking control in Brazil: a public health success story. Sao Paulo Med J. 2017;135:203–4.

7

2017 recommendations of the Brazilian Society of Rheumatology for the pharmacological treatment of rheumatoid arthritis

Licia Maria Henrique da Mota[1,16]*, Adriana Maria Kakehasi[2], Ana Paula Monteiro Gomides[1,3],
Angela Luzia Branco Pinto Duarte[4], Bóris Afonso Cruz[5], Claiton Viegas Brenol[6], Cleandro Pires de Albuquerque[7],
Geraldo da Rocha Castelar Pinheiro[8], Ieda Maria Magalhães Laurindo[9], Ivanio Alves Pereira[10],
Manoel Barros Bertolo[11], Mariana Peixoto Guimarães Ubirajara Silva de Souza[12], Max Vitor Carioca de Freitas[13],
Paulo Louzada-Júnior[14], Ricardo Machado Xavier[6] and Rina Dalva Neubarth Giorgi[15]

Abstract

The objective of this document is to provide a comprehensive update of the recommendations of Brazilian Society of Rheumatology on drug treatment of rheumatoid arthritis (RA), based on a systematic literature review and on the opinion of a panel of rheumatologists. Four general principles and eleven recommendations were approved. General principles: RA treatment should (1) preferably consist of a multidisciplinary approach coordinated by a rheumatologist, (2) include counseling on lifestyle habits, strict control of comorbidities, and updates of the vaccination record, (3) be based on decisions shared by the patient and the physician after clarification about the disease and the available therapeutic options; (4) the goal is sustained clinical remission or, when this is not feasible, low disease activity. Recommendations: (1) the first line of treatment should be a csDMARD, started as soon as the diagnosis of RA is established; (2) methotrexate (MTX) is the first-choice csDMARD; (3) the combination of two or more csDMARDs, including MTX, may be used as the first line of treatment; (4) after failure of first-line therapy with MTX, the therapeutic strategies include combining MTX with another csDMARD (leflunomide), with two csDMARDs (hydroxychloroquine and sulfasalazine), or switching MTX for another csDMARD (leflunomide or sulfasalazine) alone; (5) after failure of two schemes with csDMARDs, a bDMARD may be preferably used or, alternatively a tsDMARD, preferably combined, in both cases, with a csDMARD; (6) the different bDMARDs in combination with MTX have similar efficacy, and therefore, the therapeutic choice should take into account the peculiarities of each drug in terms of safety and cost; (7) the combination of a bDMARD and MTX is preferred over the use of a bDMARD alone; (8) in case of failure of an initial treatment scheme with a bDMARD, a scheme with another bDMARD can be used; in cases of failure with a TNFi, a second bDMARD of the same class or with another mechanism of action is effective and safe; (9) tofacitinib can be used to treat RA after failure of bDMARD; (10) corticosteroids, preferably at low doses for the shortest possible time, should be considered during periods of disease activity, and the risk-benefit ratio should also be considered; (11) reducing or spacing out bDMARD doses is possible in patients in sustained remission.

* Correspondence: liciamhmota@gmail.com
[1]Programa de Pós-graduação em Ciências Médicas, Faculdade de Medicina-Universidade de Brasília; Serviço de Reumatologia, Hospital Universitário de Brasília, Universidade de Brasília, Brasília, Brazil
[16]Rheos, Centro Médico Lúcio Costa, SGAS 610, bloco 1, salas T50- T51, L2 Sul, Asa Sul, Brasília, DF 70200700, Brazil
Full list of author information is available at the end of the article

Introduction

Rheumatoid arthritis (RA) is a systemic inflammatory autoimmune disease characterized primarily by the involvement of the synovial membrane of peripheral joints. The estimated prevalence of RA in the total population is 0.5–1.0%, and the incidence is higher in the 30–50-year-old age group and among women [1, 2]. In Brazil, a study conducted in Minas Gerais found a prevalence of 0.46% [3]. The past few decades have introduced a substantial increase in the number of RA treatments due to advances in knowledge concerning the pathophysiological mechanisms of the disease and the development of new drugs. Moreover, new monitoring and treatment strategies have been implemented, including comprehensive disease control and early intervention, during the onset of symptoms [4]. In 2012 and 2013, the RA Committee of the Brazilian Society of Rheumatology (Sociedade Brasileira de Reumatologia–SBR) published recommendations on RA diagnosis and treatment in Brazil to provide support to Brazilian rheumatologists, based upon scientific evidence combined with the experience of a panel of specialists, while safeguarding the necessary autonomy of physicians in choosing among the available therapeutic strategies [5–8]. In 2015, the recommendations were updated to include the use of target-specific synthetic disease-modifying antirheumatic drugs [9].

The objective of the current document is to provide a comprehensive update of the recommendations of SBR on drug treatment of RA in Brazil considering the advances accrued since the last revision. The scope of this work is limited to adult disease because juvenile idiopathic arthritis requires distinct and specific approaches.

Methods

The present recommendations were based on a Systematic Literature Review (SLR) and on the opinion of a panel of rheumatologists specialized in RA. In September 2016, the RA Committee met to develop questions to guide the SLR based on real-life scenarios, and these questions were improved by multiple subsequent rounds of online discussion. At the end of the interactive process, ten questions considered essential for the preparation of the recommendations were selected (Table 1). Furthermore, four general principles that should guide the entire RA treatment based on concepts widely established in the literature were formulated.

An SLR was undertaken to answer the proposed questions. Randomized clinical trials and systematic reviews of randomized clinical trials were considered eligible primarily, but controlled observational studies were also considered acceptable when interventional studies with those designs were not available. The MEDLINE, EMBASE, and SCOPUS databases were searched using specific search strategies (Table 2). In addition, the references of the

Table 1 Questions based on clinical scenarios, selected by the rheumatoid arthritis committee of the brazilian society of rheumatology to guide the development of the recommendations

Questions about possible clinical scenarios for treating rheumatoid arthritis in Brazil, considering safety, effectiveness, and cost.

Question 1: Should the first line of treatment be csDMARD (methotrexate, hydroxychloroquine, leflunomide, or sulfasalazine), tsDMARD (tofacitinib), or bDMARD (adalimumab, certolizumab, etanercept, infliximab, golimumab, abatacept, rituximab, or tocilizumab)?

Question 2: Is there evidence that a particular csDMARD is more effective than other csDMARDs?

Question 3: Is there evidence that the use of combination therapy with two or more csDMARDs is more effective than csDMARD monotherapy as the first line of treatment?

Question 4: Is there evidence that after failure of a csDMARD monotherapy as the first line of treatment, the best option is to switch to a second monotherapy regimen rather than using combination therapy with two or more csDMARDs?

Question 5: Is there evidence that a particular TNFi (adalimumab, certolizumab, etanercept, golimumab, or infliximab) or non-TNFi (abatacept, rituximab, or tocilizumab) bDMARD is more effective than other biological agents?

Question 6: Is there evidence that bDMARD (adalimumab, certolizumab, etanercept, golimumab, infliximab, abatacept, rituximab, or tocilizumab) combined with methotrexate is more effective than bDMARD monotherapy?

Question 7: In the case of failure of a first bDMARD scheme, is there evidence that a second bDMARD scheme is effective?

Question 8: Is there evidence that tsDMARD (tofacitinib) is more effective than bDMARD (adalimumab, certolizumab, etanercept, golimumab, infliximab, abatacept, rituximab, or tocilizumab)?

Question 9: Is there evidence that oral, parenteral, or intra-articular use of corticosteroids improves prognosis when combined with DMARD?

Question 10: Is there evidence that it is possible to reduce the dose or increase the dose intervals for bDMARD in patients in remission?

csDMARD conventional synthetic disease-modifying drugs – methotrexate, leflunomide, sulfasalazine and antimalarials (hydroxychloroquine and chloroquine) tsDMARD: synthetic target-specific disease-modifying drugs – tofacitinib bDMARD: biological disease-modifying drugs – tumor necrosis factor inhibitors/TNFi (adalimumab, certolizumab, etanercept, golimumab, infliximab), T-lymphocyte costimulation modulator (abatacept), anti-CD20 (rituximab), and IL-6 receptor blocker (tocilizumab)

selected studies, as well as relevant publications in the area, and the annals of congresses most relevant to the specialty were also searched. The search included the period from 2006 to October 2016 without language restrictions and was updated monthly until March 2017.

The studies were selected using the Covidence system (www.covidence.org). Two independent researchers analyzed the retrieved publications based on the titles and abstracts. Cases of disagreement were resolved by consensus. The risk of bias in clinical trials was assessed using the tool proposed by the Cochrane Collaboration [10]. Systematic reviews were evaluated using the AMSTAR tool [11]. The quality of evidence for each outcome (high, moderate, low, or very low) was evaluated using the GRADE tool (https://gradepro.org) [12]. The risk of publication bias was assessed by consulting the protocols of the clinical trials registered in ClinicalTrials.gov (https://clinicaltrials.gov)

Table 2 Search strategies used in the MEDLINE, EMBASE and SCOPUS databases for obtaining evidence on drug therapies for rheumatoid arthritis

Database	Strategy
MEDLINE (via PubMed)	((((meta analysis[ptyp] OR meta-analysis[tiab] OR meta-analysis[mh] OR (systematic[tiab] AND review[tiab]) NOT ((case[ti] AND report[ti]) OR editorial[ptyp] OR comment[ptyp] OR letter[ptyp] OR newspaper article [ptyp])) OR (randomized controlled trial[Publication Type] OR (randomized[Title/Abstract] AND controlled[Title/Abstract] AND trial[Title/Abstract])))))) AND ((arthritis, rheumatoid[mh:noexp]) or (rheumatoid arthriti*[text word])) Filters: Publication date from 2006/01/01
EMBASE	'rheumatoid arthritis'/mj AND ([cochrane review]/lim OR [systematic review]/lim OR [controlled clinical trial]/lim OR [randomized controlled trial]/lim OR [meta analysis]/lim) AND [2006–2016]/py NOT [medline]/lim
SCOPUS	TITLE-ABS-KEY(rheumatoid arthritis) AND((TITLE-ABS-KEY(randomized) AND TITLE-ABS-KEY(controlled) AND TITLE-ABS-KEY(trial)) OR (TITLE-ABS-KEY(meta-analysis) OR (TITLE-ABS-KEY(systematic) AND TITLE-ABS-KEY(review)))) AND (PUBYEAR > 2006) AND NOT (INDEX(medline) or INDEX(embase))

and WHO International Clinical Trials Registry Platform (http://www.who.int/ictrp/en) when available and by asymmetry analysis of funnel plots.

The methodological details of the SLR that supported the present recommendations and the expanded results, together with the rationale of the answers to the formulated questions, will be available as Additional file 1. In the present document, a predominantly clinical approach was adopted, in which the SLR findings were summarized in a technically accessible language as the basis for the recommendations.

Based on the results of the SLR, the RA Committee met in June and August 2017 in São Paulo and Belo Horizonte to establish the level of agreement with each general principle and recommendation according to the methodology described below. After presenting each statement, a secret ballot was held, in which the participants could agree or disagree with the general proposition of each statement. In cases of agreement by at least 70% of the participants present, a new vote was conducted to assess the level of agreement with the text using a numerical scale from 0 ("completely disagree") to 10 ("completely agree"). The general principles and recommendations that did not reach a minimum rate of agreement of 70% initially were subjected to repeated steps of reformulation and voting until this rate was reached, and the level of agreement was then determined.

This process resulted in the approval of four general principles and eleven recommendations for drug treatment of RA in Brazil, which are presented in Table 3 and discussed below. This document also includes a section on therapeutic strategies, and this section serves as the basis for the understanding and practical application of the recommendations. The therapeutic strategies were graphically summarized into the new flowchart for drug treatment of RA in Brazil (Fig. 1).

The following abbreviations and nomenclature for disease-modifying antirheumatic drugs (DMARDs) were used in this document:

csDMARD: conventional synthetic disease-modifying antirheumatic drugs – methotrexate, leflunomide, sulfasalazine, and antimalarial drugs (hydroxychloroquine and chloroquine).

tsDMARD: synthetic target-specific disease-modifying antirheumatic drug – tofacitinib.

bDMARD: biological disease-modifying antirheumatic drugs – tumor necrosis factor inhibitors/TNFi (adalimumab, certolizumab, etanercept, golimumab, infliximab), T-lymphocyte co-stimulation modulator (abatacept), anti-CD20 (rituximab), and IL-6 receptor blocker (tocilizumab).

boDMARD: original biological disease-modifying antirheumatic drugs.

bsDMARD: biosimilar biological disease-modifying antirheumatic drugs.

General principles

General principle 1: Treatment of patients with RA should preferably consist of a multidisciplinary approach coordinated by a rheumatologist. (level of agreement: 9.87)
Patients with RA should be preferably monitored by a multidisciplinary team, including a physician, physiotherapist, occupational therapist, psychologist, and nutritionist, among others. The rheumatologist, as a specialist in RA, should be responsible for coordinating the treatment.

General principle 2: Treatment of patients with RA should include counseling on lifestyle habits, strict control of comorbidities, and updates of the vaccination record. (level of agreement: 10)
Smoking, excessive intake of alcoholic beverages, obesity, and a sedentary lifestyle should be strongly discouraged. The active search and appropriate management of comorbidities, particularly systemic arterial hypertension, diabetes mellitus, dyslipidemia, and osteoporosis, are part of the care of patients with RA. The patient's vaccination record should be updated

Table 3 General principles and recommendations of the Brazilian Society of Rheumatology for pharmacological treatment of rheumatoid arthritis in Brazil

General principles

General principle 1: Treatment of patients with RA should preferably consist of a multidisciplinary approach coordinated by a rheumatologist.
Level of agreement: 9.87

General principle 2: RA treatment should include counseling on lifestyle habits, strict control of comorbidities, and updates of the vaccination record.
Level of agreement: 10

General principle 3: RA treatment should be based on decisions shared by the patient and physician after clarification about the disease and the available therapeutic options.
Level of agreement: 9.93

General Principle 4: The goal of RA treatment is sustained clinical remission or, when this is not feasible, low disease activity.
Level of agreement: 9.87

Recommendations for drug treatment of RA

Recommendation 1: The first line of treatment should be a csDMARD, started as soon as the diagnosis of RA is established.
Level of agreement: 9.93

Recommendation 2: Methotrexate is the first-choice csDMARD.
Level of agreement: 10

Recommendation 3: Combination of two or more csDMARDs, including methotrexate, may be used as the first line of treatment.
Level of agreement: 9.62

Recommendation 4: After failure of first-line therapy with MTX, the therapeutic strategies include combining MTX with another csDMARD (leflunomide), with two csDMARDs (hydroxychloroquine and sulfasalazine), or switching MTX for another csDMARD (leflunomide or sulfasalazine) alone.
Level of agreement: 9.12

Recommendation 5: After failure of two schemes with csDMARD, a bDMARD may be preferably used or, alternatively, a tsDMARD, preferably combined, in both cases, with a csDMARD.
Level of agreement: 9.5

Recommendation 6: The different bDMARDs in combination with MTX have similar efficacy, and therefore, the therapeutic choice should take into account the peculiarities of each drug in terms of safety and cost.
Level of agreement: 9.31

Recommendation 7: The combination of bDMARD and methotrexate is preferred over the use of bDMARD alone.
Level of agreement: 9.87

Recommendation 8: In case of failure of an initial treatment scheme with bDMARD, a scheme with another bDMARD can be used. In cases of failure with a TNFi, a second bDMARD of the same class or with another mechanism of action is effective and safe.
Level of agreement: 9.37

Recommendation 9: Tofacitinib can be used to treat RA after failure of bDMARD.
Level of agreement: 9.81

Recommendation 10: Corticosteroids, preferably at low doses for the shortest possible time, should be considered during periods of disease activity, and the risk-benefit ratio should also be considered.
Level of agreement: 9.81

Recommendation 11: Reducing or spacing out bDMARD doses is possible in patients in sustained remission.
Level of agreement: 9.31

csDMARD: Conventional synthetic disease-modifying antirheumatic drugs (methotrexate, leflunomide, sulfasalazine) and antimalarials (hydroxychloroquine and chloroquine)
tsDMARD: Synthetic target-specific disease-modifying antirheumatic drugs – tofacitinib
bDMARD: biological disease-modifying drugs – tumor necrosis factor inhibitors/TNFi (adalimumab, certolizumab, etanercept, golimumab, infliximab), T-lymphocyte costimulation modulator (abatacept), anti-CD20 (rituximab), and IL-6 receptor blocker (tocilizumab)

preferably before the initiation of treatment and kept updated during follow-up.

General principle 3: Treatment of patients with RA should be based on decisions that are shared by the patient and the physician after clarification about the disease and the available therapeutic options. (level of agreement: 9.93)

Patients with RA should be informed about the nature and prognosis of the disease. Moreover, patients should be informed about the available therapeutic options, their benefits, potential adverse effects, and costs.

General principle 4: The goal of RA treatment is sustained clinical remission or, when this is not feasible, low disease activity. (level of agreement: 9.83)

The rheumatologist and the patient should acknowledge that the goal of treatment is sustained clinical remission or, in cases where this is not feasible, low disease activity. In the long term, these outcomes are related to the best clinical, structural, and functional evolution [13–15].

Regular monitoring of clinical, laboratory, and imaging parameters is necessary to achieve this goal. In the initial stage of RA (the first 6 months of symptoms) and whenever the disease presents with significant inflammatory activity, follow-up should be performed monthly to allow dosage adjustment or changes in medication for disease management.

Recommendations

Recommendation 1: The first line of treatment should be a csDMARD started as soon as the diagnosis of RA is established. (level of agreement: 9.93)

The efficacy (ACR50 response) of methotrexate (MTX) monotherapy is similar to that of bDMARD monotherapy, except for tocilizumab, which was more effective than MTX [16–23].

Although monotherapy with tofacitinib has been shown more effective than with MTX, the limited availability of long-term safety data on the former requires caution and precludes its use as the first line of treatment, until more data become available [24].

In addition, the lower cost of csDMARD should be taken into account, although few cost-effectiveness

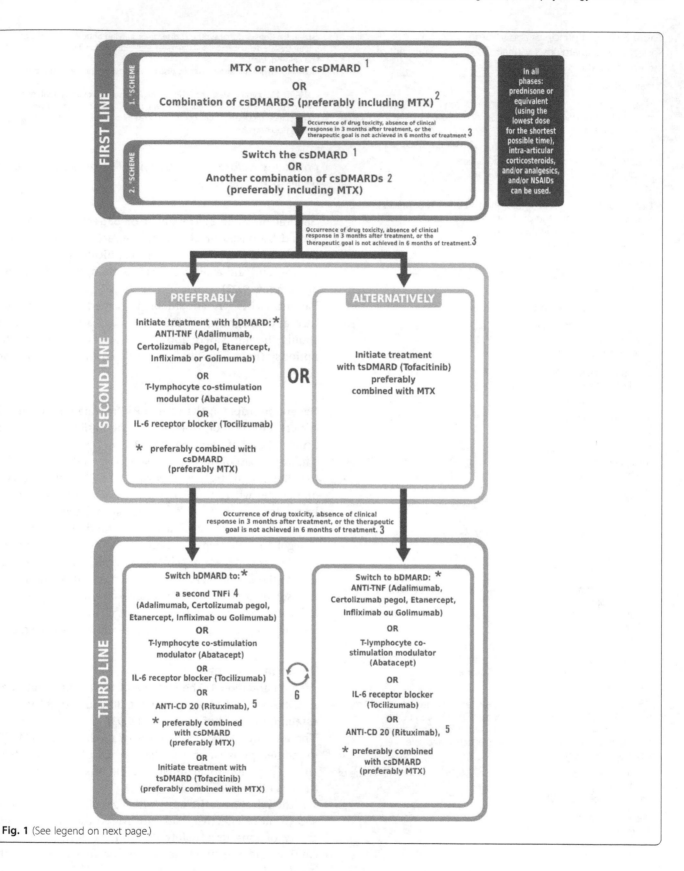

Fig. 1 (See legend on next page.)

studies have evaluated the use of csDMARD as the first line of treatment. The quality of evidence for this recommendation is low to moderate.

Recommendation 2: Methotrexate is the first-choice csDMARD. (level of agreement: 10)

There were no significant differences in the efficacy of csDMARD for most of the relevant outcomes (ACR50 and ACR70 response, number of painful and swollen joints, disease activity, pain, and functional capacity – moderate evidence) [25–36].

Compared with MTX, leflunomide causes more adverse events (discontinuation of treatment, rashes, and systemic arterial hypertension– high evidence) [30–33].

However, MTX has the highest risk of hepatic and pulmonary adverse events (low to very low evidence) [37, 38].

Subcutaneous MTX was shown to be superior to oral MTX in ACR70 and pain control, with fewer gastrointestinal adverse reactions (moderate evidence) [39].

MTX remains the first-choice drug for the RA treatment because of its efficacy and safety, possibility of individualizing the dose and route of administration, and relatively low cost [30, 40].

Recommendation 3: Combination of two or more csDMARD, including MTX, may be used as the first line of treatment. (level of agreement: 9.62)

As a first line of treatment, among the possible combinations of csDMARD, triple therapy with MTX + sulfasalazine + hydroxychloroquine, and MTX + leflunomide, both schemes compared with MTX monotherapy, showed an improved ACR response (high to moderate evidence) [25, 41, 42]. However, the cost of combination therapy is higher [43], and there is no evidence of a clinically significant difference between MTX alone and the combination of DMARDs (MTX + leflunomide, and triple therapy) in other disease activity indices [25, 42, 44–47] (moderate to low evidence), radiographic progression [41, 42, 48] (moderate to low evidence), and therapeutic safety [25, 41, 47, 49] (moderate to low evidence).

Recommendation 4: After failure of first-line therapy with MTX, therapeutic strategies include combining MTX with another csDMARD (leflunomide), with two csDMARDs (hydroxychloroquine and sulfasalazine), or switching MTX for another csDMARD (leflunomide or sulfasalazine) alone. (level of agreement: 9.12)

After failure of MTX as the first line of treatment, leflunomide (20 mg/day, without a loading dose) or sulfasalazine (with an increase in dosage to 3 g/day) are monotherapy alternatives [31, 50, 51]. Both the combination of MTX with leflunomide or with hydroxychloroquine + sulfasalazine provided better ACR50 response rates compared with MTX alone (moderate evidence), with no significant difference in radiographic progression and discontinuation of treatment due to adverse events (low evidence) [50]. The combination of sulfasalazine with MTX (without hydroxychloroquine) compared to MTX alone did not show an incremental benefit (low evidence) [41].

After failure of leflunomide, replacement with sulfasalazine or the combination of sulfasalazine and leflunomide had no additional benefit in ACR50 response, pain, quality of life, and treatment dropout (moderate evidence) [52].

After failure of sulfasalazine, the inclusion of MTX did not provide additional benefits in ACR20, ACR50, and ACR70 (moderate evidence), although an improvement of the disease activity score (DAS) with the combination of csDMARDs was observed after 18 months of treatment [53].

Recommendation 5: After failure of two schemes with csDMARD, a bDMARD may be preferably used or, alternatively, a tsDMARD, preferably combined, in both cases, with a csDMARD. (level of agreement: 9.5)

The combination of bDMARD and MTX produces higher ACR20, ACR50, and ACR70 response rates after 6 months of treatment compared with MTX monotherapy [54]. Higher ACR70 response rates at 6 to 12 months of treatment were also observed with the combination of bDMARD and csDMARD (not necessarily MTX) versus csDMARD alone [18]. The addition of bDMARD in cases of a poor response to csDMARD was effective

[24]. In cases of poor response to a csDMARD, the addition of a bDMARD was effective.

The tsDMARD tofacitinib in monotherapy or in combination with MTX was effective and safe in patients with a poor response to csDMARD, with improvement in disease activity and physical function and a reduction of radiographic progression [55, 56].

However, long-term safety and real-life data are not yet available for tsDMARD, and thus, a preference for bDMARD over tofacitinib after csDMARD failure has been proposed.

Recommendation 6: The different bDMARDs in combination with MTX have similar efficacy, and therefore, the therapeutic choice should take into account the peculiarities of each drug in terms of safety and cost. (level of agreement: 9.31)

The available bDMARDs have similar levels of effectiveness for the number of painful or swollen joints, disease activity, quality of life, functional capacity, and pain control [16, 57–62]. However, total annual costs of treatment vary among the different bDMARDs and these differences need to be taken into consideration at the time of drug selection (low to moderate evidence) [63]. All bDMARDs have consistently demonstrated superior efficacy when used in combination with MTX compared with MTX monotherapy [24, 40].

Patients using bDMARDs compared with those using csDMARDs have an increased risk of severe infections [64–68]. In general, different bDMARDs have similar levels of safety. Some SLRs of randomized trials have reported a possible increase in the incidence of severe infections with the use of certolizumab in the (indirect) comparison with other bDMARDs (moderate evidence), but this result has not been observed in registry studies [65–67, 69]. Lower intestinal perforation was more common in patients treated with tocilizumab (moderate evidence) [70]. Tuberculosis (TB) was more common in TNFi users than non-TNFi users. Among TNFi users, TB was more common in patients treated with adalimumab and infliximab compared with those treated with etanercept (moderate evidence) [68]. There were no differences among the bDMARD in the incidence of herpes zoster or neoplasia except for a possible increase in the rate of melanoma with the use of TNFi (very low evidence) [64, 71].

Recommendation 7: The combination of bDMARD and MTX is preferred over the use of bDMARD alone. (level of agreement: 9.87)

bDMARDs are more effective when combined with csDMARDs, particularly MTX [19, 72–75].

Adalimumab + MTX improved ACR20, ACR50, ACR70, and ACR90 responses and functional capacity and pain

(high evidence) and did not significantly increase the rate of treatment dropout due to adverse effects compared with adalimumab monotherapy (moderate evidence) [72].

Etanercept + MTX provided a better ACR50 response and lower radiographic progression compared with etanercept monotherapy (high evidence) and did not significantly affect the ACR70 response and dropout due to adverse events (moderate evidence) [73].

Golimumab + MTX improved the ACR50 response rate and did not significantly affect the ACR70 response, dropout due to adverse events, severe adverse events, and functional capacity compared with golimumab monotherapy (moderate evidence) [76].

Abatacept + MTX increased the remission rates (DAS28 < 2.6) compared with abatacept monotherapy [19].

Higher ACR50 and ACR70 response rates were observed with rituximab + MTX compared with rituximab alone (the groups were compared with MTX monotherapy) [75].

In a randomized trial, tocilizumab monotherapy was not significantly different from tocilizumab + MTX for ACR50 and ACR70 responses, dropout due to adverse events, severe adverse events, and functional capacity after 24 weeks of treatment. However, other randomized trial found higher remission rates (DAS28 < 2.6) and lower radiographic progression with tocilizumab + MTX compared with tocilizumab monotherapy [77–79].

The use of csDMARD in combination with bDMARD appears to reduce the formation of antibodies against the biological agent, secondary failure. Studies that used bDMARDs combined with csDMARDs, such as leflunomide, confirmed the efficacy of this combination strategy, particularly in patients who presented adverse events or contraindications to MTX [80, 81].

Recommendation 8: In case of failure of an initial treatment scheme with bDMARD, a scheme with another bDMARD can be used. In cases of failure with TNFi, a second bDMARD of the same class or with another mechanism of action is effective and safe. (level of agreement: 9.37)

The use of another bDMARD is safe and effective after therapeutic failure of an initial treatment with bDMARD [24, 82]. When the first bDMARD was an TNFi agent, the use of another TNFi agent was safe and effective in cases of treatment failure [83, 84].

Abatacept (high evidence), rituximab (high evidence), golimumab (moderate evidence), and tocilizumab (moderate evidence) were better than placebo for decreasing the number of painful and swollen joints after failure of TNFi treatment [82, 85–87].

Indirect comparisons did not allow the determination of superiority among abatacept, golimumab, rituximab, or tocilizumab in ACR50 and ACR70 responses when used after failure of the first bDMARD [88]. The risk of adverse events, including severe ones, and severe infections caused by these four biologicals after failure of the first bDMARD, was similar to placebo.

Although the use of a second TNFi agent after failure of the first is safe and effective, some studies suggest superior results for the ACR20 response, EULAR response criterion, and disease activity reduction when switching to a bDMARD with a different mechanism of action [82, 87, 89, 90]. These data must be confirmed in further studies. In other countries, rituximab has been shown to be the most cost-effective alternative among bDMARDs for the treatment of patients with previous failure to TNFi (very low evidence) [82, 85–87, 89, 91].

However, these results cannot be directly applied to the Brazilian context.

Recommendation 9: Tofacitinib can be used to treat RA after failure of bDMARD. (level of agreement: 9.81)

Tofacitinib + MTX is effective after failure of TNFi, promoting a rapid and favorable ACR20 response and improving functional capacity and disease remission [92–97].

There are no available radiographic progression data for the use of tofacitinib after failure of bDMARD.

Recommendation 10: Corticosteroids, preferably at low doses for the shortest possible time, should be considered during periods of disease activity, and the risk-benefit ratio should also be considered. (level of agreement: 9.81)

Corticosteroids are effective in treating RA when combined with csDMARD. Most of the analyzed studies used oral prednisone. The use of corticosteroids in RA reduced pain [98] (moderate evidence) and radiographic progression (high to low evidence) [99–102]. Prednisone + MTX compared with MTX alone reduced the need to switch treatment to bDMARD and did not increase the rate of adverse events [103]. However, low doses (≤10 mg/day of prednisone or equivalent) for the shortest possible time are recommended for managing periods of increased disease activity and minimizing adverse events. Special caution is necessary in patients with comorbidities that are potentially aggravated by corticosteroids.

Recommendation 11: Reducing or spacing out bDMARD doses is possible in patients in sustained remission. (level of agreement: 9.31)

Patients using bDMARD combined with csDMARD and in sustained remission (for at least 6 months) according to any composite disease activity index may receive lower bDMARD doses or the dose interval may be increased (moderate to low evidence) [104–112].

Patients with recent-onset RA (less than 6 months of symptoms) and low disease activity, suggestive of residual inflammation, rather than undergoing bDMARD

dose reduction or dose interval increase, should be treated with another bDMARD or tsDMARD [113].

However, in patients with established RA and low disease activity or remission, bDMARD dose reduction or a dose interval increase should be evaluated on an individual basis [107–112, 114–116].

Lowering the bDMARD dose reduces costs (high evidence) [114, 117].

Therapeutic strategies for treating RA in Brazil

Treatment with DMARDs should be initiated as soon as the diagnosis of RA is established. Treatment should be adjusted as necessary by frequent clinical reassessments at 30–90-day intervals. Therapeutic strategies based on specific goals produce better outcomes for disease activity and functional capacity, with less radiographic structural damage compared with conventional treatments [4, 6, 113]. The goal is sustained remission [118, 119] or at least low disease activity, as assessed by a composite measure of disease activity, also taking into consideration the absolute decrease in the composite measure score (Tables 4, 5, and 6) [7, 113].

First-line treatment: csDMARD
First scheme

MTX is the first-choice csDMARD [6, 40, 120]. MTX may be initially prescribed as monotherapy or in combination with other csDMARD (example: MTX + leflunomide) [17]. Subcutaneous MTX is an alternative to cases of drug intolerance or poor response to oral MTX before changing or adding other csDMARD. Subcutaneous MTX is better tolerated and has greater bioavailability, potentially improving clinical efficacy compared with oral administration at the same dose [39].

In cases in which MTX is contraindicated, sulfasalazine [28] or leflunomide [25] may be used as the first option. Hydroxychloroquine (or when unavailable, chloroquine) may be used in monotherapy in cases of undifferentiated arthritis or disease with low potential for the development of radiographic erosions [6].

Second scheme

In cases in which there is no clinical response in 3 months or the therapeutic goal (sustained remission or low disease activity according to a composite measure of disease activity) is not achieved within 6 months with an optimum dose of MTX or in the presence of adverse effects, it is recommended to switch MTX for another csDMARD in monotherapy, such as leflunomide [25] or sulfasalazine [28], or a combination of MTX and other csDMARDs [41, 46]. The suggested combinations are MTX + hydroxychloroquine + sulfasalazine [41] or MTX + leflunomide [121]. Therapeutic progression should be rapid, with monthly assessments in the first 6 months of treatment and adjustment of doses and schedules as needed.

Table 4 Composite measures of disease activity used in rheumatoid arthritis: components, calculation formula, and range of results

Components	SDAI	CDAI	DAS28 (with 4 variables)
Number of swollen joints	(0–28) Simple sum	(0–28) Simple sum	Square root of the simple sum
Number of painful joints	(0–28) Simple sum	(0–28) Simple sum	Square root of the simple sum
Acute phase reagents	CRP (0.1–10 mg/dL)	–	ESR 2–100 mm or CRP 0.1–10 mg/dL logarithmic transformation
Global health assessment (Patient)		–	0–100 mm
Assessment of disease activity (Patient)	(0–10 cm)	(0–10 cm)	–
Assessment of disease activity (Examiner)	(0–10 cm)	(0–10 cm)	–
Total index	Simple sum	Simple sum	Calculation formula (requires a calculator)
Index variation	(0.1–86.0)	(0–76)	(0.49–9.07)

CDAI, clinical disease activity index; DAS28, disease activity index (28 joints); CRP, C-reactive protein; SDAI, simplified disease activity index; ESR, erythrocyte sedimentation rate. Assuming a variation of 2 to 100 mm/h for ESR and of 0.1 to 10 mg/dL for CRP [6, 142].

Corticosteroids, analgesics, and non-steroidal anti-inflammatory drugs

Low doses of corticosteroids (maximum of 10 mg/day of prednisone or equivalent) may be used at the beginning of treatment or when disease worsens. However, treatment for the shortest possible time is recommended to reduce the occurrence of adverse events. Intra-articular corticosteroids may be used when necessary for symptom control, particularly for monoarticular or oligoarticular arthritis [6]. Common analgesics (paracetamol and dipyrone) and weak opioids (tramadol and codeine) may be used on demand for the control of pain symptoms [6].

Non-steroidal anti-inflammatory drugs (NSAIDs) reduce pain (low to moderate evidence) and disease activity (low evidence) and improve functional capacity (low evidence) in RA [122–127]. NSAIDs may be useful primarily at disease onset (because DMARDs do not have immediate action) and in cases of RA exacerbation [128, 129].

The choice of NSAID should be individualized because there is no demonstrated superior efficacy of one NSAID over another. Use for the shortest possible time is recommended. Additional caution is necessary in cases of risk factors for adverse events caused by NSAIDs, including advanced age, systemic arterial hypertension, heart failure, renal or hepatic dysfunction, gastrointestinal disease, arterial insufficiency, and coagulation disorders [130].

Table 5 Definition of the status of activity of rheumatoid arthritis and respective cutoff points using composite disease activity indices

Index	Disease activity status	Cutoff points
SDAI	Remission	≤5
	Low	> 5 and ≤ 20
	Moderate	> 20 and ≤ 40
	High	> 40
CDAI	Remission	≤2.8
	Low	≤10
	Moderate	> 10 and ≤ 22
	High	> 22
DAS28	Remission	≤2.6
	Low	> 2.6 and ≤ 3.2
	Moderate	> 3.2 and ≤ 5.1
	High	> 5.1

CDAI, clinical disease activity index; DAS28, disease activity index (28 joints); SDAI, simplified disease activity index [142].

Second-line treatment: bDMARD or tsDMARD

The use of bDMARD or tsDMARD is recommended in cases in which there is no clinical response after 3 months using the second scheme of the first-line treatment, the therapeutic goal is not achieved in 6 months (remission or low disease activity according to a composite measure of disease activity), or in cases of drug toxicity or intolerance.

The bDMARD drugs used in the second-line treatment are TNFi (adalimumab, certolizumab, etanercept, golimumab, or infliximab), T-lymphocyte costimulation modulator (abatacept), and IL-6 receptor blocker (tocilizumab), combined with csDMARD (preferably MTX) [24, 41, 58, 94, 95].

Tocilizumab demonstrated similar efficacy in monotherapy compared to tocilizumab + MTX for most of the relevant clinical outcomes [58, 77, 131].

Adalimumab, etanercept, certolizumab, golimumab, and abatacept can be used in monotherapy [16], but their efficacy may be lower compared with the combinations with csDMARDs [17].

Table 6 Classification of the therapeutic response in rheumatoid arthritis according to the variation in scores of the composite disease activity indices

Index	Response classification
EULAR-DAS28 response	Good: drop ≥ 1.2 points, reaching DAS28 ≤ 3.2 Moderate: drop > 1.2 points, maintenance of DAS28 > 3.2; or drop > 0.6 and ≤ 1.2 points, reaching DAS28 ≤ 5.1 Unresponsive: drop > 0.6 and ≤ 1.2 points, maintenance of DAS28 > 5.1; or drop ≤0.6 points
SDAI and CDAI response	Good: drop ≥ 85% in the score value Moderate: decrease ≥70 and < 85% in the score value Weak: drop ≥ 50% and < 70% in the score value Unresponsive: drop < 50% in the score value

CDAI, clinical disease activity index; DAS28, disease activity index (28 joints); SDAI, simplified disease activity index [142–144].

Different bDMARDs have similar levels of clinical efficacy and safety [24, 42, 120]. Therefore, bDMARDs should be chosen on an individual basis, taking into account the costs and the presence of comorbidities that may be positively or negatively affected by the treatment choice. There is not necessarily a preference for one mechanism of action relative to another for treating RA.

The tsDMARD tofacitinib may be prescribed as the second line of treatment, preferably in combination with MTX [41] or in monotherapy in cases of contraindication to MTX. However, because of the higher availability of long-term safety and real-life data for bDMARDs, at present these regimens are preferred as the second-line treatment, and tsDMARDs are considered an alternative to bDMARDs [9]. Although evidence supports the use of the bDMARD rituximab after failure of csDMARD, anti-CD20 is formally approved for treating RA only after TNFi failure and has been used as the third-line treatment in this therapeutic strategy. Nonetheless, rituximab may be considered as the first choice among bDMARDs for patients with rheumatoid factor (RF) or antibodies against citrullinated cyclic peptide (anti-CCP), with contraindications to other bDMARDs, or an associated diagnosis of lymphoma [132]. Patients with poor prognosis factors [5], including high disease activity, high number of painful or swollen joints, high RF and/or anti-CCP titers, and early occurrence of radiographic erosions, may benefit from a more aggressive treatment, including indication of a bDMARD after failure of the first csDMARD scheme, although more evidence is required to support this indication.

There is no evidence of cost-effectiveness supporting the use of bDMARD as the first-line treatment for RA in Brazil. The concomitant use of two bDMARDs or one bDMARD combined with a tsDMARD is not recommended [42].

Third-line treatment: After failure of the first bDMARD or tsDMARD

The third-line treatment is used in cases the therapeutic goal (sustained remission or low disease activity according to a composite measure of disease activity) is not achieved in 6 months using the second-line treatment

(indicating primary failure to bDMARD or tsDMARD), or loss of the previous response (secondary failure to bDMARD or tsDMARD), or cases of drug toxicity or intolerance.

The drugs available for the third-line treatment are the bDMARDs TNFi (adalimumab, certolizumab, etanercept, golimumab, or infliximab), T-lymphocyte co-stimulation modulator (abatacept), IL-6 receptor blocker (tocilizumab), anti-CD20 (rituximab), and the tsDMARD tofacitinib, combined with csDMARD (preferably MTX) [96]. Rituximab, when considered, should be indicated to patients with positive RF or anti-CCP [96, 132].

When a bDMARD is used as the second-line treatment, switching to another bDMARD or to a tsDMARD is recommended as the third-line treatment. A second TNFi drug (particularly in cases of secondary failure), switching to a bDMARD with a different mechanism of action (abatacept, tocilizumab, or rituximab) [82] or switching to a tsDMARD (tofacitinib) is recommended in cases in which the first bDMARD is a TNFi [82, 97]. Patients with failure to a first TNFi show improvements with a second TNFi [24, 59, 84, 91]. However, there are uncertainties about the cost-effectiveness of this strategy because it can result in lower response rates compared with switching the mechanism of action [87, 90, 91]. If the first bDMARD is not a TNFi, the options include prescribing another bDMARD with a mechanism of action distinct from that of the first bDMARD (including TNFi) or the use of tsDMARD.

When a tsDMARD is used as the second-line treatment, the option for the third-line treatment is switching to bDMARDs. However, this strategy requires careful clinical observation because there is no available evidence to date on the efficacy and safety of the sequential use of bDMARDs after failure of tsDMARD (tofacitinib). Until specific information is available, caution is advised on the sequential use of drugs that interfere with IL-6 (tocilizumab) and the JAK-STAT signaling pathway (tofacitinib) in patients with toxicity to any of these medications because the effects of IL-6 are mediated by the JAK-STAT pathway [40].

The treatment sequence depends on the specificities of each case and the discretion of the physician. In the case of failure or toxicity to a drug used in the third line of treatment, the next step is to switch to another (bDMARD or tsDMARD) with the same level of complexity and that has not been used previously. A minimum of 3 months and maximum of 6 months of clinical evaluation are recommended before switching a therapeutic regimen due to poor clinical response.

Gradual reduction of medication dose and treatment discontinuation

There are no data to support setting any limit for the RA treatment duration. However, patients using bDMARD in sustained remission may receive a bDMARD dose reduction or dose interval increase. Although disease reactivation may occur in some cases, disease control is usually reestablished with the return to the previous dose schedule (moderate to low evidence) [19, 23, 104, 105, 114, 133]. In cases of complete and sustained remission (at least 6 months), gradual and careful treatment withdrawal may be attempted in the following sequence: first NSAIDs, followed by corticosteroids, and bDMARD or tsDMARD, but maintaining the use of csDMARD. After the withdrawal of bDMARD, if sustained clinical remission is maintained, reduction of the csDMARD dose can be carefully attempted. Exceptionally, withdrawal of csDMARD might be feasible in cases in which clinical remission continues to be sustained [40, 116].

Sustained drug-free remission is rare, and the probability of disease exacerbation (flares) is higher in patients with long-standing disease, the presence of synovitis on ultrasound (gray scale or power Doppler), and a positive anti-CCP [116].

Biosimilar drugs

Biosimilar bDMARDs (bsDMARDs) are very similar to their original bDMARDs (boDMARDs) regarding quality, molecular structure, biological activity, clinical efficacy, safety, and immunogenicity in comparability tests, and these drugs fulfill strict regulatory criteria [134].

bsDMARDs have been shown to be safe and effective when used as an alternative to boDMARDs (moderate evidence). There were no differences in ACR20 and ACR70 response rates, disease activity (moderate evidence), or severe adverse events of the bsDMARDs adalimumab, etanercept, infliximab, and rituximab compared with their respective boDMARDs [134–140]. The development of anti-drug antibodies was similar between bsDMARDs and boDMARDs (moderate evidence), and lower for the bsDMARD of etanercept compared with the boDMARD (high evidence) [134].

However, the demonstration of biosimilarity should not be understood as evidence of interchangeability. Interchangeability, when referring to bsDMARDs, is defined by the simultaneous presence of two requirements [1]: the expected clinical outcome using the bsDMARD is similar to that produced by the corresponding boDMARD in any patient [2]; repeated switching between the boDMARD and the bsDMARD presents no additional safety or efficacy risk compared with the continued use of the reference product [141].

The SBR advocates the need for an objective demonstration of interchangeability between any boDMARD and its correspondent bsDMARD using studies specifically designed for this purpose. Until such studies are available and interchangeability conditions are regulated in Brazil, boDMARDs should not be automatically replaced with bsDMARDs without the consent of the prescriber and patient.

Pharmacological treatment flowchart for RA in Brazil

The therapeutic strategies proposed by the RA Committee of the SBR for RA treatment in Brazil are summarized in Fig. 1.

Treatment monitoring

For patients with active disease, especially in the initial phase of the disease (first 6 months of manifestations), intensive follow-up with monthly visits and, when necessary, rapid treatment escalation are recommended [6].

The efficacy and safety of the therapeutic intervention should be evaluated at each visit considering the comorbidities of the patient and aiming to achieve the lowest possible disease activity (if remission is not possible), as well as improve function and quality of life. Visits can be spaced out for patients with established disease, particularly those with controlled disease [6].

The clinical history of patients who are eligible for treatment with bDMARD should be analyzed for the presence of severe active infection, TB, or untreated latent TB, moderate to severe heart failure, multiple sclerosis or optic neuritis, previous hypersensitivity to TNFi, malignancy or lymphoma, and congenital or acquired immunodeficiency. Complementary examinations to identify hepatitis B virus, hepatitis C virus, and HIV, as well as chest X-ray and the tuberculin test, should be part of the pretreatment evaluation [6].

Conclusions

Advances in RA diagnosis and treatment have allowed improvements in disease outcome. The presence of a rheumatologist is critical in evaluating and treating patients with RA because these professionals are trained to make an early diagnosis and are familiar with the available drug therapies, indications, management, and adverse events.

The Brazilian scenario has specificities that require attention, including the local availability of medications and the socioeconomic status of the population. Brazil is a large country with a growing population, requiring rational allocation of resources to allow broad and equitable access of the population to medications and other health technologies.

The recommendations presented herein seek to provide scientific evidence to Brazilian rheumatologists, considering the therapeutic efficacy, safety, and costs, together with the critical assessment and experience of a panel of experts to standardize the management of RA in the national socioeconomic context, but maintaining the autonomy of the physician in choosing different therapeutic options. These recommendations should be updated periodically because of the rapid development of this field of knowledge. The 2017 SBR recommendations and supporting documents could be accessed online

Additional file

Additional file 1: Methodological details, expanded results and rationale of the answers to the formulated questions of the SLR that supported the present recommendations.

Acknowledgements
The authors wish to acknowledge the researchers Tais Freire Galvão and Marcus Tolentino Silva, who performed the systematic review that is presented in detail in the Additional file 1, funded by the Brazilian Society of Rheumatology.

Authors' contributions
All authors made substantial contributions to the acquisition of data, have been involved in drafting the manuscript or revising it critically for important intellectual content, gave final approval of the version to be published and have participated sufficiently in the work to take public responsibility for appropriate portions of the content; and agreed to be accountable for all aspects of the work in ensuring that questions related to the accuracy or integrity of any part of the work are appropriately investigated and resolved.

Competing interests
Licia Maria Henrique da Mota Has received personal or institutional support from Abbvie, Janssen, Pfizer and Roche; has delivered speeches at events related to this work and sponsored by Abbvie, Janssen, Pfizer, Roche and UCB. Financial competing interest: none.
Adriana Maria Kakehasi Research funds: CNPq, SBR, FAPEMIG Support for Scientific Events: Abbvie, BMS, Janssen Lecture Fees: UCB, Janssen, Pfizer, Roche, BMS Clinical research: Roche, Pfizer Advisory board: Janssen, Roche, BMS, Pfizer.
Ana Paula Monteiro Gomides Assistance for participation in events: Pfizer.
Angela Luzia Branco Pinto Duarte Lecture Fees: Janssen, BMS.
Bóris Afonso Cruz Support for Scientific Events and Lecture Fees: Abbvie, BMS, Janssen, Novartis, Pfizer, Roche.
Claiton Viegas Brenol Has participated in clinical and/or experimental studies related to this work and sponsored by the PI (Abbvie, BMS, Janssen, Pfizer and Roche); has received personal or institutional support from the PI (Abbvie, BMS, Janssen, Pfizer and Roche); has delivered speeches at events related to this work and sponsored by the PI (Abbvie, Janssen, Pfizer and

Roche). Financial competing interest: none. Non-financial competing interest: none.
Cleandro Pires de Albuquerque Personal fees and/or non-financial support from Pfizer, Abbvie, AstraZeneca, Janssen, Bristol-Myers-Squibb, Roche, Novartis and UCB, outside the submitted work.
Geraldo da Rocha Castelar Pinheiro Consultants for: Abbvie, Bristol-Myers Squibb, Eli Lilly, Glaxo Smith Kline, Janssen, Pfizer, Sanofi Genzyme and Roche.

Ieda Maria Magalhães Laurindo Consultants for Abbvie, Bristol, GSK, Janssen, Lilly, Pfizer and UCB; has received personal or institutional support from Abbvie, Bristol, Janssen, Lilly, Pfizer, UCB; has delivered speeches at events related to this work and sponsored by Abbvie, Bristol, Janssen, Lilly, Pfizer, Roche and UCB.

Ivanio Alves Pereira Has received consulting fees,speaking fees and supporting for internationals congresses from Roche,Pfizer, Janssen, Novartis, Bristol-Myers-Squibb, UCB Pharma, Eli-Lilly, AbbVie, and EMS.
Manoel Barros Bertolo Has participated in clinical and/or experimental studies related to this work and sponsored by the PI (Roche); has delivered speeches at events related to this work and sponsored by the PI (Abbvie, Pfizer). Financial competing interest: none. Non-financial competing interest: none.

Mariana Peixoto Guimarães Ubirajara Silva de Souza Support in Congresses: UCB, Roche, Janssen Lectures with fee: UCB, Janssen, Abbvie, Pfizer, Roche, BMS Clinical research: GSK, UCB, Abbvie Advisory Board: Janssen.
Max Vitor Carioca Freitas Speaker at events related to this work and sponsored by Abbvie, Novartis, Roche, Pfizer and UCB. Managing Partner of Integrare Therapeutics.

Paulo Louzada Júnior Sponsored by: Bristol-Myers Squibb, UCB, Pfizer Board Participation: Pfizer.

Ricardo Machado Xavier Lectures, consultancies: Abbvie, BMS, GSK, Janssen, Lilly, Novartis, Pfizer, Roche, UCB Clinical trials: Abbvie, UCB, Pfizer, GSK, Lilly.
Rina Dalva Neubarth Giorgi Has received consulting fees,speaking fees and supporting for internationals congresses from Roche,Pfizer,Bristol-Myers-Squibb, UCB Pharma, Eli-Lilly,AbbVie,Abbott and EMS.

Author details
[1]Programa de Pós-graduação em Ciências Médicas, Faculdade de Medicina-Universidade de Brasília; Serviço de Reumatologia, Hospital Universitário de Brasília, Universidade de Brasília, Brasília, Brazil. [2]Disciplina de Reumatologia, Faculdade de Medicina, Universidade Federal de Minas Gerais, Belo Horizonte, Brazil. [3]Centro Universitário de Brasília- UniCEUB, Brasília, Brazil. [4]Universidade Federal de Pernambuco, Recife, Brazil. [5]Hospital Vera Cruz, Belo Horizonte, Brazil. [6]Serviço de Reumatologia, Departamento de Medicina Interna, Serviço de Reumatologia, Hospital de Clínicas de Porto Alegre, Universidade Federal do Rio Grande do Sul, Porto Alegre, Brazil. [7]Serviço de Reumatologia, Hospital Universitário de Brasília, Universidade de Brasília, Brasília, Brazil. [8]Disciplina de Reumatologia, Departamento de Medicina Interna, Universidade do Estado do Rio de Janeiro, Rio de Janeiro, Brazil. [9]Universidade Nove de Julho, São Paulo, Brazil. [10]Universidade do Sul de Santa Catarina, Florianópolis, Brazil. [11]Disciplina de Reumatologia, Faculdade de Ciências Médicas, Universidade Estadual de Campinas, Campinas, Brazil. [12]Santa Casa de Belo Horizonte, Belo Horizonte, Brazil. [13]Universidade de Fortaleza, Fortaleza, Brazil. [14]Disciplina de Reumatologia, Faculdade de Medicina de Universidade de Ribeirão Preto, Universidade de São Paulo, Ribeirão Preto, Brazil. [15]Serviço de Reumatologia, Hospital do Servidor Público Estadual de São Paulo, Instituto de Assistência Médica ao Servidor Público Estadual, São Paulo, Brazil. [16]Rheos, Centro Médico Lúcio Costa, SGAS 610, bloco 1, salas T50- T51, L2 Sul, Asa Sul, Brasília, DF 70200700, Brazil.

References
1.   Silman A HM. Epidemiology of rheumatic diseases. Oxford University Press; 2000.

2. Minichiello E, Semerano L, Boissier M-C. Time trends in the incidence, prevalence, and severity of rheumatoid arthritis: a systematic literature review. Joint Bone Spine. 2016;83(6):625–30.

3. Senna ER, De Barros ALP, Silva EO, Costa IF, Pereira LVB, Ciconelli RM, et al. Prevalence of rheumatic diseases in Brazil: a study using the COPCORD approach. J Rheumatol. 2004;31(3):594–7.

4. Burmester GR, Bijlsma JWJ, Cutolo M, McInnes IB. Managing rheumatic and musculoskeletal diseases - past, present and future. Nat Rev Rheumatol. 2017;13(7):443–8.

5. Mota LMH, Cruz BA, Brenol CV, Pereira IA, Fronza LSR, Bertolo MB, et al. Consenso da Sociedade Brasileira de Reumatologia 2011 para o diagnóstico e avaliação inicial da artrite reumatoide. Rev Bras Reumatol. 2011;51(3):207–19.

6. Mota LMH, Cruz BA, Brenol CV, Pereira IA, Rezende-fronza LS, Bertolo MB, et al. Consenso 2012 da Sociedade Brasileira de Reumatologia para o tratamento da artrite reumatoide. Rev Bras Reumatol [Internet]. 2012;52(2):152–74.

7. Pereira IA, Mota LMH, Cruz BA, Brenol CV, LSR F, Bertolo MB, et al. Consenso 2012 da Sociedade Brasileira de Reumatologia sobre o manejo de comorbidades em pacientes com artrite reumatoide. Rev Bras Reumatol Bras Reumatol. 2012;52(4):474–95.

8. Brenol CV, da Mota LMH, Cruz BA, Pileggi GS, Pereira IA, Rezende LS, et al. 2012 Brazilian society of rheumatology consensus on vaccination of patients with rheumatoid arthritis. Rev Bras Reumatol [Internet]. 2013;53(1): 13–23. Elsevier.

9. Mota LMH, Cruz BA, de ACP, Gonçalves DP, IMM L, Pereira IA, et al. Posicionamento sobre o uso de tofacitinibe no algoritmo do Consenso 2012 da Sociedade Brasileira de Reumatologia para o tratamento da artrite reumatoide. Rev Bras Reumatol [Internet]. 2015;55(6):512–21.

10. Cochrane Handbook for Systematic Reviews of Interventions. The Cochrane Collaboration.; 2011.

11. Shea BJ, Grimshaw JM, Wells GA, Boers M, Andersson N, Hamel C, et al. Development of AMSTAR: a measurement tool to assess the methodological quality of systematic reviews. BMC Med Res Methodol. 2007;7:10.

12. Schünemann H, Brożek J, Guyatt G, Oxman A. Handbook for grading the quality of evidence and the strength of recommendations using the GRADE approach. 2013.

13. Einarsson JT, Geborek P, Saxne T, Kristensen LE, Kapetanovic MC. Sustained remission improves physical function in patients with established rheumatoid arthritis, and should be a treatment goal: a prospective observational cohort study from southern Sweden. J Rheumatol. 2016;43(6):1017–23.

14. Radner H, Alasti F, Smolen JS, Aletaha D. Physical function continues to improve when clinical remission is sustained in rheumatoid arthritis patients. Arthritis Res Ther. 2015;17(1):203.

15. Ruyssen-Witrand A, Guernec G, Nigon D, Tobon G, Jamard B, Rat A-C, et al. Aiming for SDAI remission versus low disease activity at 1 year after inclusion in ESPOIR cohort is associated with better 3-year structural outcomes. Ann Rheum Dis. 2015;74(9):1676–83.

16. Tarp S, Furst DE, Dossing A, Ostergaard M, Lorenzen T, Hansen MS, et al. Defining the optimal biological monotherapy in rheumatoid arthritis: a systematic review and meta-analysis of randomised trials. Semin Arthritis Rheum. 2017;46(6):699–708.

17. Stevenson M, Archer R, Tosh J, Simpson E, Everson-Hock E, Stevens J, et al. Adalimumab, etanercept, infliximab, certolizumab pegol, golimumab, tocilizumab and abatacept for the treatment of rheumatoid arthritis not previously treated with disease-modifying antirheumatic drugs and after the failure of conventional disease-modifying antirheumatic drugs only: systematic review and economic evaluation. Health Technol Assess. 2016;20(35):1–610.

18. Nam JL, Ramiro S, Gaujoux-Viala C, Takase K, Leon-Garcia M, Emery P, et al. Efficacy of biological disease-modifying antirheumatic drugs: a systematic literature review informing the 2013 update of the EULAR recommendations for the management of rheumatoid arthritis. Ann Rheum Dis. 2014;73(3):516–28.

19. Emery P, Burmester GR, Bykerk VP, Combe BG, Furst DE, Barre E, et al. Evaluating drug-free remission with abatacept in early rheumatoid arthritis: results from the phase 3b, multicentre, randomised, active-controlled AVERT study of 24 months, with a 12-month, double-blind treatment period. Ann Rheum Dis. 2015;74(1):19–26.

20. Lethaby A, Lopez-Olivo MA, Maxwell L, Burls A, Tugwell P, Wells GA. Etanercept for the treatment of rheumatoid arthritis. Cochrane Database Syst Rev. 2013;5:CD004525.

21. Emery P, Fleischmann RM, Strusberg I, Durez P, Nash P, Amante EJB, et al. Efficacy and safety of subcutaneous Golimumab in methotrexate-naive patients with rheumatoid arthritis: five-year results of a randomized clinical trial. Arthritis Care Res (Hoboken). 2016;68(6):744–52.

22. Lopez-Olivo MA, Amezaga Urruela M, McGahan L, Pollono EN, Suarez-Almazor ME. Rituximab for rheumatoid arthritis. Cochrane Database Syst Rev. 2015;1:CD007356.

23. Ruiz Garcia V, Jobanputra P, Burls A, Cabello JB, Vela Casasempere P, Bort-Marti S, et al. Certolizumab pegol (CDP870) for rheumatoid arthritis in adults. Cochrane database Syst Rev. 2014;9:CD007649.

24. Nam JL, Takase-Minegishi K, Ramiro S, Chatzidionysiou K, Smolen JS, van der Heijde D, et al. Efficacy of biological disease-modifying antirheumatic drugs: a systematic literature review informing the 2016 update of the EULAR recommendations for the management of rheumatoid arthritis. Ann Rheum Dis. 2017;76(6):1102–7.

25. Osiri M, Shea B, Robinson V, Suarez-Almazor M, Strand V, Tugwell P, et al. Leflunomide for treating rheumatoid arthritis. Cochrane database Syst Rev. 2003;1:CD002047.

26. Donahue KE, Gartlehner G, Jonas DE, Lux LJ, Thieda P, Jonas BL, et al. Systematic review: comparative effectiveness and harms of disease-modifying medications for rheumatoid arthritis. Ann Intern Med. 2008; 148(2):124–34.

27. Lopez-Olivo MA, Siddhanamatha HR, Shea B, Tugwell P, Wells GA, Suarez-Almazor ME. Methotrexate for treating rheumatoid arthritis. Cochrane Database Syst Rev. 2014;6:CD000957.

28. Suarez-Almazor ME, Belseck E, Shea B, Wells G, Tugwell P. Sulfasalazine for rheumatoid arthritis. Cochrane Database Syst Rev. 2000;2:CD000958.

29. Zeb S, Wazir N, Waqas M, Taqweem A, Taqweem A. Comparison of short-term efficacy of leflunomide and methotrexate in active rheumatoid arthritis. J Postgrad Med Inst. 2016;30(2):177–80.

30. Ishaq M, Muhammad JS, Hameed K, Mirza AI. Leflunomide or methotrexate? Comparison of clinical efficacy and safety in low socio-economic rheumatoid arthritis patients. Mod Rheumatol. 2011;21(4):375–80.

31. Emery P, Breedveld FC, Lemmel EM, Kaltwasser JP, Dawes PT, Gomor B, et al. A comparison of the efficacy and safety of leflunomide and methotrexate for the treatment of rheumatoid arthritis. Rheumatology (Oxford). 2000;39(6):655–65.

32. Strand V, Cohen S, Schiff M, Weaver A, Fleischmann R, Cannon G, et al. Treatment of active rheumatoid arthritis with leflunomide compared with placebo and methotrexate. Leflunomide rheumatoid arthritis investigators group. Arch Intern Med. 1999;159(21):2542–50.

33. Jaimes-Hernandez J, Melendez-Mercado CI, Mendoza-Fuentes A, Aranda-Pereira P, Castaneda-Hernandez G. Efficacy of leflunomide 100mg weekly compared to low dose methotrexate in patients with active rheumatoid arthritis. Double blind, randomized clinical trial. Reumatol Clin. 2012;8(5):243–9.

34. Smolen JS, Kalden JR, Scott DL, Rozman B, Kvien TK, Larsen A, et al. Efficacy and safety of leflunomide compared with placebo and sulphasalazine in active rheumatoid arthritis: a double-blind, randomised, multicentre trial. European Leflunomide Study Group Lancet (London, England). 1999; 353(9149):259–66.

35. Haagsma CJ, van Riel PL, de Jong AJ, van de Putte LB. Combination of sulphasalazine and methotrexate versus the single components in early rheumatoid arthritis: a randomized, controlled, double-blind, 52 week clinical trial. Br J Rheumatol. 1997;36(10):1082–8.

36. Dougados M, Combe B, Cantagrel A, Goupille P, Olive P, Schattenkirchner M, et al. Combination therapy in early rheumatoid arthritis: a randomised, controlled, double blind 52 week clinical trial of sulphasalazine and methotrexate compared with the single components. Ann Rheum Dis. 1999;58(4):220–5.

37. Conway R, Low C, Coughlan RJ, O'Donnell MJ, Carey JJ. Risk of liver injury among methotrexate users: a meta-analysis of randomised controlled trials. Semin Arthritis Rheum. 2015;45(2):156–62.

38. Conway R, Low C, Coughlan RJ, O'Donnell MJ, Carey JJ. Methotrexate and lung disease in rheumatoid arthritis: a meta-analysis of randomized controlled trials. Arthritis Rheumatol (Hoboken, NJ). 2014;66(4):803–12.

39. Li D, Yang Z, Kang P, Xie X. Subcutaneous administration of methotrexate at high doses makes a better performance in the treatment of rheumatoid arthritis compared with oral administration of methotrexate: a systematic review and meta-analysis. Semin Arthritis Rheum. 2016;45(6):656–62.

40. Smolen JS, Landewe R, Bijlsma J, Burmester G, Chatzidionysiou K, Dougados M, et al. EULAR recommendations for the management of rheumatoid

arthritis with synthetic and biological disease-modifying antirheumatic drugs: 2016 update. Ann Rheum Dis. 2017;76(6):960–77.

41. Hazlewood GS, Barnabe C, Tomlinson G, Marshall D, Devoe D, Bombardier C. Methotrexate monotherapy and methotrexate combination therapy with traditional and biologic disease modifying antirheumatic drugs for rheumatoid arthritis: abridged Cochrane systematic review and network meta-analysis. BMJ. 2016;353:i1777.

42. Donahue K, Jonas D, Hansen R, Roubey R, Jonas B, Lux L, et al. Drug therapy for rheumatoid arthritis in adults: an update. Comp Eff Rev [Internet]. 2012;55:1–1073.

43. De Cock D, De Saedeleer A, Van der Elst K, Stouten V, Joly J, Westhovens R, et al. A Cost-Effectiveness Analysis of Different Intensive Combination Therapies for Early Rheumatoid Arthritis: 1 Year Results of The Carera Trial. Ann Rheum Dis [Internet]. 2016;75(Suppl 2):121. Available from: https://doi.org/10.1136/annrheumdis-2016-eular.4139

44. Shashikumar NS, Shivamurthy MC, Chandrashekara S. Evaluation of efficacy of combination of methotrexate and hydroxychloroquine with leflunomide in active rheumatoid arthritis. Indian J Pharmacol. 2010;42(6):358–61.

45. Verschueren P, De Cock D, Corluy L, Joos R, Langenaken C, Taelman V, et al. Methotrexate in combination with other DMARDs is not superior to methotrexate alone for remission induction with moderate-to-high-dose glucocorticoid bridging in early rheumatoid arthritis after 16 weeks of treatment: the CareRA trial. Ann Rheum Dis. 2015;74(1):27–34.

46. Makinen H, Kautiainen H, Hannonen P, Mottonen T, Leirisalo-Repo M, Laasonen L, et al. Sustained remission and reduced radiographic progression with combination disease modifying antirheumatic drugs in early rheumatoid arthritis. J Rheumatol. 2007;34(2):316–21.

47. den Uyl D, ter Wee M, Boers M, Kerstens P, Voskuyl A, Nurmohamed M, et al. A non-inferiority trial of an attenuated combination strategy ('COBRA-light') compared to the original COBRA strategy: clinical results after 26 weeks. Ann Rheum Dis. 2014;73(6):1071–8.

48. Verschueren P, De Cock D, Corluy L, Joos R, Langenaken C, Taelman V, et al. Effectiveness of methotrexate with step-down glucocorticoid remission induction (COBRA slim) versus other intensive treatment strategies for early rheumatoid arthritis in a treat-to-target approach: 1-year results of CareRA, a randomised pragmatic open-la. Ann Rheum Dis. 2017;76(3):511–20.

49. Karstila KL, Rantalaiho VM, Mustonen JT, Mottonen TT, Hannonen PJ, Leirisalo-Repo M, et al. Renal safety of initial combination versus single DMARD therapy in patients with early rheumatoid arthritis: an 11-year experience from the FIN-RACo trial. Clin Exp Rheumatol. 2010;28(1):73–8.

50. Gaujoux-Viala C, Smolen JS, Landewe R, Dougados M, Kvien TK, Mola EM, et al. Current evidence for the management of rheumatoid arthritis with synthetic disease-modifying antirheumatic drugs: a systematic literature review informing the EULAR recommendations for the management of rheumatoid arthritis. Ann Rheum Dis. 2010;69(6):1004–9.

51. Klarenbeek NB, Guler-Yuksel M, van der Kooij SM, Han KH, Ronday HK, Kerstens PJSM, et al. The impact of four dynamic, goal-steered treatment strategies on the 5-year outcomes of rheumatoid arthritis patients in the BeSt study. Ann Rheum Dis. 2011;70(6):1039–46.

52. Dougados M, Emery P, Lemmel EM, Zerbini CAF, Brin S, van Riel P. When a DMARD fails, should patients switch to sulfasalazine or add sulfasalazine to continuing leflunomide? Ann Rheum Dis. 2005;64(1):44–51.

53. Capell HA, Madhok R, Porter DR, Munro RAL, McInnes IB, Hunter JA, et al. Combination therapy with sulfasalazine and methotrexate is more effective than either drug alone in patients with rheumatoid arthritis with a suboptimal response to sulfasalazine: results from the double-blind placebo-controlled MASCOT study. Ann Rheum Dis. 2007;66(2):235–41.

54. Nam JL, Winthrop KL, van Vollenhoven RF, Pavelka K, Valesini G, Hensor EMA, et al. Current evidence for the management of rheumatoid arthritis with biological disease-modifying antirheumatic drugs: a systematic literature review informing the EULAR recommendations for the management of RA. Ann Rheum Dis. 2010;69(6):976–86.

55. Chatzidionysiou K, Emamikia S, Nam J, Ramiro S, Smolen J, van der Heijde D, et al. Efficacy of glucocorticoids, conventional and targeted synthetic disease-modifying antirheumatic drugs: a systematic literature review informing the 2016 update of the EULAR recommendations for the management of rheumatoid arthritis. Ann Rheum Dis. 2017;76(6):1102–7.

56. Gaujoux-Viala C, Nam J, Ramiro S, Landewe R, Buch MH, Smolen JS, et al. Efficacy of conventional synthetic disease-modifying antirheumatic drugs, glucocorticoids and tofacitinib: a systematic literature review informing the 2013 update of the EULAR recommendations for management of rheumatoid arthritis. Ann Rheum Dis. 2014;73(3):510–5.

57. Guyot P, Taylor P, Christensen R, Pericleous L, Poncet C, Lebmeier M, et al. Abatacept with methotrexate versus other biologic agents in treatment of patients with active rheumatoid arthritis despite methotrexate: a network meta-analysis. Arthritis Res Ther. 2011;13(6):R204.

58. Jansen JP, Buckley F, Dejonckheere F, Ogale S. Comparative efficacy of biologics as monotherapy and in combination with methotrexate on patient reported outcomes (PROs) in rheumatoid arthritis patients with an inadequate response to conventional DMARDs–a systematic review and network meta-analysis. Health Qual Life Outcomes. 2014;12:102.

59. Schiff M, Weinblatt ME, Valente R, van der Heijde D, Citera G, Elegbe A, et al. Head-to-head comparison of subcutaneous abatacept versus adalimumab for rheumatoid arthritis: two-year efficacy and safety findings from AMPLE trial. Ann Rheum Dis. 2014;73(1):86–94.

60. Porter D, van Melckebeke J, Dale J, Messow CM, McConnachie A, Walker A, et al. Tumour necrosis factor inhibition versus rituximab for patients with rheumatoid arthritis who require biological treatment (ORBIT): an open-label, randomised controlled, non-inferiority, trial. Lancet (London, England). 2016;388(10041):239–47.

61. Schiff M, Keiserman M, Codding C, Songcharoen S, Berman A, Nayiager S, et al. Efficacy and safety of abatacept or infliximab vs placebo in ATTEST: a phase III, multi-Centre, randomised, double-blind, placebo-controlled study in patients with rheumatoid arthritis and an inadequate response to methotrexate. Ann Rheum Dis. 2008;67(8):1096–103.

62. Benucci M, Stam WB, Gilloteau I, Sennfalt K, Leclerc A, Maetzel A, et al. Abatacept or infliximab for patients with rheumatoid arthritis and inadequate response to methotrexate: an Italian trial-based and real-life cost-consequence analysis. Clin Exp Rheumatol. 2013;31(4):575–83.

63. Nobre MRC, Costa FM, Taino B, Kiyomoto HD, Rosa GF. Annual Expenditure on Anti-Tnf Treatment of Rheumatoid Arthritis for the Public Health System in Brazil. Value Heal [Internet]. 2013;16(7):A561. Elsevier.

64. Che H, Lukas C, Morel J, Combe B. Risk of herpes/herpes zoster during anti-tumor necrosis factor therapy in patients with rheumatoid arthritis. Systematic review and meta-analysis. Joint Bone Spine. 2014;81(3):215–21.

65. Singh JA, Wells GA, Christensen R, Tanjong Ghogomu E, Maxwell L, Macdonald JK, et al. Adverse effects of biologics: a network meta-analysis and Cochrane overview. Cochrane Database Syst Rev. 2011;2:CD008794.

66. de La Forest Divonne M, Gottenberg JE, Salliot C. Safety of biologic DMARDs in RA patients in real life: a systematic literature review and meta-analyses of biologic registers. Joint Bone Spine. 2017;84(2):133–40.

67. Tarp S, Eric Furst D, Boers M, Luta G, Bliddal H, Tarp U, et al. Risk of serious adverse effects of biological and targeted drugs in patients with rheumatoid arthritis: a systematic review meta-analysis. Rheumatology (Oxford). 2017;56(3):417–25.

68. Ai J-W, Zhang S, Ruan Q-L, Yu Y-Q, Zhang B-Y, Liu Q-H, et al. The risk of tuberculosis in patients with rheumatoid arthritis treated with tumor necrosis factor-alpha antagonist: a Metaanalysis of both randomized controlled trials and registry/cohort studies. J Rheumatol. 2015;42(12):2229–37.

69. Ramiro S, Gaujoux-Viala C, Nam JL, Smolen JS, Buch M, Gossec L, et al. Safety of synthetic and biological DMARDs: a systematic literature review informing the 2013 update of the EULAR recommendations for management of rheumatoid arthritis. Ann Rheum Dis. 2014;73(3):529–35.

70. Strangfeld A, Richter A, Siegmund B, Herzer P, Rockwitz K, Demary W, et al. Risk for lower intestinal perforations in patients with rheumatoid arthritis treated with tocilizumab in comparison to treatment with other biologic or conventional synthetic DMARDs. Ann Rheum Dis. 2017;76(3):504–10.

71. Suissa S, Baker N, Kawabata H, Ray NST. Comparative risk of malignancy with initiation of Abatacept and other biologics in patients with rheumatoid arthritis: a cohort analysis of a United States claims database. Ann Rheum Dis. 2016;75:719–20.

72. Breedveld FC, Weisman MH, Kavanaugh AF, Cohen SB, Pavelka K, van Vollenhoven R, et al. The PREMIER study: a multicenter, randomized, double-blind clinical trial of combination therapy with adalimumab plus methotrexate versus methotrexate alone or adalimumab alone in patients with early, aggressive rheumatoid arthritis who had not had previo. Arthritis Rheum. 2006;54(1):26–37.

73. van der Heijde D, Klareskog L, Rodriguez-Valverde V, Codreanu C, Bolosiu H, Melo-Gomes J, et al. Comparison of etanercept and methotrexate, alone and combined, in the treatment of rheumatoid arthritis: two-year clinical

and radiographic results from the TEMPO study, a double-blind, randomized trial. Arthritis Rheum. 2006;54(4):1063–74.

74. Hyrich KL, Watson KD, Silman AJ, Symmons DPM. Predictors of response to TNFi-alpha therapy among patients with rheumatoid arthritis: results from the British Society for Rheumatology biologics register. Rheumatology (Oxford). 2006;45(12):1558–65.

75. Edwards JCW, Szczepanski L, Szechinski J, Filipowicz-Sosnowska A, Emery P, Close DR, et al. Efficacy of B-cell-targeted therapy with rituximab in patients with rheumatoid arthritis. N Engl J Med. 2004;350(25):2572–81.

76. Emery P, Fleischmann RM, Doyle MK, Strusberg I, Durez P, Nash P, et al. Golimumab, a human anti-tumor necrosis factor monoclonal antibody, injected subcutaneously every 4 weeks in patients with active rheumatoid arthritis who had never taken methotrexate: 1-year and 2-year clinical, radiologic, and physical function findings. Arthritis Care Res (Hoboken). 2013;65(11):1732–42.

77. Burmester GR, Rigby WF, van Vollenhoven RF, Kay J, Rubbert-Roth A, Kelman A, et al. Tocilizumab in early progressive rheumatoid arthritis: FUNCTION, a randomised controlled trial. Ann Rheum Dis. 2016;75(6): 1081–91.

78. Burmester GR, Rigby WF, van Vollenhoven RF, Kay J, Rubbert-Roth A, Kelman A, et al. Tocilizumab in combination therapy and monotherapy versus methotrexate in methotrexate-naive patients with early rheumatoid arthritis: clinical and radiographic outcomes from a randomized, placebo-controlled trial. Arthritis Rheum [Internet]. 2013;65:S1182–3.

79. Kaneko Y, Atsumi T, Tanaka Y, Inoo M, Kobayashi-Haraoka H, Amano K, et al. Comparison of adding tocilizumab to methotrexate with switching to tocilizumab in patients with rheumatoid arthritis with inadequate response to methotrexate: 52-week results from a prospective, randomised, controlled study (SURPRISE study). Ann Rheum Dis. 2016;75(11):1917–23.

80. Chatzidionysiou K, Lie E, Nasonov E, Lukina G, Hetland ML, Tarp U, et al. Effectiveness of disease-modifying antirheumatic drug co-therapy with methotrexate and leflunomide in rituximab-treated rheumatoid arthritis patients: results of a 1-year follow-up study from the CERERRA collaboration. Ann Rheum Dis. 2012;71(3):374–7.

81. Wendler J, Sørensen H, Tony H, Richter C, Krause A, Rubbert-Roth A, Effectiveness BMBG. Safety of rituximab (RTX) monotherapy compared to RTX combination therapy with methotrexate or leflunomide in the German RTX-treatment of active rheumatoid arthritis in daily practice trial. Ann Rheum Dis. 2009;68:76.

82. Lee YH, Bae S-C. Comparative efficacy and safety of tocilizumab, rituximab, abatacept and tofacitinib in patients with active rheumatoid arthritis that inadequately responds to tumor necrosis factor inhibitors: a Bayesian network meta-analysis of randomized controlled tri. Int J Rheum Dis. 2016;19(11):1103–11.

83. Smolen JS, Burmester G-R, Combe B, Curtis JR, Hall S, Haraoui B, et al. Head-to-head comparison of certolizumab pegol versus adalimumab in rheumatoid arthritis: 2-year efficacy and safety results from the randomised EXXELERATE study. Lancet (London, England). 2016;388(10061):2763–74.

84. Smolen JS, Kay J, Doyle MK, Landewe R, Matteson EL, Wollenhaupt J, et al. Golimumab in patients with active rheumatoid arthritis after treatment with tumour necrosis factor alpha inhibitors (GO-AFTER study): a multicentre, randomised, double-blind, placebo-controlled, phase III trial. Lancet (London, England). 2009;374(9685):210–21.

85. Mease PJ, Cohen S, Gaylis NB, Chubick A, Kaell AT, Greenwald M, et al. Efficacy and safety of retreatment in patients with rheumatoid arthritis with previous inadequate response to tumor necrosis factor inhibitors: results from the SUNRISE trial. J Rheumatol. 2010;37(5):917–27.

86. Gonzalez-Vacarezza N, Aleman A, Gonzalez G, Perez A. Rituximab and tocilizumab for the treatment of rheumatoid arthritis. Int J Technol Assess Health Care. 2014;30(3):282–8.

87. Kim H-L, Lee M-Y, Park S-Y, Park S-K, Byun J-H, Kwon S, et al. Comparative effectiveness of cycling of tumor necrosis factor-alpha (TNF-alpha) inhibitors versus switching to non-TNF biologics in rheumatoid arthritis patients with inadequate response to TNF-alpha inhibitor using a Bayesian approach. Arch Pharm Res. 2014;37(5):662–70.

88. Schoels M, Aletaha D, Smolen JS, Wong JB. Comparative effectiveness and safety of biological treatment options after tumour necrosis factor alpha inhibitor failure in rheumatoid arthritis: systematic review and indirect pairwise meta-analysis. Ann Rheum Dis England. 2012;71(8):1303–8.

89. Joensuu JT, Huoponen S, Aaltonen KJ, Konttinen YT, Nordstrom D, Blom M. The cost-effectiveness of biologics for the treatment of rheumatoid arthritis: a systematic review. PLoS One. 2015;10(3):e0119683.

90. Gottenberg J-E, Brocq O, Perdriger A, Lassoued S, Berthelot J-M, Wendling D, et al. Non-TNF-targeted biologic vs a second TNFi drug to treat rheumatoid arthritis in patients with insufficient response to a first TNFi drug: a randomized clinical trial. JAMA. 2016;316(11):1172–80.

91. Malottki K, Barton P, Tsourapas A, Uthman AO, Liu Z, Routh K, et al. Adalimumab, etanercept, infliximab, rituximab and abatacept for the treatment of rheumatoid arthritis after the failure of a tumour necrosis factor inhibitor: a systematic review and economic evaluation. Health Technol Assess. 2011;15(14):1–278.

92. Kremer J, Li Z-G, Hall S, Fleischmann R, Genovese M, Martin-Mola E, et al. Tofacitinib in combination with nonbiologic disease-modifying antirheumatic drugs in patients with active rheumatoid arthritis: a randomized trial. Ann Intern Med. 2013;159(4):253–61.

93. van Vollenhoven RF, Fleischmann R, Cohen S, Lee EB, Garcia Meijide JA, Wagner S, et al. Tofacitinib or adalimumab versus placebo in rheumatoid arthritis. N Engl J Med. 2012;367(6):508–19.

94. Kremer JM, Cohen S, Wilkinson BE, Connell CA, French JL, Gomez-Reino J, Gruben D, Kanik KS, Krishnaswami S, Pascual-Ramos V, Wallenstein G, Zwillich SH. A phase IIb dose-ranging study of the oral JAK inhibitor tofacitinib (CP-690,550) versus placebo in combination with background methotrexate in patients with active rheumatoid arthritis and an inadequate response to methotrexate alone. Arthritis Rheum. 2012;64(4):970–81.

95. Singh JA, Hossain A, Tanjong Ghogomu E, Mudano AS, Tugwell P, Wells GA. Biologic or tofacitinib monotherapy for rheumatoid arthritis in people with traditional disease-modifying anti-rheumatic drug (DMARD) failure: a Cochrane systematic review and network meta-analysis (NMA). Cochrane Database Syst Rev. 2016;11:CD012437.

96. Singh JA, Hossain A, Tanjong Ghogomu E, Mudano AS, Maxwell LJ, Buchbinder R, et al. Biologics or tofacitinib for people with rheumatoid arthritis unsuccessfully treated with biologics: a systematic review and network meta-analysis. Cochrane Database Syst Rev. 2017;3:CD012591.

97. Burmester GR, Blanco R, Charles-Schoeman C, Wollenhaupt J, Zerbini C, Benda B, et al. Tofacitinib (CP-690,550) in combination with methotrexate in patients with active rheumatoid arthritis with an inadequate response to tumour necrosis factor inhibitors: a randomised phase 3 trial. Lancet (London, England). 2013;381(9865):451–60.

98. Montecucco C, Todoerti M, Sakellariou G, Scire CA, Caporali R. Low-dose oral prednisone improves clinical and ultrasonographic remission rates in early rheumatoid arthritis: results of a 12-month open-label randomised study. Arthritis Res Ther. 2012;14(3):R112.

99. Choy EHS, Smith CM, Farewell V, Walker D, Hassell A, Chau L, et al. Factorial randomised controlled trial of glucocorticoids and combination disease modifying drugs in early rheumatoid arthritis. Ann Rheum Dis. 2008;67(5):656–63.

100. Kirwan JR, Bijlsma JWJ, Boers M, Shea BJ. Effects of glucocorticoids on radiological progression in rheumatoid arthritis. Cochrane Database Syst Rev. 2007;1:CD006356.

101. van der Goes MC, Jacobs JW, Boers M, Kirwan JR, Hafström I, Svensson B, et al. AT0217 long term effects of glucocorticoid therapy on radiological progression of joint damage in rheumatoid arthritis: an individual patient Meta-analysis. Ann Rheum Dis. 2015;74:736.

102. Kume K, Amano K, Yamada S, Kanazawa T, Ohta H, Hatta 2K. THU0211 combination of intra-articular steroid injection and Etanercept more effective than Etanercept in rapid radiographic progression patients with rheumatoid arthritis: a randomized, open label, X ray reader blinded study. Ann Rheum Dis. 2013;72:A235–6.

103. Bakker MF, Jacobs JWG, Welsing PMJ, Verstappen SMM, Tekstra J, Ton E, et al. Low-dose prednisone inclusion in a methotrexate-based, tight control strategy for early rheumatoid arthritis: a randomized trial. Ann Intern Med. 2012;156(5):329–39.

104. Fautrel B, Pham T, Alfaiate T, Gandjbakhch F, Foltz V, Morel J, et al. Step-down strategy of spacing TNF-blocker injections for established rheumatoid arthritis in remission: results of the multicentre non-inferiority randomised open-label controlled trial STRASS: spacing of TNF-blocker injections in rheumatoid ArthritiS St. Ann Rheum Dis. 2016;75(1):59–67.

105. Haschka J, Englbrecht M, Hueber AJ, Manger B, Kleyer A, Reiser M, et al. Relapse rates in patients with rheumatoid arthritis in stable remission tapering or stopping antirheumatic therapy: interim results from the prospective randomised controlled RETRO study. Ann Rheum Dis. 2016;75(1):45–51.

106. van Herwaarden N, van der Maas A, Minten MJM, van den Hoogen FHJ, Kievit W, van Vollenhoven RF, et al. Disease activity guided dose reduction and withdrawal of adalimumab or etanercept compared with usual care in

rheumatoid arthritis: open label, randomised controlled, non-inferiority trial. BMJ. 2015;350:h1389.

107. Smolen JS, Nash P, Durez P, Hall S, Ilivanova E, Irazoque-Palazuelos F, et al. Maintenance, reduction, or withdrawal of etanercept after treatment with etanercept and methotrexate in patients with moderate rheumatoid arthritis (PRESERVE): a randomised controlled trial. Lancet (London, England). 2013;381(9870):918–29.

108. Kuijper TM, Lamers-Karnebeek FBG, Jacobs JWG, Hazes JMW, Luime JJ. Flare rate in patients with rheumatoid arthritis in low disease activity or remission when tapering or stopping synthetic or biologic DMARD: a systematic review. J Rheumatol. 2015;42(11):2012–22.

109. Jiang M, Ren F, Zheng Y, Yan R, Huang W, Xia N, et al. Efficacy and safety of down-titration versus continuation strategies of biological disease-modifying anti-rheumatic drugs in patients with rheumatoid arthritis with low disease activity or in remission: a systematic review and meta-analysis. Clin Exp Rheumatol. 2017;35(1):152–60.

110. Emery P, Hammoudeh M, FitzGerald O, Combe B, Martin-Mola E, Buch MH, et al. Sustained remission with etanercept tapering in early rheumatoid arthritis. N Engl J Med. 2014;371(19):1781–92.

111. Smolen JS, Emery P, Fleischmann R, van Vollenhoven RF, Pavelka K, Durez P, et al. Adjustment of therapy in rheumatoid arthritis on the basis of achievement of stable low disease activity with adalimumab plus methotrexate or methotrexate alone: the randomised controlled OPTIMA trial. Lancet (London, England). 2014;383(9914):321–32.

112. Tanaka Y, Takeuchi T, Mimori T, Saito K, Nawata M, Kameda H, et al. Discontinuation of infliximab after attaining low disease activity in patients with rheumatoid arthritis: RRR (remission induction by Remicade in RA) study. Ann Rheum Dis England. 2010;69(7):1286–91.

113. Smolen JS, Breedveld FC, Burmester GR, Bykerk V, Dougados M, Emery P, et al. Treating rheumatoid arthritis to target: 2014 update of the recommendations of an international task force. Ann Rheum Dis. 2016;75(1):3–15.

114. Kievit W, van Herwaarden N, van den Hoogen FH, van Vollenhoven RF, Bijlsma JW, van den Bemt BJ, et al. Disease activity-guided dose optimisation of adalimumab and etanercept is a cost-effective strategy compared with non-tapering tight control rheumatoid arthritis care: analyses of the DRESS study. Ann Rheum Dis. 2016;75(11):1939–44.

115. van Herwaarden N, den Broeder AA, Jacobs W, van der Maas A, Bijlsma JWJ, van Vollenhoven RF, et al. Down-titration and discontinuation strategies of tumor necrosis factor-blocking agents for rheumatoid arthritis in patients with low disease activity. Cochrane database Syst Rev. 2014;9:CD010455.

116. Schett G, Emery P, Tanaka Y, Burmester G, Pisetsky DS, Naredo E, et al. Tapering biologic and conventional DMARD therapy in rheumatoid arthritis: current evidence and future directions. Ann Rheum Dis England. 2016;75(8):1428–37.

117. Kobelt G. Treating to target with etanercept in rheumatoid arthritis: cost-effectiveness of dose reductions when remission is achieved. Value Heal J Int Soc Pharmacoeconomics Outcomes Res. 2014;17(5):537–44.

118. Felson DT, Smolen JS, Wells G, Zhang B, van Tuyl LHD, Funovits J, et al. American College of Rheumatology/European league against rheumatism provisional definition of remission in rheumatoid arthritis for clinical trials. Arthritis Rheum. 2011;63(3):573–86.

119. Anderson J, Caplan L, Yazdany J, Robbins ML, Neogi T, Michaud K, et al. Rheumatoid arthritis disease activity measures: American College of Rheumatology recommendations for use in clinical practice. Arthritis Care Res (Hoboken). 2012;64(5):640–7.

120. Singh JA, Cameron DR. Summary of AHRQ's comparative effectiveness review of drug therapy for rheumatoid arthritis (RA) in adults–an update. J Manag Care Pharm. 2012;18(4 Supp C):S1–18.

121. Ding C-Z, Yao Y, Feng X-B, Fang Y, Zhao C, Wang Y. Clinical analysis of chinese patients with rheumatoid arthritis treated with leflunomide and methotrexate combined with different dosages of glucocorticoid. Curr Ther Res Clin Exp. 2012;73(4–5):123–33.

122. Colebatch AN, Marks JL, Edwards CJ. Safety of non-steroidal anti-inflammatory drugs, including aspirin and paracetamol (acetaminophen) in people receiving methotrexate for inflammatory arthritis (rheumatoid arthritis, ankylosing spondylitis, psoriatic arthritis, other spondyloarthritis). Cochrane Database Syst Rev. 2011;11:CD008872.

123. Chen Y-F, Jobanputra P, Barton P, Bryan S, Fry-Smith A, Harris G, et al. Cyclooxygenase-2 selective non-steroidal anti-inflammatory drugs (etodolac, meloxicam, celecoxib, rofecoxib, etoricoxib, valdecoxib and lumiracoxib) for

124. Bickham K, Kivitz AJ, Mehta A, Frontera N, Shah S, Stryszak P, et al. Evaluation of two doses of etoricoxib, a COX-2 selective non-steroidal anti-inflammatory drug (NSAID), in the treatment of rheumatoid arthritis in a double-blind, randomized controlled trial. BMC Musculoskelet Disord. 2016;17:331.

125. Kvien TK, Greenwald M, Peloso PM, Wang H, Mehta A, Gammaitoni A. Do COX-2 inhibitors provide additional pain relief and anti-inflammatory effects in patients with rheumatoid arthritis who are on biological disease-modifying anti-rheumatic drugs and/or corticosteroids? Post-hoc analyses from a randomized clinical trial. BMC Musculoskelet Disord. 2015;16:26.

126. van Walsem A, Pandhi S, Nixon RM, Guyot P, Karabis A, Moore RA. Relative benefit-risk comparing diclofenac to other traditional non-steroidal anti-inflammatory drugs and cyclooxygenase-2 inhibitors in patients with osteoarthritis or rheumatoid arthritis: a network meta-analysis. Arthritis Res Ther. 2015;17:66.

127. Adams K, Bombardier C, van der Heijde D. Safety and efficacy of on-demand versus continuous use of nonsteroidal antiinflammatory drugs in patients with inflammatory arthritis: a systematic literature review. J Rheumatol Suppl. 2012;90:56–8.

128. American College of Rheumatology Subcommittee on Rheumatoid Arthritis Guidelines. Guidelines for the management of rheumatoid arthritis: 2002 Update. Arthritis Rheum. 2002;46(2):328–46.

129. Katchamart W, Johnson S, Lin H-JL, Phumethum V, Salliot C, Bombardier C. Predictors for remission in rheumatoid arthritis patients: a systematic review. Arthritis Care Res (Hoboken). 2010;62(8):1128–43.

130. Ferraz-Amaro I, Machin S, Carmona L, Gonzalez-Alvaro I, Diaz-Gonzalez F. Pattern of use and safety of non-steroidal anti-inflammatory drugs in rheumatoid arthritis patients. A prospective analysis from clinical practice. Reumatol Clin. 2009;5(6):252–8.

131. Dougados M, Kissel K, Sheeran T, Tak PP, Conaghan PG, Mola EM, et al. Adding tocilizumab or switching to tocilizumab monotherapy in methotrexate inadequate responders: 24-week symptomatic and structural results of a 2-year randomised controlled strategy trial in rheumatoid arthritis (ACT-RAY). Ann Rheum Dis. 2013;72(1):43–50.

132. Buch MH, Smolen JS, Betteridge N, Breedveld FC, Burmester G, Dorner T, et al. Updated consensus statement on the use of rituximab in patients with rheumatoid arthritis. Ann Rheum Dis. 2011;70(6):909–20.

133. van Vollenhoven RF, Ostergaard M, Leirisalo-Repo M, Uhlig T, Jansson M, Larsson E, et al. Full dose, reduced dose or discontinuation of etanercept in rheumatoid arthritis. Ann Rheum Dis. 2016;75(1):52–8.

134. Komaki Y, Yamada A, Komaki F, Kudaravalli P, Micic D, Ido A, et al. Efficacy, safety and pharmacokinetics of biosimilars of anti-tumor necrosis factor-alpha agents in rheumatic diseases; a systematic review and meta-analysis. J Autoimmun. 2017;79:4–16.

135. Yoo DH, Racewicz A, Brzezicki J, Yatsyshyn R, Arteaga ET, Baranauskaite A, et al. A phase III randomized study to evaluate the efficacy and safety of CT-P13 compared with reference infliximab in patients with active rheumatoid arthritis: 54-week results from the PLANETRA study. Arthritis Res Ther. 2016;18:82.

136. Yoo DH, Suh CH, Shim SC, Jeka S, Molina FFC, Hrycaj P, et al. Efficacy, Safety and Pharmacokinetics of Up to Two Courses of the Rituximab Biosimilar CT-P10 Versus Innovator Rituximab in Patients with Rheumatoid Arthritis: Results up to Week 72 of a Phase I Randomized Controlled Trial. BioDrugs. 2017;31(4):357–367.

137. Cohen S, Emery P, Greenwald M, Yin D, Becker J-C, Melia LA, et al. A phase I pharmacokinetics trial comparing PF-05280586 (a potential biosimilar) and rituximab in patients with active rheumatoid arthritis. Br J Clin Pharmacol. 2016;82(1):129–34.

138. Eremeeva A, Chernyaeva E, Ivanov R, Nasonov E, Knyazeva L. FRI0224 comparison of efficacy and safety of rituximab biosimilar, BCD-020, and innovator rituximab in patients with active rheumatoid arthritis refractory to TNFA inhibitors. Ann Rheum Dis. 2016;75:513–4.

139. Jacobs I, Petersel D, Isakov L, Lula S, Lea Sewell K. Biosimilars for the treatment of chronic inflammatory diseases: a systematic review of published evidence. BioDrugs. 2016;30(6):525–70.

140. Chingcuanco F, Segal JB, Kim SC, Alexander GC. Bioequivalence of biosimilar tumor necrosis factor-alpha inhibitors compared with their reference biologics: a systematic review. Ann Intern Med. 2016;165(8):565–74.

osteoarthritis and rheumatoid arthritis: a systematic review and economic evaluation. Health Technol Assess. 2008;12(11):1–278, iii.

141. Tothfalusi L, Endrenyi L, Chow S-C. Statistical and regulatory considerations in assessments of interchangeability of biological drug products. Eur J Health Econ. 2014;15(Suppl 1):S5–11.

142. Aletaha D, Smolen JS. The Simplified Disease Activity Index (SDAI) and Clinical Disease Activity Index (CDAI) to monitor patients in standard clinical care. Best Pract Res Clin Rheumatol. 2007;21(4):663–75.

143. Aletaha D, Funovits J, Ward MM, Smolen JS, Kvien TK. Perception of improvement in patients with rheumatoid arthritis varies with disease activity levels at baseline. Arthritis Rheum. 2009;61(3):313–20.

144. Smolen JS, Aletaha D. Scores for all seasons: SDAI and CDAI. Clin Exp Rheumatol. 2014;32(5 Suppl 85):S-75–9.

8

Adipokines in rheumatoid arthritis

Elis Carolina de Souza Fatel[1,5][*] (iD), Flávia Troncon Rosa[2], Andréa Name Colado Simão[3] and Isaias Dichi[4]

Abstract

Rheumatoid arthritis affects millions of people worldwide and is considered a chronic multisystem disease whose causes are unknown. In general, the main objective of rheumatoid arthritis treatment is to improve the quality of life of patients by relieving pain, maintaining or improving functional capacity, preventing thus, disability. In recent years the role of adipokines in the pathogenesis of rheumatoid arthritis has been discussed but results are still conflicting. Although results from some studies have shown the implications of adipokines in the pathophysiology of autoimmune diseases, including rheumatoid arthritis, their role in the pathogenesis of disease progression is not clear. Thus, this review aimed to describe the association of key adipokines (leptin, resistin, visfatin and adiponectin) and rheumatoid arthritis, given the high prevalence of this disease and the important social impact caused by this chronic disabling disease.

Keywords: Adipokines, Rheumatoid arthritis, Cytokines

Background

Rheumatoid arthritis (RA) is a chronic multisystem disease whose causes are unknown [1]. This disease presents a variety of systemic manifestations being the persistent inflammatory synovitis the most typical feature, compromising peripheral joints in a symmetric distribution. Mateen et al. (2016) [2] highlights RA as a disease, which is characterized in the majority of patients by the presence of rheumatoid factor (RF) and anti–citrullinated protein antibody (ACPA). The authors reinforce that cytokines such as tumor necrosis factor (TNF)-α, interleukin (IL)-1 and IL-17 have an important role in the pathophysiology of RA since serum concentrations of these substances may indicate the severity of the disease.

The diagnosis of RA must be at earlier stages of disease and treatment should aim to relieve pain, maintain or improve functional capacity, preventing thus, disability, and improving patients quality of life [3].

Barbosa et al. (2012) [4] reported the important role of mediators synthesized in adipose tissue, named adipokines, in RA. Hutcheson (2015) [5] points out that knowledge about adiposity has changed and currently it appears as an important regulator of several key processes, including inflammation. Furthermore, adipokines have hormonal action supporting the regulation of appetite and glucose metabolism, and some of them such as leptin, resistin, adiponectin and visfatin have been associated to RA development. However the results are still conflicting [4, 5].

Thus, this review aimed to describe the association of key adipokines (leptin, resistin, visfatin and adiponectin) and RA, given the high prevalence of this disease and the important social impact caused by chronic disabling diseases of the articular system.

Methods
Study selection

This review is in accordance with the guidelines of the Preferred Reporting Items for Systematic Reviews and Meta-Analyses (PRISMA) [6]. The search string was restricted to humans, including clinical studies, controlled clinical trials, meta-analysis, multicentric, observational studies, and randomized controlled trials. Relevant articles that were not retrieved in the main search but were cited in the publications were carefully reviewed and included if they met the criteria. As the main objective was to verify the association of adipokines with rheumatoid arthritis, most of the studies analyzed refer to observational studies such as cross-sectional, case-control and cohort studies presenting quantitative information regarding plasma or serum adipokines concentrations. The on line databases U.S. National Library of Medicine PUBMED, Periódicos

---
* Correspondence: elis.fatel@uffs.edu.br; elis.fatel@hotmail.com
[1]Postgraduate Program, Health Sciences Center, State University of Londrina, Londrina, Paraná, Brazil
[5]Department of Nutrition, University of Fronteira Sul, Rodovia PR 182 Km 466, CEP 85770-000, Realeza, Paraná Postal Code 253, Brazil
Full list of author information is available at the end of the article

Capes, Science Direct, and Scientific Electronic Library Online (SciELO) were searched for English, Spanish or Portuguese-language articles. The crossing of "rheumatoid arthritis" with the following descriptors separately was used to accomplish this review: "adipokines", "leptin", "resistin", "visfatin", and "adiponectin". No exclusion criteria were established in view of the small number of articles regarding this current issue. The study selection process is described in Fig. 1.

Data extraction

The information sources were the results described in the articles selected. The following data were extracted from articles included in this review: authors, year of publication, study design, number of participants, disease characteristics, control groups and results regarding associations between each adipokine and markers of disease activity.

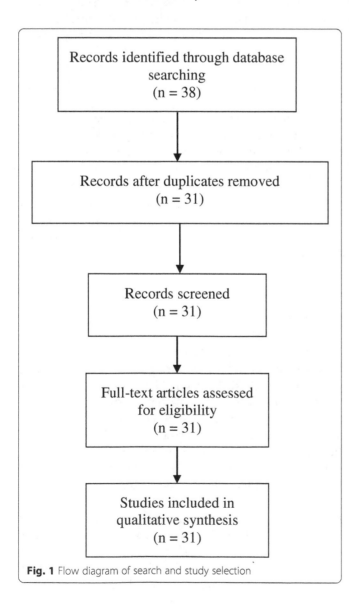

Fig. 1 Flow diagram of search and study selection

Results and discussion
Adipokines

Adipose tissue is a multifunctional organ responsible for lipid storage, thermogenesis, structural components and support of many organs such as joints, gastrointestinal tract and skin and nowadays also described as secretory and endocrine functions [7]. It is noteworthy in this context its role as an endocrine organ by synthesizing and secreting adipokines, which play an important role in the pathophysiology of insulin resistance, inflammation and atherogenesis [8, 9].

Leptin

Leptin is an adipokine produced in white adipose tissue. Discovered in 1994 [10], it is an *Ob* gene product [11], cloned and sequenced in mice and considered the adipokine responsible for the regulation of energy metabolism and homeostasis, as well as neuroendocrine functions [12]. It also assists the immunity and inflammation control through its receptor [13]. Thus, leptin is responsible for the regulation of various biological processes, being involved in the pathophysiology of many diseases. Leptin is considered a proinflammatory adipokine since it stimulates production of cytokines such as TNF-α, IL-6 and reactive oxygen species, and induces the production of CC chemokines by macrophages and alters the T helper (Th)1 / Th2 profile [13].

Paz-Filho et al. (2012) [14] described molecular mechanisms and pro-inflammatory systemic effects of leptin. It acts through its Ob receptor triggering inflammatory responses together with infectious and inflammatory stimuli of cytokines such as IL-1, lipopolysaccharide (LPS), and TNF-α, which may, in turn, increase levels of leptin. The interaction between leptin and inflammation are bidirectional, but all pro inflammatory since cytokines increases the synthesis and release of leptin, which in turn perpetuates the cycle of inflammation.

Leptin showed a significant effect on increasing the expression of Th1 cytokines. Experimental studies on mice demonstrated that these animals showed less severe stages of induced RA with lower levels of IL-1B and TNF-α in the synovial fluid and reduction in T-cell proliferative response induced by antigen [14]. However, clinical studies revealed paradoxical results about the effects of endogenous leptin in protecting joints in severe forms of erosive RA in humans [15].

In the last two decades, several studies have described the action of leptin in RA [16], leading researchers near to assume the hypothesis that this hormone has a key role in rheumatic diseases. [17] Thus, leptin levels may be a risk factor for the pathogenesis of RA [18].

Olama et al. (2012) [15] evaluated the ratio of synovial and serum leptin in patients with RA and found that the local utilization of leptin at the joint cavity has a protector role against the destructive course of RA. Rho et al. (2010) [19] also examined the hypothesis that the adipokines could influence insulin resistance and coronary atherosclerosis in patients with RA. Leptin was positively associated with insulin resistance assessed by Homeostasis Model Assessment - Insulin Resistance (HOMA-IR), even after adjusting for age, race, sex, body mass index (BMI), traditional cardiovascular risk factors and inflammation mediators. Targońska-Stepniak et al. (2010) [20] assessed leptin levels in patients with RA and demonstrated positive correlation between leptin levels and Disease Activity Score (DAS)-28. Yoshino et al. (2011) [21] found leptin levels significantly higher in RA patients compared to controls, and this adipokine correlated positively with C-Reactive Protein (CRP) levels, suggesting that leptin can act as a proinflammatory in this disease. On the other hand, Kontunen et al. (2011) [22] showed that leptin levels were increased only in patients with RA and concomitant diagnosis of metabolic syndrome (MetS).

Kang et al. (2013) [23] demonstrated that TNF-α was positively associated to leptin and the latter was associated with various metabolic risk factors, including insulin resistance. Bustos Rivera-Bahena et al. (2015) [24] evidenced that circulating levels of leptin correlate positively with clinical activity of RA, regardless of BMI. However, Xibille-Friedmann et al. (2015) [25] concluded that in a short term basal levels of leptin may predict disease activity independent of BMI. However, when submitted to treatment, this only occurred in patients with normal body weight.

Tian et al. (2014) [26] reported a review in which 23 studies were analyzed. The following results were obtained: 13 studies showed increased leptin levels; 8 studies did not demonstrate any significant difference and 2 had reduced leptin levels when compared to control subjects. Therefore, most of the studies have found higher levels of leptin in patients with RA, showing a possible role in the regulation of joint damage, and suggested that more studies are needed to understand the mechanisms of action of this adipokine. A meta-analysis conducted by Lee e Bae (2016) [27] confirmed these data showing that circulating levels of leptin were significantly higher in patients with RA with a positive correlation between this hormone and RA activity.

Despite the evidence demonstrated, some studies do not corroborate these associations. Allam e Radwan (2012) [28] and Abdalla et al. (2014) [29] found that although serum leptin level was significantly higher in RA patients than in control group, there was no correlation with clinical and laboratory markers of disease activity. Mirfeizi et al. (2014) [30] also stated that leptin has no effect on the process of joint damage in RA patients. Oner et al. (2015) [31] did not find any correlation between disease activity and serum leptin levels, indicating that this adipokine is not a good biomarker to monitor inflammation in RA.

Thus, leptin seems to have a role in the pathophysiology of RA and comorbidities associated, such as obesity and metabolic syndrome. Leptin is considered a pro inflammatory adipokine by the great majority of authors who suggest a predominantly deleterious action on the joint. Only one survey showed that increased levels of leptin can act as a protective factor against the destructive course of RA.

Table 1 summarizes the main findings of leptin in RA patients.

Resistin

Isolated in rodents, resistin was first described in 2001. It is a protein rich in cysteine, compounded by 108 amino acids, called RELMs (resistin-like molecules) also known as FIZZ 332 [32]. In humans, it is originated mainly from circulating monocytes and macrophages [33].

It was initially correlated to the pathogenesis of insulin resistance in obesity and some cardiovascular diseases (CVD) but now is also considered an important link between obesity and inflammation [34]. Resistin has been found in areas of inflammation and seems to be mediated by IL-6 and TNF α [35].

Due to its implication in inflammation processes, the involvement of resistin in the pathogenesis of RA has been investigated. Kassem et al. (2010) [36] studied if there is a role of resistin in the pathogenesis of RA by investigating possible correlations between resistin concentration in serum and synovial fluid with disease activity and radiographic joint damage. The authors' results supported the hypothesis that resistin is involved in the pathogenesis of RA and suggested serum resistin as a good marker of prognosis of the disease in RA patients. Yoshino et al. (2011) [21] compared serum resistin levels from RA patients and healthy control subjects. The authors found that the level of resistin in serum did not differ between patients and controls, but observed that serum resistin were positively associated with CRP levels in RA patients, suggesting a pro inflammatory action of this cytokine.

Kontunen et al. (2011) [22] reported that high levels of resistin are associated with RA, regardless of the presence of MetS. Fadda et al. (2013) [37] compared resistin levels in serum and synovial fluid of patients with RA and osteoarthritis and found higher levels in patients with RA. This result indicates a possible role of resistin in the pathogenesis of inflammatory rheumatic diseases. The high levels of this adipokine in the synovial fluid could suggest a

Table 1 Studies investigating the association of leptin and rheumatoid arthritis in humans

Authors	Study design	Subjects	Results/outcomes
Rho et al. (2010) [19]	Cross-sectional study evaluating correlation between HOMA-IR and serum adipokine levels.	169 RA patients	Positive correlation between serum leptin and insulin resistance.
Targońska-Stepniak et al. (2010) [20]	Cross-sectional study evaluating correlation between disease activity and serum adipokine levels.	80 RA patients	Positive correlation between serum leptin and DAS28.
Yoshino et al. (2011) [21]	Case-control study evaluating correlation between inflammation markers and serum adipokine levels.	141 RA patients 146 controls without RA	Positive correlation between serum leptin and CRP.
Kontunen et al. (2011) [22]	Cross-sectional study evaluating correlation between serum adipokines levels and markers of inflammation and MetS.	54 RA patients, 20 with MetS	Increased levels of serum leptin observed only in patients with MetS.
Olama et al. (2012) [15]	Case-control study evaluating differences between serum leptin and synovial/serum leptin ratio.	40 RA patients 30 controls without RA	Inverse correlation between leptin concentration and protection of joints in severe RA.
Allam e Radwan (2012) [28]	Case-control study evaluating correlation between serum leptin levels and disease activity.	37 RA patients 34 controls without RA	No correlation between leptin levels and disease activity.
Kang et al. (2013) [23]	Cross-sectional study evaluating correlation between adipokine levels, inflammation markers, insulin resistance and atherosclerosis.	192 RA patients	Positive correlation between serum leptin and TNF-α and metabolic risk, including insulin resistance
Mirfeizi et al. (2014) [30]	Cross-sectional study evaluating correlation between adipokine levels and radiographic joint damage.	54 RA patients (29 with erosion and 25 without erosion)	No differences in serum leptin between the two groups.
Abdalla et al. (2014) [29]	Case-control study evaluating correlation between serum leptin levels and clinical manifestations of disease activity.	60 RA patients 30 healthy controls	No correlation between leptin levels and clinical and laboratorial markers of disease activity.
Bustos Rivera-Bahena et al. (2015) [24]	Cross-sectional study evaluating correlation between adipokine levels and disease activity.	121 RA patients	Positive correlation between serum leptin and disease activity.
Xibille-Friedmann et al. (2015) [25]	Cohort study evaluating if baseline levels of adipokines may predict disease activity or response to treatment.	127 RA patients after 6 months of follow up; 91 after 1 year of follow up; 52 after 2 years of follow up	Positive correlation between serum leptin and prevention of disease activity progression.
Oner et al. (2015) [31]	Case-control study evaluating correlation between serum leptin levels and disease activity.	106 RA patients 52 healthy controls 37 osteoarthritis patients	No correlation between serum leptin and disease activity.
Lee e Bae (2016) [27]	Meta-analysis evaluating correlation between serum leptin levels and disease activity.	13 studies: 648 RA patients 426 controls without RA	Leptin levels significantly higher in RA patients and weak positive correlation between leptin levels and disease activity.

RA = rheumatoid arthritis; HOMA-IR = homeostatic model assessment-insulin resistance; DAS28 = Disease Activity Score-28; CRP = C-reactive protein; TNF-α = tumor necrosis factor-α; Metabolic Syndrome = MetS

bad prognosis for progression of RA, but the authors point out that more studies are needed to confirm if resistin is a good marker to evaluate the progression of this disease. Kang et al. (2013) [23] reinforced this hypothesis. The authors found an association between resistin levels and inflammatory markers in patients with RA. Recently, Bustos Rivera-Bahena et al. (2015) [24] demonstrated that resistin levels correlated positively with clinical manifestations of disease activity in patients with RA, albeit of patient body mass index. Huang et al. (2015) [38] in a meta-analysis concluded that serum resistin levels were significantly higher in RA patients compared to control group.

However, some authors did not show significant associations between serum resistin and HOMA-IR, nor differences between serum and synovial fluid resistin levels between RA patients and controls [19]. Al-Kady et al. (2010) [39] after studying the levels of resistin in of RA patients found no significant differences in resistin levels between RA patients and controls. Hammad et al. (2014) [40] also found no correlation between serum levels of resistin with clinical or laboratory markers in RA patients.

Thus, there is an important role of adipokines in the pathogenesis of obesity, CVD and inflammatory processes. The pro inflammatory action of resistin was observed in most studies of patients with RA, which suggest that this adipokines is a good marker to assess the progression of this disease.

Table 2 summarizes the main findings of resistin in RA patients.

Visfatin

Also known as PBEF (pre-B-cell colony-enhancing factor) or Nicotinamide Phosphoribosyltransferase (Nampt) [41], visfatin is a protein with molecular weight of 52 kDa, first described by Samal et al. (1994) [42]. It is primarily found in liver, bone marrow and muscle tissue, but also produced by adipose tissue and secreted by macrophage [43]. Its production is influenced by TNF-α, IL-6, Toll-like receptor (TLR) and chemokines [44]. Stofkova (2010) [45] reports that visfatin may contribute to inflammation processes, triggering production of cytokines and activation of nuclear factor kappa beta (NF-κβ). Thus, some studies have suggested some relation between this adipokine and the pathogenesis of type 2 diabetes and obesity [46] and increased cardiovascular risk [47].

Other studies have demonstrated a correlation between serum and synovial fluid levels of visfatin and the pathogenesis of RA [13, 41, 48, 49]. This adipokine can act as a regulator of inflammation and the destruction process of joints [35] and induce stimulation of great quantities of chemokines [50], thus possibly contributing to the inflammatory state of RA. However, its association to disease activity is not yet fully known [51].

Alkady et al. (2011) [52] showed that visfatin levels correlated with disease activity and may be involved in the progression of RA. Khalifa et al. (2013) [53] suggested that visfatin has a role in the pathogenesis of RA, and it may be considered as a marker of the disease and the radiographic bone lesion score. Therefore, it can be a potential therapeutic target for RA. El-Hini et al. (2013) [54] demonstrated positive and significant correlation between visfatin and insulin resistance and also with serum cholesterol, low density lipoprotein cholesterol (LDL-c) and triglycerides.

Table 2 Studies investigating the association of resistin and rheumatoid arthritis in humans

Authors	Study design	Subjects	Results/outcomes
Kassem et al. (2010) [36]	Case-control study evaluating correlation between serum and synovial resistin and inflammation markers, disease activity and radiographic joint damage.	30 RA patients 15 healthy controls	Significant correlation between serum resistin levels and CRP, ESR, rheumatoid factor and disease activity. Also considered a good prognostic marker of RA.
Rho et al. (2010) [19]	Cross-sectional study evaluating correlation between HOMA-IR and serum adipokine levels.	169 RA patients	No significant correlation between serum resistin and insulin resistance.
Al-Kady et al. (2010) [39]	Case-control study evaluating correlation between serum and synovial liquid adipokines and disease activity.	70 RA patients 30 controls	No differences between groups in serum resistin, but it was observed synovial liquid resistin levels significantly higher in patients with active disease.
Yoshino et al. (2011) [21]	Case-control study evaluating correlation between inflammation markers and serum adipokines levels.	141 RA patients 146 controls	No differences in serum resistin between groups, but in RA patients it was positively associated with CRP levels.
Kontunen et al. (2011) [22]	Cross-sectional study evaluating correlation between serum adipokine levels and markers of inflammation and MetS in RA.	54 RA patients, 20 with MetS	Increased levels of resistin were associated with RA irrespective of the presence of MetS.
Fadda et al. (2013) [37]	Case-control study comparing serum and synovial liquid resistin in patients with RA and osteoarthritis.	25 RA patients 25 osteoarthritis patients	Significant correlation between synovial liquid resistin and rheumatoid factor and ACPA, indicating a bad prognosis of disease.
Kang et al. (2013) [23]	Cross-sectional study evaluating correlation between adipokines levels, inflammation markers, insulin resistance and atherosclerosis.	192 RA patients	Significant correlation between serum resistin and inflammation markers ESR and CRP and disease duration.
Hammad et al. (2014) [40]	Case-control study comparing serum resistin in RA patients and a control group and its association to disease activity.	30 RA patients 30 controls	No correlation between serum resistin levels and clinical and laboratorial markers of disease activity.
Bustos Rivera-Bahena et al. (2015) [24]	Cross-sectional study evaluating correlation between adipokines levels and disease activity.	121 RA patients	Positive correlation between resistin levels and disease activity.
Huang et al. (2015) [38]	Meta-analysis evaluating correlation between serum resistin levels and RA.	8 studies with RA: 620 RA patients 460 controls	Serum resistin levels were significantly higher in patients with RA.

RA = rheumatoid arthritis; CRP = C-reactive protein; TNF-α = tumor necrosis factor-α; ESR = erythrocyte sedimentation rate; ACPA = anti-citrullinated protein antibody; HOMA-IR = homeostatic model assessment-insulin resistance; Metabolic Syndrome = MetS

Additionally, the disease activity score was positively correlated with visfatin.

Sglunda et al. (2014) [55] observed that visfatin levels in serum were significantly higher in RA patients compared to healthy individuals and suggested that reduction in visfatin concentrations could reduce disease activity in patients at early stage of RA. They also found positive association between this adipokine and elevated levels of total cholesterol, but not with the atherogenic index. Mirfeizi et al. (2014) [30] found that serum levels of visfatin in RA patients with radiographic joint damage were significantly higher than in patients without joint damage.

Nonetheless, Rho et al. (2010) [19] did not evidence relationship between visfatin and insulin resistance nor coronary atherosclerosis in patients with RA and Meyer et al. (2013) [56] did not show any correlation between serum levels of visfatin and radiographic progression of the disease.

Table 3 summarizes the main findings of visfatin in RA patients.

Adponectin

Adiponectin is an anti-inflammatory adipokine compounded by 244 amino acids and is produced and secreted mainly by adipocytes. [57, 58] Studies suggest that monomeric form of adiponectin appears to occur only in adipocytes, but there are three forms of adiponectin circulating in the body: trimmers (low molecular weight, LMW), hexamers (middle molecular weight, MMW) and multimers (high molecular weight, HMW) are the plasma circulating forms of adiponectin [58]. The receptors are AdipoR1and AdipoR2, respectively present at skeletal muscles and liver [59].

Several studies have demonstrated the role of this important anti-inflammatory cytokine in obesity, diabetes mellitus type 2, atherosclerosis and metabolic syndrome, being the highest levels a protective factor for these diseases [35, 60–62].

Paradoxically, in the pathogenesis of rheumatoid arthritis adiponectin seems to have proinflammatory effects in the joints, because its ability to stimulate the secretion of inflammatory mediators [63] and may also be associated to disease activity [52]. Scotece et al. (2012) [64] described the major effects of increased synovial and circulating levels of adiponectin in RA. They concluded that adiponectin in synovial fibroblasts induced prostaglandin (PG)E2, IL-6, IL-8, matrix metalloproteinase (MMP)-1 and MMP-13; in human chondrocytes induced nitric oxide (NO), IL-6, MMP-3, MMP-9, monocyte chemoattractant protein (MCP)-1 and IL-8 and promoted inflammation by increasing TNF-α, IL-6 and IL-8.

Krysiak et al. (2012) [65] suggested that these different actions can be explained by different mechanisms: LMW adiponectin has anti-inflammatory activities, while the HMW adiponectin has proinflammatory activities. However, Frommer et al. (2012) [66] showed a proinflammatory and destructive role of all isoforms

Table 3 Studies investigating the association of visfatin and rheumatoid arthritis in humans

Authors	Study design	Subjects	Results/outcomes
Rho et al. (2010) [19]	Cross-sectional study evaluating correlation between HOMA-IR and serum adipokine levels.	169 RA patients	No correlation between visfatin levels and IR
Alkady et al. (2011) [52]	Case-control study evaluating correlation between serum and synovial liquid adipokines and disease activity.	70 RA patients 30 controls	Positive correlation between serum visfatin levels and disease activity.
Khalifa et al. (2013) [53]	Case-control study evaluating correlation between serum visfatin and inflammation markers.	60 RA patients 20 controls	Positive correlation between visfatin levels and IL-6, CRP, ERS, TNF-α and DAS-28 in RA.
El-Hini et al. (2013) [54]	Case-control study evaluating metabolic disorder and its association with clinical characteristics of RA patients.	40 RA patients 40 controls	Positive correlations between serum visfatin levels and IR, cholesterol, triglycerides and LDL-C.
Meyer et al. (2013) [56]	Cohort study evaluating serum adipokine levels and radiographic progression of RA.	632 RA patients at early stage of disease and 159 with unspecific arthritis	No correlation between visfatin levels and progression of RA.
Sglunda et al. (2014) [55]	Prospective study evaluating visfatin level and its relationship with disease activity and serum lipids.	40 patients with early, treatment-naïve RA 30 controls	Correlation between visfatin levels and disease activity and reduced levels after treatment.
Mirfeizi et al. (2014) [30]	Cross-sectional study evaluating correlation between serum adipokines levels and radiographic joint damage.	54 RA patients (29 with erosion and 25 without erosion)	The levels of visfatin were higher in patients with radiographic joint damage and dependent on the duration of the disease.

RA = rheumatoid arthritis; IR = insulin resistance; MetS = metabolic syndrome; IL-6 = interleukin-6; CRP = C-reactive protein; ESR = erythrocyte sedimentation rate; DAS28 = Disease Activity Score-28; TNF-α = tumor necrosis factor α; LDL-C = low-density lipoprotein cholesterol of adiponectin in patients with RA, suggesting a much more harmful than beneficial action of adiponectin in chronic inflammatory diseases. Several studies evidenced association of adiponectin in radiographic progression of RA [67, 68]. Thus, serum adiponectin levels could be a good biomarker to evaluate the early stages of disease progression [56]. However, this association was not mediated by the selective effect of HMW adiponectin. [69] Recently, Skalska and Kontny (2016) [18] observed that HMW and MMW adiponectins potentially stimulated the secretion of rheumatoid ASC (adipose-derived stem cells) in patients with RA, but did not exert a strong impact on ASC towards RA-FLS (fibroblast-like synoviocytes) and peripheral blood mononuclear cells.

Furthermore, Rho et al. (2010) [19] did not find any association between adiponectin levels and insulin resistance or coronary artery calcium score. Yoshino et al. (2011) [21] also observed higher levels of adiponectin in serum of RA patients, but it was negatively associated with CRP levels. Bustos Rivera-Bahena et al. (2015) [24] did not evidenced association between adiponectin and disease activity and Chennareddy et al. (2016) [70] reported that despite serum levels of adiponectin are higher in RA patients than in controls there was no correlation with disease activity, duration, BMI and waist-to-hip ratio.

Despite the protective effect of adiponectin in the pathogenesis of obesity, diabetes mellitus, atherosclerosis, and metabolic syndrome, it is unclear whether this effect is reproduced in RA. Several studies emphasize that adiponectin appears to play a pro inflammatory role in the pathogenesis of RA, particularly in the joints, by stimulating the secretion of inflammatory mediators. In this scenario, it highlights the importance of developing new research elucidating the real role of adipokines in the pathogenesis of RA.

Table 4 summarizes the main findings of adipnectin in RA patients.

Conclusion

In recent years, it has been studied the importance of adipokines in the pathogenesis of RA, however the results are still conflicting and the exactly role of adipose tissue in RA is not yet fully understood. Despite studies have been demonstrating the implications of adipokines in the pathophysiology of autoimmune diseases, including RA, it is not yet clear their role in the progression of disease. It is noteworthy the complex pathophysiology of this disease, thus requiring better knowledge about the mechanisms of action of these adipokines in RA as well as the changes that drugs can promote in the circulating levels of these adipokines in these patients.

Table 4 Studies investigating the association of adiponectin and rheumatoid arthritis in humans

Authors	Study design	Subjects	Results/outcomes
Rho et al. (2010) [19]	Cross-sectional study evaluating correlation between HOMA-IR and serum adipokine levels.	169 RA patients	No correlation between adiponectin and insulin resistance.
Alkady et al. (2011) [52]	Case-control study evaluating correlation between serum and synovial liquid adipokines and disease activity.	70 RA patients 30 controls	Positive correlation between serum and synovial adiponectin levels and disease activity.
Yoshino et al. (2011) [21]	Case-control study evaluating correlation between inflammation markers and serum adipokine levels.	141 RA patients 146 controls	No correlation between serum adiponectin levels and CRP.
Giles et al. (2011) [67]	Prospective study evaluating association of serum adipokine levels with progression of radiographic joint damage in patients with rheumatoid arthritis.	152 RA patients	Positive correlation between serum adiponectin levels and erosive joint destruction.
Klein-Wieringa et al. (2011) [68]	Cohort study evaluating baseline adipokine levels to predict radiographic progression of RA over a period of 4 years.	253 RA patients	Positive correlation between serum levels of adiponectin and radiographic progression of 4 RA.
Meyer et al. (2013) [56]	Cohort study evaluating serum adipokines levels and radiographic progression of RA.	632 RA patients at early stage of disease and 159 with unspecific arthritis	Positive association between serum adiponectin levels and radiographic progression of RA at early stage.
Bustos Rivera-Bahena et al. (2015) [24]	Cross-sectional study evaluating correlation between adipokines levels and disease activity.	121 RA patients	No correlation between serum adiponectin and clinical activity of RA, but negative correlation with TNFα and positive correlation with IL-1β.
Chennareddy et al. (2016) [70]	Cross-sectional study evaluating the serum concentrations of adiponectin and its impact on disease activity and radiographic joint damage.	43 RA patients 25 controls	Increased levels of serum adiponectin in RA, but no correlation with erosive and non-erosive disease, disease duration, BMI, waist-hip ratio and disease activity.

RA = rheumatoid arthritis; IR = insulin resistance; CRP = C-reactive protein; BMI = body mass index

Abbreviations

ACPA: Anti–citrullinated protein antibody; ASC: Adipose-derived stem cells; BMI: Body mass index; CRP: C-reactive protein; CVD: Cardiovascular diseases; DAS: Disease Activity Score; FLS: Fibroblast-like synoviocytes; HMW: High molecular weight; HOMA-IR: Homeostasis Model Assessment - Insulin Resistance; IL: Interleukin; LDL-c: Low density lipoprotein cholesterol; LMW: Low molecular weight; LPS: Lipopolysaccharide; MCP: Monocyte chemoattractant protein; MetS: Metabolic syndrome; MMP: Matrix metalloproteinase; MMW: Middle molecular weight; Nampt: Nicotinamide phosphoribosyltransferase; NF-κβ: Nuclear factor kappa beta; NO: Nitric oxide; PBEF: Pre-B-cell colony-enhancing factor; PG: Prostaglandina; PRISMA: Preferred Reporting Items for Systematic Reviews and Meta-Analyses; RA: Rheumatoid arthritis; RELM: Resistin-like molecules; RF: Rheumatoid factor; SciELO: Scientific Electronic Library Online; Th: T helper; TLR: Toll-like receptor; TNF: Tumor necrosis factor

Authors' contributions

ECSF and FTR made substantial contributions to acquisition and interpretation of data, and writing the manuscript. ANCS and ID contributed to conception of the study, and revising it critically. All authors read and approved the final manuscript.

Author details

[1]Postgraduate Program, Health Sciences Center, State University of Londrina, Londrina, Paraná, Brazil. [2]Postgraduate Program, Experimental Pathology, State University of Londrina, Londrina, Paraná, Brazil. [3]Department of Pathology, Clinical Analysis and Toxicology, University Londrina, Londrina, Paraná, Brazil. [4]Department of Internal Medicine, University of Londrina, Londrina, Paraná, Brazil. [5]Department of Nutrition, University of Fronteira Sul, Rodovia PR 182 Km 466, CEP 85770-000, Realeza, Paraná Postal Code 253, Brazil.

References

1. Lipsky PE. Artrite Reumatoide. In: Medicina interna de Harrison. 14th ed. Rio de Janeiro: Amgh Editora; 1998. p. 1996–7.
2. Mateen S, Zafar A, Moin S, Khan AQ, Zubair S. Understanding the role of cytokines in the pathogenesis of rheumatoid arthritis. Clin Chim Acta. 2016; 455:161–71.
3. American College of Rheumatology Subcommittee on Rheumatoid Arthritis Guidelines. Guidelines for the management of rheumatoid arthritis: 2002 update. Arthritis Rheum. 2002;46(2):328–46. http://www.ncbi.nlm.nih.gov/pubmed/11840435
4. Barbosa VDS, Rêgo J, Antônio N. Possível papel das adipocinas no lúpus eritematoso sitêmico e na artrite reumatoide. Rev Bras Reumatol. 2012;52(2):278–87.
5. Hutcheson J. Adipokines influence the inflammatory balance in autoimmunity. Cytokine. 2015;75(2):272–9.
6. Shamseer L, Moher D, Clarke M, Ghersi D, Liberati A, Petticrew M, et al. Preferred reporting items for systematic review and meta-analysis protocols (PRISMA-P) 2015: elaboration and explanation. BMJ. 2015;349 http://www.bmj.com/content/349/bmj.g7647
7. Neumann E, Frommer KW, Vasile M, Müller-Ladner U. Adipocytokines as driving forces in rheumatoid arthritis and related inflammatory diseases? Arthritis Rheum. 2011;63(5):1159–69.
8. Freitas Lima LC, Braga VA, do Socorro de França Silva M, Cruz JC, Sousa Santos SH, de Oliveira Monteiro MM, et al. Adipokines, diabetes and atherosclerosis: an inflammatory association. Front Physiol. 2015;6:1–15.
9. Dichi I, Simão ANC. Metabolic syndrome: new targets for an old problem. Expert Opin Ther Targets. 2012;16(2):147–50. http://www.tandfonline.com/doi/full/10.1517/14728222.2012.648924
10. Zhang Y, Proenca R, Maffei M, Barone M, Leopold L, Friedman JM. Positional cloning of the mouse obese gene and its human homologue. Nature. 1994;372(6505):425–32. http://www.ncbi.nlm.nih.gov/pubmed/7984236
11. Guimarães DED, Sardinha FL DC, Mizurini D DM, Das GT Do CM. Adipocitocinas: uma nova visão do tecido adiposo. Rev Nutr. 2007;20(5):

549–59. http://www.scielo.br/scielo.php?script=sci_arttext&pid=S1415-52732007000500010&lng=pt&nrm=iso&tlng=pt
12. Mantzoros CS, Magkos F, Brinkoetter M, Sienkiewicz E, Dardeno TA, Kim S, et al. Leptin in human physiology and pathophysiology. AJP Endocrinol Metab. 2011;301:567–84.
13. Del Prete A, Salvi V, Sozzani S. Adipokines as potential biomarkers in rheumatoid arthritis. Mediat Inflamm. 2014;2014:1–12.
14. Paz-Filho G, Mastronardi C, Franco CB, Wang KB, Wong M-L, Licinio J. Leptin: molecular mechanisms, systemic pro-inflammatory effects, and clinical implications. Arq Bras Endocrinol Metabol. 2012;56(9):597–607. http://www.ncbi.nlm.nih.gov/pubmed/23329181
15. Olama SM, Senna MK, Elarman M. Synovial/serum leptin ratio in rheumatoid arthritis: the association with activity and erosion. Rheumatol Int. 2012;32(3):683–90. http://www.ncbi.nlm.nih.gov/pubmed/21140264
16. Toussirot É, Michel F, Binda D, Dumoulin G. The role of leptin in the pathophysiology of rheumatoid arthritis. Life Sci. 2015;140:29–36. http://linkinghub.elsevier.com/retrieve/pii/S002432051500257X
17. Scotece M, Conde J, López V, Lago F, Pino J, Gómez-Reino JJ, et al. Adiponectin and leptin: new targets in inflammation. Basic Clin Pharmacol Toxicol. 2014;114(1):97–102.
18. Skalska U, Kontny E. Adiponectin isoforms and Leptin impact on rheumatoid adipose Mesenchymal stem cells function. Stem Cells Int. 2016;2016:1–7.
19. Rho YH, Chung CP, Solus JF, Raggi P, Oeser A, Gebretsadik T, et al. Adipocytokines, insulin resistance, and coronary atherosclerosis in rheumatoid arthritis. Arthritis Rheum. 2010;62(5):1259–64.
20. Targońska-Stepniak B, Dryglewska M, Majdan M. Adiponectin and leptin serum concentrations in patients with rheumatoid arthritis. Rheumatol Int. 2010;30:731–7.
21. Yoshino T, Kusunoki N, Tanaka N, Kaneko K, Kusunoki Y, Endo H, et al. Elevated serum levels of resistin, leptin, and adiponectin are associated with C-reactive protein and also other clinical conditions in rheumatoid arthritis. Intern Med. 2011;50(4):269–75. https://www.ncbi.nlm.nih.gov/pubmed/21325757
22. Kontunen P, Vuolteenaho K, Nieminen R, Lehtimäki L, Kautiainen H, Kesäniemi Y, et al. Resistin is linked to inflammation, and leptin to metabolic syndrome, in women with inflammatory arthritis. Scand J Rheumatol. 2011; 40(4):256–62. http://www.ncbi.nlm.nih.gov/pubmed/21453187
23. Kang Y, Park H-J, Kang M-I, Lee H-S, Lee S-W, Lee S-K, et al. Adipokines, inflammation, insulin resistance, and carotid atherosclerosis in patients with rheumatoid arthritis. Arthritis Res Ther. 2013;15(6):1–7. http://www.ncbi.nlm.nih.gov/pubmed/24245495
24. Bustos Rivera-Bahena C, Xibillé-Friedmann DX, González-Christen J, Carrillo-Vázquez SM, Montiel-Hernández JL. Peripheral blood Leptin and Resistin levels as clinical activity biomarkers in Mexican rheumatoid arthritis patients. Reumatol Clin. 2016;12(6):323–6.
25. Xibille-Friedmann DX, Ortiz-Panozo E, Bustos Rivera-Bahena C, Sandoval-Rios M, Hernandez-Gongora SE, Dominguez-Hernandez L, et al. Leptin and adiponectin as predictors of disease activity in rheumatoid arthritis. Clin Exp Rheumatol. 2015;33(4):471–7.
26. Tian G, Liang J-N, Wang Z-Y, Zhou D. Emerging role of leptin in rheumatoid arthritis. Clin Exp Immunol. 2014;177(3):557–70. http://www.pubmedcentral.nih.gov/articlerender.fcgi?artid=4137840&tool=pmcentrez&rendertype=abstract
27. Lee YH, Bae S-C. Circulating leptin level in rheumatoid arthritis and its correlation with disease activity: a meta-analysis. Z Rheumatol. 2016;75(10):1021–7.
28. Allam A, Radwan A. The relationship of serum leptin levels with disease activity in Egyptian patients with rheumatoid arthritis. Egypt Rheumatol. 2012;34(4):185–90.
29. Abdalla M, Effat D, Sheta M, Hamed WE. Serum Leptin levels in rheumatoid arthritis and relationship with disease activity. Egypt Rheumatol. 2014;36(1):1–5.
30. Mirfeizi Z, Noubakht Z, Rezaie AE, Jokar MH, Sarabi ZS. Plasma levels of leptin and visfatin in rheumatoid arthritis patients; is there any relationship with joint damage? Iran J Basic Med Sci. 2014;17(9):662–6. http://www.ncbi.nlm.nih.gov/pubmed/25691942
31. Oner SY, Volkan O, Oner C, Mengi A, Direskeneli H, Tasan DA. Serum leptin levels do not correlate with disease activity in rheumatoid arthritis. Acta Reumatol Port. 2015;40(1):50–4.
32. Steppan CM, Bailey ST, Bhat S, Brown EJ, Banerjee RR, Wright CM, et al. The hormone resistin links obesity to diabetes. Nature. 2001;409(6818):307–12. http://www.ncbi.nlm.nih.gov/pubmed/11201732

33. Lee JH, Chan JL, Yiannakouris N, Kontogianni M, Estrada E, Seip R, et al. Circulating resistin levels are not associated with obesity or insulin resistance in humans and are not regulated by fasting or leptin administration: cross-sectional and interventional studies in normal, insulin-resistant, and diabetic subjects. J Clin Endocrinol Metab. 2003;88(10):4848–56. http://www.ncbi.nlm.nih.gov/pubmed/14557464

34. Codoñer-Franch P, Alonso-Iglesias E. Resistin: insulin resistance to malignancy. Clin Chim Acta. 2015;438:46–54.

35. Abella V, Scotece M, Conde J, López V, Lazzaro V, Pino J, et al. Review article Adipokines. Metabolic Syndrome and Rheumatic Diseases J Immunol Researc. 2014;2014:1–15.

36. Kassem E, Mahmoud L, Salah W. Study of Resistin and YKL-40 in rheumatoid arthritis. J Am Sci. 2010;6(10):1004–12.

37. Fadda SMH, Gamal SM, Elsaid NY, Mohy AM. Resistin in inflammatory and degenerative rheumatologic diseases: relationship between resistin and rheumatoid arthritis disease progression. Z Rheumatol. 2013;72(6): 594–600.

38. Huang Q, Tao S-S, Zhang Y-J, Zhang C, Li L-J, Zhao W, et al. Serum resistin levels in patients with rheumatoid arthritis and systemic lupus erythematosus: a meta analysis. Clin Rheumatol. 2015:1713–20. http://link.springer.com/10.1007/s10067-015-2955-5

39. Al-kady EA, Ahmed HM, Tag L, Adel M, Al-Kady EA. Adipocytokines: Adiponectin, Resistin and Visfatin in serum and synovial fluid of rheumatoid arthritis patients and their relation to disease activity. Med J Cairo Univ. 2010;78(2):723–9.

40. Hammad MH, Nasef S, Musalam D, Ahmed MM, Osman I, Hammad MH. Resistin, an adipokine , its relation to inflammation in Systemic Lupus Erythematosus and Rheumatoid Arthritis. Middle East J Intern Med. 2014;7(3):3–9.

41. Bao JP, Chen WP, Wu LD. Visfatin: a potential therapeutic target for rheumatoid arthritis. J Int Med Res. 2009;37(6):1655–61. http://www.ncbi.nlm.nih.gov/entrez/query.fcgi?cmd=Retrieve&db=PubMed&dopt=Citation&list_uids=20146863

42. Samal B, Sun Y, Stearns G, Xie C, Suggs S, McNiece I. Cloning and characterization of the cDNA encoding a novel human pre-B-cell Colony-enhancing. Mol Cell Biol. 1994;14(2):1431–7.

43. Fukuhara A, Matsuda M, Nishizawa M, Segawa K, Tanaka M, Kishimoto K, et al. Visfatin: a protein secreted by visceral fat that mimics the effects of insulin. Science. 2005;307(5708):426–30. http://www.ncbi.nlm.nih.gov/pubmed/15604363

44. Kerekes G, Nurmohamed MT, González-Gay MA, Seres I, Paragh G, Kardos Z, et al. Rheumatoid arthritis and metabolic syndrome. Nat Rev Rheumatol. 2014;10(11):691–6. http://www.ncbi.nlm.nih.gov/pubmed/25090948

45. Stofkova A. Resistin and visfatin: regulators of insulin sensitivity, inflammation and immunity. Endocr Regul. 2010;44(1):25–36. http://www.ncbi.nlm.nih.gov/pubmed/20151765

46. Haider DG, Schindler K, Schaller G, Prager G, Wolzt M, Ludvik B. Increased plasma visfatin concentrations in morbidly obese subjects are reduced after gastric banding. J Clin Endocrinol Metab. 2006;91(4):1578–81. http://www.ncbi.nlm.nih.gov/pubmed/16449335

47. Romacho T, Sánchez-ferrer CF, Peiró C. Review article Visfatin / Nampt: an Adipokine with cardiovascular impact. Mediat Inflamm. 2013;2013:1–16.

48. Naguib A, Elsawy N, Aboul-enein F, Hossam N. The relation between serum visfatin levels and cardiovascular involvement in rheumatoid arthritis. Alexandria J Med. 2011;47(2):117–24. https://doi.org/10.1016/j.ajme.2011.07.005%5Cnhttp://linkinghub.elsevier.com/retrieve/pii/S2090506811000479

49. Gómez R, Suarez A, Villalvilla A, Herrero-Beaumont G, Largo R, Young DA. Visfatin: a new player in rheumatic diseases. Immunometabolism. 2013;1:10–5. http://www.degruyter.com/view/j/immun.2013.1.issue/immun-2013-0002/immun-2013-0002.xml

50. Meier FMP, Frommer KW, Peters MA, Brentano F, Lefèvre S, Schröder D, et al. Visfatin/pre-B-cell colony-enhancing factor (PBEF), a proinflammatory and cell motility-changing factor in rheumatoid arthritis. J Biol Chem. 2012;287(34):28378–85.

51. Kim KS, Choi HM, Ji HI, Song R, Yang HI, Lee SK, et al. Serum adipokine levels in rheumatoid arthritis patients and their contributions to the resistance to treatment. Mol Med Rep. 2014;9(1):255–60.

52. Alkady EAM, Ahmed HM, Tag L, Abdou MA. Adiponectin, Resistin und Visfatin in Serum und Gelenkflüssigkeit bei Patienten mit rheumatoider Arthritis. Z Rheumatol. 2011;70(7):602–8. http://link.springer.com/10.1007/s00393-011-0834-2

53. Khalifa IA, Abdelfattah A. Relation between serum visfatin and clinical severity in different stages of rheumatoid arthritis. Egypt Rheumatol Rehabil. 2013;40(1):1–8.

54. El-Hini SH, Mohamed FI, Hassan AA, Ali F, Mahmoud A, Ibraheem HM. Visfatin and adiponectin as novel markers for evaluation of metabolic disturbance in recently diagnosed rheumatoid arthritis patients. Rheumatol Int. 2013;33(9):2283–9.

55. Sglunda O, Mann H, Hulejová H, Kuklová M, Pecha O, Pleštilová L, et al. Decreased circulating visfatin is associated with improved disease activity in early rheumatoid arthritis: data from the PERAC cohort. PLoS One. 2014;9(7):1–5.

56. Meyer M, Sellam J, Fellahi S, Kotti S, Bastard J-P, Meyer O, et al. Serum level of adiponectin is a surrogate independent biomarker of radiographic disease progression in early rheumatoid arthritis: results from the ESPOIR cohort. Arthritis Res Ther. 2013;15(6):1–13.

57. Scherer PE, Williams S, Fogliano M, Baldini G, Lodish HF. A novel serum protein similar to C1q, produced exclusively in adipocytes. J Biol Chem. 1995;270(45):26746–9. http://www.ncbi.nlm.nih.gov/pubmed/7592907

58. Garaulet M, Hernández-Morante JJ, de Heredia FP, Tébar FJ. Adiponectin, the controversial hormone. Public Health Nutr. 2007;10(10A):1145–50. http://www.ncbi.nlm.nih.gov/pubmed/17903323

59. Yamauchi T, Nio Y, Maki T, Kobayashi M, Takazawa T, Iwabu M, et al. Targeted disruption of AdipoR1 and AdipoR2 causes abrogation of adiponectin binding and metabolic actions. Nat Med. 2007;13(3):332–9. http://www.ncbi.nlm.nih.gov/pubmed/17268472

60. Ohashi K, Ouchi N, Matsuzawa Y. Anti-inflammatory and anti-atherogenic properties of adiponectin. Biochimie. 2012;94(10):2137–42.

61. Fantuzzi G. Adiponectin in inflammatory and immune-mediated diseases. Cytokine. 2013;64(1):1–10. http://www.ncbi.nlm.nih.gov/pubmed/23850004

62. Simão TNC, Lozovoy MAB, Simão ANC, Oliveira SR, Venturini D, Morimoto HK, et al. Reduced-energy cranberry juice increases folic acid and adiponectin and reduces homocysteine and oxidative stress in patients with the metabolic syndrome. Br J Nutr. 2013;110(10):1885–94. http://www.journals.cambridge.org/abstract_S0007114513001207

63. Chen X, Lu J, Bao J, Guo J, Shi J, Wang Y. Adiponectin: a biomarker for rheumatoid arthritis? Cytokine Growth Factor Rev. 2013;24(1):83–9.

64. Scotece M, Conde J, Gómez R, López V, Pino J, González A, et al. Role of adipokines in atherosclerosis: interferences with cardiovascular complications in rheumatic diseases. Mediat Inflamm. 2012;2012:1–14.

65. Krysiak R, Handzlik-Orlik G, Okopien B. The role of adipokines in connective tissue diseases. Eur J Nutr. 2012;51(5):513–28.

66. Frommer KW, Schäffler A, Büchler C, Steinmeyer J, Rickert M, Rehart S, et al. Adiponectin isoforms: a potential therapeutic target in rheumatoid arthritis? Ann Rheum Dis. 2012;71(10):1724–32. http://www.ncbi.nlm.nih.gov/pubmed/22532632

67. Giles JT, van der Heijde DM, Bathon JM. Association of circulating adiponectin levels with progression of radiographic joint destruction in rheumatoid arthritis. Ann Rheum Dis [Internet]. 2011;70(9):1562–8. http://www.ncbi.nlm.nih.gov/pubmed/21571734

68. Klein-Wieringa IR, Van Der Linden MPM, Knevel R, Kwekkeboom JC, Van Beelen E, Huizinga TWJ, et al. Baseline serum adipokine levels predict radiographic progression in early rheumatoid arthritis. Arthritis Rheum. 2011;63(9):2567–74.

69. Klein-Wieringa IR, Andersen SN, Herb-Van Toorn L, Kwekkeboom JC, Van Der Helm-Van Mil AHM, Meulenbelt I, et al. Are baseline high molecular weight adiponectin levels associated with radiographic progression in rheumatoid arthritis and osteoarthritis? J Rheumatol. 2014;41(5):853–7.

70. Chennareddy S, Kishore Babu KV, Kommireddy S, Varaprasad R, Rajasekhar L. Serum adiponectin and its impact on disease activity and radiographic joint damage in early rheumatoid arthritis – a cross-sectional study. Indian J Rheumatol. 2016;11(2):82–5.

9

Hand strength in patients with RA correlates strongly with function but not with activity of disease

Graziela Sferra da Silva* iD, Mariana de Almeida Lourenço and Marcos Renato de Assis

Abstract

Background: Rheumatoid arthritis (RA) is a systemic autoimmune disease characterized by chronic inflammation of the joints, especially of the hands. The evaluation of handgrip strength (HS) and pinch strength can be useful to detect reduction in hand function in RA patients. The aim of the study was to compare HS and pinch strength between RA patients (RA Group - RAG) and a non-RA control group (CG) and to relate HS and pinch strength to functional capacity, duration and disease activity in the RAG.

Methods: A cross-sectional case control study. The RAG was assessed for disease activity by the Disease Activity Score (DAS-28); for functional capacity by the Health Assessment Questionnaire (HAQ), the Cochin Hand Functional Scale (CHFS) questionnaire, and the Disability of the Arm, Shoulder, and Hand (DASH) questionnaire; and for HS and pinch strength (2-point tip-to-tip, lateral or key, and 3-point) using Jamar® and pinch gauge dynamometers, respectively. Associations were analyzed by Pearson and Spearman tests, and groups were compared by the independent samples t test, with a significance level of $P < 0.05$.

Results: The convenience sample included 121 rheumatoid patients and a control group matched by age, sex, and body mass index. The RAG showed lower strength values compared with the CG in all measurements ($P < 0.01$, 95% CI) and these values were associated with worse performance in the functional questionnaires and greater disease activity and duration. There was a strong correlation among the functional assessment instruments.

Conclusions: The decrease in grip and pinch strength, easily measured by portable dynamometers, is a strong indicator of functional disability in RA patients.

Keywords: Rheumatoid arthritis, Hand strength, Pinch strength, Muscle weakness, Disability evaluation

Background

Rheumatoid arthritis (RA) is a chronic inflammatory joint disease that preferentially affects the hands, resulting in reductions in muscle strength and mobility and deformities associated with considerable functional impairment [1, 2]. Loss of muscle strength, made worse by lack of use [3], can impair the basic grip and pinch functions of the hands. Some studies conducted with portable dynamometers have shown reductions in hand strength in patients with RA compared with healthy controls and correlated with functional ability [4–8]. However, such studies exhibit several limitations, such

as small sample size, lack of control groups, and poor description of the measurement protocols.

The aims of the present study were to measure the hand grip strength (HS) and pinch strength of individuals with RA, compared with a control group, and to correlate hand strength with functional ability and length and activity of disease.

Methods

This cross-sectional, case-control study was conducted with individuals with RA (RA group - RAG) followed up at the rheumatology outpatient clinic, School of Medicine of Marilia, interior of the state of São Paulo, Brazil. Controls (Control group - CG), matched by sex, age, and body mass index (BMI), were selected among escorts of

* Correspondence: gra_sferra@hotmail.com
Faculty of Medicine of Marilia (Famema), Marília, SP, Brazil

patients at the rheumatology outpatient clinic and at the internal medicine, obstetrics, and otorhinolaryngology outpatient clinics.

The Institutional Ethics Committee, under Certificate of Presentation for Ethical Appraisal (CAAE) 45,124,815.0000.5413, approved the study. Participants were included in the study after signing an informed consent form. The study was conducted from September 2015 to September 2016.

Sample size was calculated using a two-tailed test with the significance level set to 5, 90% power, standard deviation 9.8 kgf [9] for handgrip strength, and a clinically significant difference of 4.5 kgf. To compensate for eventual losses, the calculated sample size was increased by 20%, resulting in 121 participants per group.

Individuals 18 years old or older were included. RAG members had to meet the classification criteria formulated by the American College of Rheumatology in 1987 (ACR 1987) or the criteria formulated by the American College of Rheumatology and the European League Against Rheumatism in 2010 (ACR/ EULAR 2010) [10, 11]. Exclusion criteria for both groups were understanding, cognition, or sensory deficits hindering participation in interviews; skin or neurological lesions impairing the grip and pinch functions; and amputation of the upper limbs. Individuals with hand joint complaints were excluded from CG.

Patients with RA were subjected to assessment of activity of disease. All participants were subjected to measurements of body mass and height (Filizola mechanical scale with stadiometer, 100-g and 0.1-cm precision), functional ability questionnaires, and hand dynamometry.

Disease activity was assessed by means of the Disease Activity Score (DAS28) and the measurement of C-reactive protein (CRP; immunoturbidimetric method) [12–14]. The DAS28 final score was interpreted according to the following classification: remission ≤ 2.4; low disease activity ≤ 3.2; moderate activity ≤ 5.5; and high activity > 5.5, and according to the Boolean definition of remission (2010 ACR/EULAR remission criteria): tender and swollen joint count < 1, CRP ≤ 1 mg/dl, and visual analog scale (VAS) score ≤ 1 or Simplified Disease Activity Index (SDAI) ≤ 3 [15, 16].

Functional ability was assessed by means of 3 questionnaires: a) the Health Assessment Questionnaire (HAQ), one of the most widely used for patients with RA and that was translated to and validated for the Portuguese language [17–19]; b) the Cochin Hand Functional Scale (CHFS), developed in France initially for assessment of patients with RA and then extended to other conditions, and translated and adapted for Brazilian populations [20, 21]; and c) the Disability of the Arm, Shoulder, and Hand (DASH) questionnaire, developed for assessment of the upper limb functional ability in various

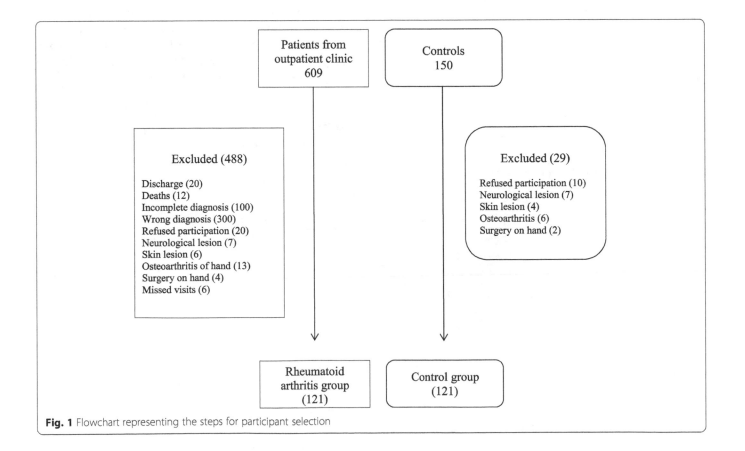

Fig. 1 Flowchart representing the steps for participant selection

Table 1 Characteristics of the rheumatoid arthritis group (RAG) and the control group (CG)

Variables	RAG $n = 121$	CG $n = 121$
Age (years)	57.50 ± 10.75	57.48 ± 10.48
BMI (kg/m ^{2})	28.26 ± 5.84	29.74 ± 6.08
Sex (%)		
Male	14 (11.6)	14 (11.2)
Female	107 (88.4)	107 (88.4)
Ethnicity (%)		
White	81 (66.9)	67 (55.4)
Black	3 (2.5)	12 (9.9)
Brown skin	36 (29.8)	42 (34.7)
Indian	1 (0.8)	–
Educational level (%)		
None	8 (6.6)	5 (4.1)
Incomplete elementary school	49 (40.5)	52 (43.0)
Complete elementary school	17 (14.0)	15 (12.4)
Incomplete secondary school	22 (18.2)	5 (4.1)
Complete secondary school	18 (14.9)	37 (30.6)
Higher education	7 (5.8)	7 (5.8)
Marital status (%)		
Single	19 (15.7)	10 (8.3)
Married	65 (53.7)	72 (59.5)
Divorced	19 (15.7)	14 (11.6)
Widowed	14 (11.6)	18 (14.9)
Stable union	4 (3.3)	7 (5.8)
Dominant hand (%)		
Right	114 (94.2)	115 (95.0)
Associated diseases (%)		
Systemic arterial hypertension	71 (58.7)	74 (61.2)
Osteoporosis	31 (25.6)	3 (2.5)
Diabetes	18 (14.9)	32 (26.4)

SD: standard deviation; kg/m ^{2}: kilograms per square meter

conditions and translated, validated, and adapted for the Portuguese language in 2005 [22, 23].

Hand strength was assessed with the participants sitting on an armless chair, with 90° elbow flexion, forearms in a neutral position, and 0 to 30° wrist extension. Maximum strength was assessed after a 3-s sustained contraction; the average of 3 attempts at 1-min intervals was considered for analysis. During the tests, all participants received verbal feedback by means of the sentence "strength, strength, strength" [24, 25]. Measurements included a) handgrip strength (HS) measured with a Jamar® hydraulic dynamometer at handle position 2, as established by the *American Society of Hand Therapists* (ASHT); results were recorded in kilogram-force (kgf) [24], and b) pinch strength measured using a B&L *Engineering*® PG-30 pinch gauge, including 2-point tip-to-tip pinch strength (classic, between the thumb and index finger), lateral or key pinch strength (between the pad of the thumb and the lateral surface of the middle phalanx of the index finger), and 3-point pinch strength (between the thumb, index, and middle fingers) [26].

The data were subjected to descriptive statistics; normality was assessed by means of the Kolmogorov-Smirnov test. Groups were matched 1:1 by sex, age, and BMI and were compared with the t-test. Correlations were investigated using Pearson's and Spearman's tests, and the strength of correlation was categorized as follows: 0.0 to 0.3, non-significant; 0.3 to 0.5 weak; 0.5 to 0.7 moderate; 0.7 to 0.9 strong; and 0.9 to 1.0 very strong [27]. Intergroup comparisons were performed by means of the independent t-test, with significance level $P < 0.05$. Analyses were performed with software Statistical Package for the Social Sciences (SPSS version 24) - US.

Results

Figure 1 most participants in the groups were female, married, and white (self-reported ethnicity) with a low educational level, reported arterial hypertension, and

Table 2 Hand strength of participants in the rheumatoid arthritis group (RAG) and the control group (CG)

Strength test	RAG	CG	CG-RAG difference	
	Mean ± SD (kgf)		(%)	P
Handgrip R	17.74 ± 9.23	25.94 ± 8.33	30	< 0.01
Handgrip L	17.34 ± 8.87	25.85 ± 8.32	31	< 0.01
2-point tip-to-tip pinch R	3.47 ± 1.56	5.24 ± 1.49	32	< 0.01
2-point tip-to-tip pinch L	3.33 ± 1.58	4.98 ± 1.39	31	< 0.01
3-point R	4.55 ± 1.99	6.87 ± 2.10	32	< 0.01
3-point L	4.50 ± 2.05	6.57 ± 1.95	30	< 0.01
Lateral pinch R	6.02 ± 2.40	7.79 ± 1.96	21	< 0.01
Lateral pinch L	5.60 ± 2.31	7.26 ± 1.86	21	< 0.01

kgf: kilogram-force; R: right; L: left. Independent t-test

Table 3 Length and activity of disease and functional ability of participants in the rheumatoid arthritis group (RAG)

Variables (n = 121)	Mean (±SD)	Median [P25-P75]
Length of disease (years)		10 [5–16]
DAS28	2.98 (±1.32)	
HAQ		0.87 [0.31–1.75]
Cochin Hand Functional Score		8 [1–27]
DASH		20 [7.50–43.33]

N: sample; SD: standard deviation; P25-P75: 25th and 75th percentiles; DAS28: Disease Activity Score; HAQ: Health Assessment Questionnaire; DASH: Disability of Arm, Shoulder, and Hand

were right-handed for writing and performing activities of daily living (ADL). Details on the characteristics of the participants from both groups are described in (Tables 1 and 2).

Rheumatoid factor tested positive in 78.5% (*n* = 95) of participants in the RAG; data on anti-citrullinated protein antibodies (ACPAs) were missing for 43 patients. The drug most widely used by patients was methotrexate, 71.9% (*n* = 87), followed by leflunomide, 52.9% (*n* = 64), and hydroxychloroquine, 38% (*n* = 46) (Tables 3 and 4).

Length of disease did not exhibit any significant correlations with activity of disease, scores on questionnaires, or functional ability.

In a separate analysis by age range (10-year interval) in the RAG, we found that HS decreased after 35 years of age and was more accentuated after 65 years of age. In the CG, the highest strength level was exhibited by G2, with a gradual decline with age (Table 5).

The scores on the functional ability scales showed strong mutual correlations: HAQ and CHFS 0.789 (*P* < 0.01), HAQ and DASH 0.825 (P < 0.01), and CHFS and DASH 0.820 (P < 0.01), but weak correlations with activity of disease.

There was no correlation of hand strength and functional ability with RA Boolean remission (Table 6).

Discussion

The handgrip strength and pinch strength were lower among the patients with RA compared with the controls.

Handgrip strength and pinch strength were lower among patients with poorer functional ability but showed weak correlations with activity and length of disease.

The average age of the participants was 58 years; age did not exhibit a correlation with HS, as has been described in the literature [1, 18, 28–31].

A study conducted with healthy individuals found that the peak HS occurred in the age range of 25 to 39 years; pinch strength remained stable until age 59 years, followed by a gradual decline together with age [32]. In another study performed with healthy Brazilians, peak HS occurred in the age range of 35 to 39 years, followed by a gradual decline with age [33]. A study that analyzed patients with RA did not find a difference in 2-point pinch after 5-year follow up [34]. However, the meta-analysis conducted by Beenakker et al. [31] showed a decline of HS before age 50 years, suggesting that the disease might cause premature aging. In our study, we did not find a clear-cut strength reduction gradient, but strength declined in the groups with patients older than 35 years, similar to previous studies; this variation might be attributed to the expected loss of muscle mass and strength that occurs after age 40. The group with patients older than 65 years old showed additional HS reduction, which is consistent with the frailty developed by older seniors [35].

There is controversy regarding hand strength and dominance. Some studies conducted with healthy individuals found significant differences, with the dominant hand being the strongest [36]. Two studies simultaneously analyzed patients with RA and healthy individuals. In one study, the dominant hand was 20% weaker than the non-dominant one among patients with RA and 8% stronger among healthy individuals [37]. The other study found differences among the healthy participants only [38]. In our study, we did not find a correlation between strength and dominance in either group; in addition, dominance might be influenced by several factors, such as work and leisure demands [39].

Regarding associated diseases, systemic arterial hypertension was the most prevalent in the analyzed sample. Use of cardiovascular medications has been associated

Table 4 Negative correlations among hand strength, functional ability, activity, and duration of disease in the rheumatoid arthritis group (RAG)

Variables	Handgrip		2-point tip-to-tip pinch		3-point pinch		Lateral pinch	
	D	E	D	E	D	E	D	E
HAQ	0.585*	0.528*	0.446*	0.472*	0.505*	0.501*	0.470*	0.555*
DASH	0.606*	0.559*	0.453*	0.444*	0.484*	0.486*	0.444*	0.535*
CHFS	0.606*	0.512*	0.452*	0.448*	0.496*	0.474*	0.474*	0.509*
Length of disease	0.168	0.196**	0.171	0.204**	0.189**	0.217**	0.187**	0.238*
DAS28	0.431*	0.401*	0.473*	0.436*	0.467*	0.424*	0.341*	0.336*

HAQ: *Health Assessment Questionnaire*; DASH: *Disabilities Arm, Shoulder, and Hand*; CHFS: *Cochin Hand Functional Scale*. Pearson's correlation test for DAS28; Spearman's correlation test for all others; * *P* < 0.01, ** *P* < 0.05

Table 5 Handgrip strength per age range in the rheumatoid arthritis group (RAG) and the control group (CG)

| Age range | RAG | | CG | |
	HS R Mean ± SD	HS L Mean ± SD	HS R Mean ± SD	HS L Mean ± SD
26–35 - G1	25.53 ± 14.89	20.67 ± 14.26	30.17 ± 11.49	32.33 ± 10.54
36–45 - G2	16.37 ± 8.22	18.54 ± 7.94	34.13 ± 8.51	33.75 ± 9.66
46–55 - G3	17.55 ± 8.13	17.39 ± 7.86	27.54 ± 8.20	27.67 ± 7.07
56–65 - G4	18.18 ± 9.77	18.30 ± 9.52	24.96 ± 8.44	24.90 ± 9.49
+ 65 - G5	14.75 ± 11.52	13.61 ± 10.22	22.46 ± 5.66	21.93 ± 4.45

HS R: right handgrip strength; HS L: left handgrip strength

with HS reduction in a cohort of older adults [40]. In our study, neither hypertension nor use of medications – with similar prevalence rates in both groups – showed a relationship with hand strength.

There was no difference in hand strength according to the use of synthetic drugs for disease control. An isolated correlation was detected between pinch strength and the use of a biological agent, without sufficient consistency to infer a causal relationship.

Rheumatoid factor – related to poor prognosis in RA – tested positive in 78.5% of the RAG, somewhat above the average of 70% reported in the literature [18]; however, positive rheumatoid factor was not associated with hand strength. Data on ACPAs were missing for 43 patients; therefore, we did not investigate their correlation with hand strength.

A meta-analysis performed in 2010 [31] found that the average HS of patients with RA was 17.68 kgf. Although the analyzed studies had excluded individuals with diabetes mellitus, chronic obstructive pulmonary disease, and testosterone and/or growth hormone deficiencies, the abovementioned value is similar to the one we found in the present study, in which patients with such conditions were not excluded. Alomari et al. [41] found a 30% reduction in HS among patients with RA compared with healthy individuals recruited from the local community

without ischemia, systemic arterial hypertension, angina, diabetes mellitus, anemia, dyslipidemia, kidney failure, obesity, or higher cardiovascular risk and who were non-smokers. Even without excluding participants with any of these conditions, in our study, we found a similar difference between patients and controls.

The study by Dedeoğlu et al., which correlated hand strength with pain, activity of disease, functional ability, and joint lesions in RA, found average values of 24.6 kgf for HS, 4.4 kgf for tip-to-tip pinch strength, 5.65 kgf for 3-point pinch strength, and 6.65 kgf for lateral pinch strength. These values are higher than those found in the present study; however, Dedeoğlu et al. excluded individuals with diabetes mellitus, hypo- or hyperthyroidism, and cervical disc disease [9], constituting a sample with a profile different from the one met in clinical practice. In addition, their study did not include a control group.

The data described above show that there is wide variability among studies, with the issue of the inclusion of control groups being crucial. When designing our study, we took special care to include a control group with a profile similar to the one of patients seen in clinical practice, who have several associated diseases, and to match the groups according to variables with potentially strong influences on hand strength. We believe that one strength of our study is that it has satisfactory internal quality without any impairment of its external validity.

In their study, Poole et al. [42] found that among patients with RA, HS, 2-point tip-to-tip, and 3-point pinch strength were lower with lower hand functional ability, as measured by means of the CHFS. Another study assessed HS, 2-point tip-to-tip, 3-point pinch strength, and lateral pinch strength and found the same correlations with functional ability [9]. Although utilizing a small sample of 36 patients with RA, Adams et al. [4] found that DASH showed a strong correlation with HS and 3-point pinch strength and suggested that DASH is the best instrument to discriminate the functional ability of the upper limbs. Similarly, the study by Nampei et al.

Table 6 Hand strength of patients with rheumatoid arthritis (RA) and Boolean remission or active disease

Hand strength	RA in remission ($n = 8$) Mean ± SD (kgf)	RA in activity ($n = 113$)	P
Handgrip R	18.44 ± 5.71	17.69 ± 9.44	> 0.05
Handgrip L	19.63 ± 5.88	17.18 ± 9.04	> 0.05
2-point tip-to-tip pinch R	4.03 ± 1.20	3.43 ± 1.58	> 0.05
2-point tip-to-tip pinch L	4.10 ± 1.50	3.28 ± 1.57	> 0.05
3-point R	4.82 ± 0.99	4.54 ± 2.05	> 0.05
3-point L	5.44 ± 2.14	4.43 ± 2.03	> 0.05
Lateral pinch R	6.46 ± 1.62	5.99 ± 2.45	> 0.05
Lateral pinch L	6.98 ± 1.99	5.50 ± 2.30	> 0.05

kgf: kilogram-force; R: right; L: left; Independent t-test

[43] concluded that there were significant correlations of 2-point tip-to-tip, 3-point pinch strength, and lateral pinch strength with loss of hand function among patients with RA. This is the only study that also described associations with thumb and index deformities. In addition, our study showed associations with hand function, but we did not record deformities.

The DAS28 score (2.98 ± 1.32) showed a weak correlation with grip and pinch strength. A recent study found a moderate negative correlation between DAS28 score and grip and pinch strength, as measured with a dynamometer coupled to a smartphone; the authors concluded that HS might contribute to the assessment of disease activity in the outpatient setting [44]. In addition, a recent pilot study reported a reduction of HS among patients with RA and high disease activity and a negative correlation of HS with pain and swelling [38].

In contrast, in our study, we observed a weak correlation between strength and disease activity, which was not expected because the hand joints have considerable weight on the DAS28 scores. There were correlations for some of the hand strength parameters, but those correlations were below 0.3 in all cases, i.e., they were clinically insignificant.

There was not any significant difference between patients with Boolean remission and active RA; however, the low representation of the former, just 8 patients, makes drawing robust conclusions difficult [38, 45].

Like ours, one study observed a strong correlation between CHFS and HAQ [9], which reinforces the fact that RA hand involvement impairs functional ability in a global manner [46].

In the validation study of CHFS for the Brazilian population, it showed moderate correlation with DASH. Conversely, in our study, these two instruments showed a strong correlation, which might be accounted for by the fact that RA affects not only the small but also the large joints of the upper limbs. There is considerable overlap among the items assessed with the HAQ, CHFS, and DASH, rendering their simultaneous use unnecessary. However, there is a wide diversity of parameters cited in the literature; thus, we chose to apply all three instruments to enable comparisons with other studies.

Length of disease had a significant, albeit, weak correlation with functional activity, as was the case of the study by Dedeoğlu et al., who used CHFS [9], and Toyama et al. [34], who employed DASH, which must be quite variable as a function of disease aggressiveness, early diagnosis, and intensity of treatment in each patient.

We believe that our study provides a relevant reference for the measurement of hand strength in patients with RA, as the sample size was larger compared with the studies available in the literature [37, 38, 41, 45, 47]. In addition, we used a control group composed of individuals with sociocultural profiles similar to those of the RA patients and matched per sex, age, and BMI; therefore, both the internal and external validity are satisfactory. Nevertheless, we admit some limitations, such as not having recorded radiological deformities of the hands and fingers, which might be associated with measurements of strength.

Several issues still need to be elucidated. Our sample did not have a sufficient number of patients for assessment of the hand strength impairment at baseline, which might contribute to discriminating the roles that inflammation and sequelae play in loss of strength. The sample size was also restricted for the purpose of drawing conclusions on male patients. What is the correlation between hand strength and lower limb strength and risk of falls? What are the impacts of rehabilitation programs and physical exercise on hand strength among patients with RA? These data will contribute to elucidate the potential of hand strength measurement along the follow-up of patients with RA as an additional parameter for therapeutic decision-making to contribute to improve the functional ability and quality of life of patients and disease control.

We conclude that handgrip and pinch strength were lower in patients with RA compared with individuals without disease. Grip and pinch strength were inversely correlated with global functional ability and hand and upper limb function; however, they showed weak correlations with activity and length of disease.

Acknowledgements
Jamil Natour and Anamaria Jones from the Spine, Procedures, and Rehabilitation in Rheumatology Sector at Rheumatology Division, UNIFESP, Brazil for their support and for making dynamometers available.

Authors' contributions
GSS: Main author and acted in data collection, literature review and author of the manuscript. MAL: Acted in data collection. MRA: He acted as counselor and critically reviewed the manuscript for key intellectual content. All authors read and approved the final manuscript.

Authors' information
Graziela Sferra da Silva.
Specialization in physiology of physical exercise and resitance training in health, disease and aging. Main author and acted in data collection, literature review and author of the manuscript.
Mariana de Almeida Lourenço.
PhD stundent in the Human Development and Technologies Program at Unesp Rio Claro Campus, MSc in Health and Aging at Marilia School of Medicine (Famema). Acted in data colletion.
Marcos Renato de Assis.
PhD in Sciences by the Rehabilitation Program. He acted as advisor and reviewer of the manuscript.

References

1. Louzada-Júnior P, Souza BDB, Toledo RA, Ciconelli RM. Análise descritiva das características demográficas e clínicas de pacientes com artrite reumatóide no estado de São Paulo. Brazil Rev Bras Reumatol. 2007;47(2): 84–90.

2. Sociedade Brasileira de Reumatologia. Artrite reumatoide: diagnóstico e tratamento. In: Associação Médica Brasileira e Comissão Federal. São Paulo: Projeto Diretrizes; 2002.

3. Helliwell PS, Jackson S. Relationship between weakness and muscle wasting in rheumatoid arthritis. Ann Rheum Dis. 1994;53(11):726–8.

4. Vargas A, Chiapas-Gasca K, Hernández-Díaz C, Canoso JJ, Saavedra MÁ, Navarro-Zarza JE, et al. Clinical anatomy of the hand. Reumatol Clin. 2013; 8(2):25–32.

5. Bodur H, Yilmaz O, Keskin D. Hand disability and related variables in patients with rheumatoid arthritis. Rheumatol Int. 2006;26(6):541–4.

6. Adams J, Burridge J, Mullee M, Hammond A, Cooper C. Correlation between upper limb functional ability and structural hand impairment in an early rheumatoid population. Clin Rehabil. 2004;18(4):405–13.

7. Santana FS, Nascimento DC, Freitas JPM, Miranda RF, Muniz LF, Santos Neto L, et al. Avaliação da capacidade funcional em pacientes com artrite reumatoide: implicações para a recomendação de exercícios físicos. Rev Bras Reumatol. 2014;54(5):378–85.

8. Oku EC, Pinheiro GRC, Araújo PMP. Hand functional assessment in patients with rheumatoid arthritis. Fisioter Mov. 2009;22(2):221–8.

9. Dedeoğlu M, Gafuroğlu Ü, Yilmaz Ö, Bodur H. The relationship between hand grip and pinch strengths and disease activity, articular damage, pain and disability in patients with rheumatoid arthritis. Turk J Rheumatol. 2013; 28(2):69–77.

10. Villeneuve E, Nam J, Emery P. ACR-EULAR classification criteria for rheumatoid arthritis. Rev Bras Reumatol. 2010;50(5):481–3.

11. Aletaha D, Neogi T, Silman AJ, Funovits J, Felson DT, Bingham CO 3rd, et al. 2010 rheumatoid arthritis classification criteria: an American College of Rheumatology/European league against rheumatism collaborative initiative. Arthritis Rheum. 2010;62(9):2569–81.

12. Wells G, Becker JC, Teng J, Dougados M, Schiff M, Smolen J, et al. Validation of the 28-joint disease activity score (DAS28) and European league against rheumatism response criteria based on C-reactive protein against disease progression in patients with rheumatoid arthritis, and comparison with the DAS28 based on erythrythrocyte sedimentation rate. Ann Rheum Dis. 2009; 68(6):954–60.

13. Pinheiro GRC. Instrumentos de medida da atividade da artrite reumatóide - Por que e como empregá-los. Rev Bras Reumatol. 2007;47(5):362–5.

14. Prevoo ML, Van't Hof MA, Kuper HH, van Leeuwen MA, van de Putte LB, Van RP. Modified disease activity scores that include twenty-eight-joint development and validation in a prospective longitudinal study of patients with arthritis, rheumatoid. Arthritis Rheum. 1995;38(1):44–8.

15. Felson DT, Smolen JS, Wells G, Zhang B, Van LHD, Funovits J, et al. American College of Rheumatology / European league against rheumatism provisional Defi nition of remission in rheumatoid arthritis for clinical trials. Ann Rheum Dis [Internet]. 2011;70(3):404–13.

16. Bykerk VP, Massarotti EM. The new ACR/EULAR remission criteria: rationale for developing new criteria for remission. Rheumatol (United Kingdom). 2012;51(SUPPL. 6):16–20.

17. Corbacho MI, Dapueto JJ. Avaliação da capacidade funcional e da qualidade de vida de pacientes com artrite reumatoide. Rev Bras Reum. 2010;50(1):31–43.

18. Mota LMH, Cruz BA, Brenol CV, Pereira IA, Fronza LSR, Bertolo MB, et al. Consenso da Sociedade Brasileira de Reumatologia 2011 para o diagnóstico e avaliação inicial da artrite reumatoide. Rev Bras Reumatol. 2011;51(3):199–219.

19. Bruce B, Fries JF. The health assessment questionnaire (HAQ). Clin Exp Rheumatol. 2005;23(5 Suppl 39):S14–8.

20. Chiari A, Sardim CC, Natour J. Translation, cultural adaptation and reproducibility of the cochin hand functional scale questionnaire for Brazil. Clinics (Sao Paulo). 2011;66(5):731–6.

21. Lefevre-Colau MM, Poiraudeau S, Fermanian J, Etchepare F, Alnot JY, Le Viet D, et al. Responsiveness of the cochin rheumatoid hand disability scale after surgery. Rheumatology. 2001;40(8):843–50.

22. Aktekin LA, Eser F, Başkan BM, Sivas F, Malhan S, Öksüz E, et al. Disability of arm shoulder and hand questionnaire in rheumatoid arthritis patients: relationship with disease activity, HAQ, SF-36. Rheumatol Int. 2011;31(6):823–6.

23. Orfale AG, Araújo PMP, Ferraz MB, Natour J. Translation into Brazilian Portuguese, cultural adaptation and evaluation of the reliability of the disabilities of the arm, shoulder and hand questionnaire. Brazilian J Med Biol Res. 2005;38(2):293–302.

24. Shiratori AP, Iop R, Borges Júnior NG, Domenech SC, Gevaerd MS. Protocolos de avaliação da força de preensão manual em indivíduos com artrite reumatoide: uma revisão sistemática. Rev Bras Reum. 2014;54(2):140–7.

25. Kapandji AI. Fisiologia articular: esquemas comentados de mecânica humana: membro superior. 5 ed. Panamericana São Paulo. 2000;1:140–298.

26. Häkkinen A, Kautiainen H, Hannonen P, Ylinen J, Mäkinen H, Sokka T. Muscle strength, pain, and disease activity explain individual subdimensions of the health assessment questionnaire disability index, especially in women with rheumatoid arthritis. Ann Rheum Dis. 2006;65(1):30–4.

27. Mukaka MM. Statistics corner: a guide to appropriate use of correlation coefficient in medical research. Malawi Med J. 2012;24(3):69–71.

28. Vaz AE. Perfil epidemiológico e clínico de pacientes portadores de artrite reumatóide em um hospital escola de medicina em Goiânia, Goiás, Brasil. Med (Ribeirão Preto). 2013;46(2):141–53.

29. Alamanos Y, Drosos AA. Epidemiology of adult rheumatoid arthritis. Autoimmun Rev. 2005;4(3):130–6.

30. Goeldner I, Skare T, Reason I, Utiyama S. Artrite reumatoide: uma visão atual. J Bras Patol Med Lab. 2011:495–503. [cited 2015 Feb 9]; Available from: http://www.scielo.br/pdf/jbpml/v47n5/v47n5a02.pdf

31. Beenakker KG, Ling CH, Meskers CG, de Craen AJ, Stijnen T. Westendorp RGet al. Patterns of muscle strength loss with age in the general population and patients with a chronic inflammatory state. Ageing Res Rev. 2010;9(4):431–6.

32. Mathiowetz V, Kashman N, Volland G, Weber K, Dowe M, Rogers S. Grip and pinch strength: normative data for adults. Arch Phys Med Rehabil. 1985; 66(2):69–74.

33. Caporrino FA, Faloppa F, Santos JBG, Réssio C, Soares FHC, Nakachima LR, et al. Estudo populacional da força de preensão palmar com dinamômetro Jamar. Rev Bras Ortop. 1998;33(2):150–4.

34. Toyama S, Tokunaga D, Fujiwara H, Oda R, Kobashi H, Okumura H, et al. Rheumatoid arthritis of the hand: a five-year longitudinal analysis of clinical and radiographic findings. Mod Rheumatol. 2014;24(1):69–77.

35. Lenardt MH, Binotto MA, Carneiro NHK, Cechinel C, Betiolli SE, Lourenço TM. Handgrip strength and physical activity in frail elderly. Rev Esc Enferm USP. 2016;50(1):86–92. https://doi.org/10.1590/S0080-623420160000100012.

36. Nicolay CW, Walker AL. Grip strength and endurance: influences of anthropometric variation, hand dominance, and gender. Int J Ind Ergon. 2005;35(7):605–18.

37. Fraser A, Vallow J, Preston A, Cooper RG. Predicting 'normal' grip strength for rheumatoid arthritis patients. Rheumatology. 1999;38(6):521–8.

38. Iop RR, Shiratori AP, Ferreira L. Borges Júnior, Domenech SC, Gevaerd MS. Capacidade de produção de força de preensão isométrica máxima em mulheres com artrite reumatoide : um estudo piloto. Fisioter Pesq. 2015; 22(1):11–6.

39. Figueiredo IM, Sampaio RF, Mancini MC, Silva FCM, Jamar SMAPT d f d p u o d. Acta Fisiátrica. 2007;14:104–10.

40. Ashfield TA, Syddall HE, Martin HJ, Dennison EM, Cooper C, Aihie Sayer A. Grip strength and cardiovascular drug use in older people: findings from the Hertfordshire cohort study. Age Ageing. 2009;39(2):185–91.

41. Alomari MA, Keewan EF, Shammaa RA, Alawneh K, Khatib SY, Welsch MA. Vascular function and handgrip strength in rheumatoid arthritis patients. Sci World J. 2012;2012:1–6.

42. Poole JL, Santhanam DD, Latham AL. Hand impairment and activity limitations in four chronic diseases. J Hand Ther. 2013;26(3):232–6.

43. Nampei A, Shi K, Hirao M, Murase T, Yoshikawa H, Hashimoto J. Association of pinch strength with hand dysfunction, finger deformities and contact points in patients with rheumatoid arthritis. Clin Exp Rheumatol. 2011;29(6):1061.

44. Espinoza F, Le Blay P, Coulon D, Lieu S, Munro J, Jorgensen C, et al. Handgrip strength measured by a dynamometer connected to a smartphone: a new applied health technology solution for the self-assessment of rheumatoid arthritis disease activity. Rheumatology. 2016; 55(5):897–901.

45. Sheehy C, Gaffney K, Mukhtyar C. Standardized grip strength as an outcome measure in early rheumatoid arthritis. Scand J Rheumatol. 2013;42(4):289–93.

46. Birtane M, Kabayel DD, Uzunca K, Unlu E, Tastekin N. The relation of hand functions with radiological damage and disease activity in rheumatoid arthritis. Rheumatol Int. 2008;28(5):407–12.

47. Cima SR, Barone A, Porto JM, de Abreu DC. Strengthening exercises to improve hand strength and functionality in rheumatoid arthritis with hand deformities: a randomized, controlled trial. Rheumatol Int. 2013;33(3):725–32.

10

Staying in the labor force among patients with rheumatoid arthritis and associated factors in Southern Brazil

Rafael Kmiliauskis Santos Gomes[1,2,5*], Luana Cristina Schreiner[3], Mateus Oliveira Vieira[3], Patrícia Helena Machado[3] and Moacyr Roberto Cuce Nobre[4]

Abstract

Background: Rheumatoid arthritis primarily affects the working-age population and may cause key functional and work limitations. As the disease progresses, individuals become increasingly unable to conduct daily activities, which has a substantial personal and socioeconomic impact. Fairly recent prior studies showed that patients with RA stop working 20 years earlier than age-matched controls. Factors related to sociodemographic, clinical, care and disease profiles might affect the loss of work capacity. The purpose of this study was to assess the factors associated with the prevalence of working patients with rheumatoid arthritis in the municipality of Blumenau.

Methods: A cross-sectional, population-based study was conducted between July 2014 and January 2015, with 296 individuals aged 20 years or older, male and female, living in Blumenau, Santa Catarina state, Brazil, and diagnosed with rheumatoid arthritis according to the 1987 American College of Rheumatology criteria. The prevalence of working patients with RA was assessed by employment status self-reporting during the interview. The chi-squared test, Wald test and Poisson regression analysis were used to test the possible associations between the independent variables and outcome.

Results: The prevalence of working patients with rheumatoid arthritis was 44.3%. Patients aged 20 to 59 years had a 90% higher prevalence of outcome than subjects aged 60 years or older. The prevalence of working patients was 132% and 73% higher among individuals with low income and high functional disability, measured using the Health Assessment Questionnaire (HAQ), respectively.

Conclusion: The prevalence of working RA patients was highest among adult patients with low income and high functional disability. The first variable is directly related to the individual characteristic, the second reflects the socioeconomic context of the patient, and the third reflects the degree of disability caused by the disease, which may be modifiable by health professionals.

Keywords: Rheumatoid arthritis, Occupation, Job market

Background

Rheumatoid arthritis (RA) is a chronic, autoimmune, and systemic inflammatory disease characterized by symmetrical synovitis of the peripheral joints. Inflammation of the synovial membranes causes pain, edema and stiffness and, if untreated, may lead to joint destruction and a loss of functional capacity [1, 2]. RA occurs in 0.24% to 1% of the population, predominantly among women between the fourth and sixth decades of life [3, 4]. According to a multicenter study, the prevalence of RA in Brazil is similar, ranging from 0.2 to 1% of the population [5].

RA primarily affects the working-age population and may cause key functional and work limitations [6]. As the disease progresses, individuals become increasingly unable to conduct daily activities, which has a substantial personal and socioeconomic impact [7, 8]. Studies report that 40% of patients with early-onset disease and

* Correspondence: gomesmed2002@ibest.com.br
[1]Specialty Center of the City of Blumenau, Blumenau, Santa Catarina State (SC), Brazil
[2]Specialty Center of the City of Brusque, Brusque, SC, Brazil
Full list of author information is available at the end of the article

60% of patients with advanced disease were unable to work [9, 10].

Fairly recent prior studies showed that patients with RA stop working 20 years earlier than age-matched controls [11]. Researchers who conducted a study in Germany concluded that 59% of patients continued working until 12 months after diagnosis, whereas 17% stopped working and received disability payments, and 9% lost their jobs because of RA but received no disability pension [12]. Another study, conducted in the state of São Paulo, showed that 30% of patients were actually employed and that the others were homemakers, on leaves of absence or unemployed [13].

Factors related to sociodemographic, clinical, care and disease profiles might affect the loss of work capacity. Early diagnosis combined with disease-modifying antirheumatic drugs (DMARDs) is the most effective method to reduce the prevalence of disability [13]. Other predictors, such as age, education level, the presence of comorbidities and the use of biopharmaceuticals may also be associated with disease progression [13, 14].

Studies on RA among working-age populations are increasingly conducted in developed countries. However, few studies considering this approach in Brazil were identified. Among them, a study conducted in the state of São Paulo determined that 30% of such patients were actively working, 34% were unemployed, 31% were retirees, and 5% were working retirees [15].

To collect additional data on this subject, the present study aimed to assess the percentage of and the possible factors associated with working patients with RA in Blumenau.

Methods

This cross-sectional, population-based study was conducted between July 2014 and January 2015, with 296 individuals aged 20 years or older, male and female, living in the municipality of Blumenau in the south region of Brazil and diagnosed with rheumatoid arthritis according to the 1987 American College of Rheumatology criteria. According to the United Nations Development Program (UNDP), this municipality had a Human Development Index (HDI) of 0.806 in 2010, ranking 25th among Brazilian municipalities [16]. The number of inhabitants in the study age group corresponded to 221,839 people, which is equivalent to 71.7% of the municipality population [17].

The formula for calculating the sample size required to estimate the prevalence of an event in a simple random sample was used considering the following parameters: 0.5% RA prevalence (1110 patients), 50% prevalence of exposure and unknown outcome, 5% sample error and 95% confidence level. The effective calculated sample size was 286 individuals. The participants

were recruited from all primary care centers (Unidades Básicas de Saúde – UBS), the specialty outpatient clinic and the specialty pharmacy of the municipality.

Sample loss occurred when households were visited twice, once on the weekend and again in the evening, and no resident was at home, the resident had moved or refused to participate in the study on both occasions. The data collection team consisted of a local supervisor docent and 8 medical academics of the Regional University of Blumenau (Universidade Regional de Blumenau – FURB) previously trained to conduct structured interviews at home and, if necessary, by telephone. Quality control was performed in 20% of respondents, who were interviewed for the second time using a short questionnaire.

The dependent variable analyzed was the employment status at the time of the interview, considering the prevalence of working patients with RA, in any type of occupation, the outcome. Conversely, the independent variables were selected based on the sociodemographic, clinical, care and disease profiles. The following sociodemographic variables were analyzed: sex, age in completed years, ranging from 20 to 59 years for adults and 60 years or older for the elderly, in accordance with the status of the elderly/Ministry of Health (Ministério da Saúde – MS), current monthly personal income, ranging from 0 to 2 and greater than 2 minimum wages, education in years of completed study and self-reported skin color, categorized as white, brown, black, yellow or indigenous (IBGE). The clinical variable analyzed was the presence of comorbidities. The care variables analyzed were consultations with another rheumatologist during their treatment, number of consultations with a rheumatologist in the last 12 months, type of medical care classified into two groups, the Unified Health System (Sistema Único de Saúde – SUS; free, public healthcare system) and Public-Private Healthcare (supplementary healthcare system), defined according to the MS, in addition to private healthcare (fee-for-service care), and diagnostic delay in months, which was calculated by subtracting the date of the medical diagnosis by the date of the onset of symptoms. Lastly, the disease-related variables were total disease time in months, current use of DMARDs (methotrexate, sulfasalazine, leflunomide and antimalarial drugs), current use of anti-TNF immunobiologicals (adalimumab, etanercept, infliximab), Health Assessment Questionnaire (HAQ) score, ranging from 0 to 1 (mild disability) and from 1.1 to 3 (moderate and severe disability), presence of rheumatoid factor lower than or equal to 60 (negative or low titer) or higher than 60 (high titer) and, finally, the presence of radiographic changes (joint erosion) in the hands.

The data were entered into a system developed for this study in an Excel file format, and the final file was subsequently exported to the software Stata 10.0 (Stata

Corporation, College Station, United States). The distribution of the variables of interest was analyzed using the mean, standard deviation and median for continuous variables, and the frequency and percentage for categorical variables. To test the association between the employment status and the independent variables, the chi-squared test and, where appropriate, the Wald test were used. Then, crude and Poisson regression analyses were performed to assess the association between the study factors and the dependent variables, estimating the crude and adjusted prevalence ratios (PRs), the respective 95% confidence intervals and the p value.

All variables with p value < 0.20 in the crude analysis were considered for entry into the final model. The variables that maintained a p value ≤0.05 or that fitted the final model remained in the adjusted regression model. The researchers chose to sequentially include sociodemographic, clinical, care and disease-related variables in the regression model.

This research study was submitted to the research ethics committees of the University of São Paulo (Universidade de São Paulo – USP) and of the FURB (protocol numbers 339/13 and 133/12, respectively) and approved; all participants signed the informed consent form.

Results

A total of 336 patients were identified. After excluding deceased patients and those who refused to participate in the study or patients without data for the dependent variable, 296 patients were included in the study. Those individuals who were unemployed, pensioners, housewives or regular or RA-unrelated disability retirees were excluded from the analysis of the dependent variable data, which resulted in an effective final sample of 185 patients (Fig. 1).

In the sociodemographic analysis, females (82.7%) and adults (71.9%) accounted for most individuals, with a mean age of 54.5 years, ranging from 26 to 79 years and with a standard deviation (SD) of 10.4. The mean income was 1.9 minimum wages (SD: 1.4). Approximately one-third of the subjects had education ranging from 0 to 4 years of completed study, with a mean education of 7.9 years (SD: 4.3). Regarding the care variables, the diagnostic delay was longer than or equal to 4 months in 74.1% of the sample and the mean diagnostic delay time was 27.6 months, ranging from 1 to 240 months (SD: 45). Most respondents stated that they visited another rheumatologist (72.4%), with a mean of 3.4 visits in the last 12 months (SD: 2.4). Regarding the type of care, private or public-private healthcare was predominant (55.9%). The analysis of the disease variables showed that most subjects had a disease time longer than or equal to 25 months (89.9%), with a mean of 127.8 months, ranging from 2 to 420 months (SD: 95.8; Table 1).

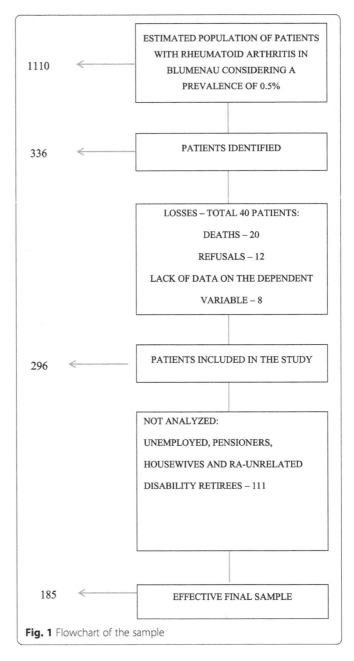

Fig. 1 Flowchart of the sample

The crude analysis showed an increase in outcome with the decrease in age and among low-income individuals. The prevalence of working patients with RA was 64%, 37% and 66% higher among patients with up to 4 years of education, comorbidities and a higher HAQ score, respectively. Due to confounding between education and income in the adjusted analysis, the variables education and comorbidities lost significance and were excluded from the final model, which consisted of age, income and HAQ. The prevalence of working patients was 90% higher among adults than among the elderly. The prevalence of working patients was 132% higher among low-income individuals than among those earning more than 2 minimum wages. The prevalence of working patients was 73% higher among individuals with

Table 1 Description of the sample and of the prevalence of working patients with rheumatoid arthritis in Blumenau, Santa Catarina state, Brazil, according to the independent variables, 2014

Variables	Sample		Working Patients	
	n^*	%	Prevalence (%) 95% CI	p
Total	185	100.0	44.3 (37.0-51.5)	
Sex (n = 185)				0.943**
Male	32	17.3	43.7 (25.5-61.9)	
Female	153	82.7	44.4 (36.4-52.4)	
Age in years (n = 185)				0.025***
20-59 (adults)	133	71.9	48.8 (40.2-57.4)	
≥ 60 (elderly)	52	28.1	32.6 (19.5-45.8)	
Income in minimum wages (n = 154)				0.001***
0-2	117	75.9	34.1 (25.5-42.9)	
> 2	37	24.1	64.8 (48.2-81.0)	
Education in completed years (n = 176)				0.000***
0-4	60	34.1	25.0 (13.7-36.2)	
> 4	116	65.9	54.3 (45.1-63.5)	
Self-reported skin color (n = 178)				0.686**
White	165	92.7	44.2 (36.5-51.9)	
Brown and black	13	7.3	38.4 (7.8-69.0)	
Presence of comorbidities (n = 181)				0.016**
No	87	48.1	52.8 (42.1-63.5)	
Yes	94	51.9	35.1 (25.2-44.9)	
Consultation with another rheumatologist (n = 181)				0.900**
No	50	27.6	44.0 (29.7-58.2)	
Yes	131	72.4	45.0 (36.4-53.6)	
Number of visits in the last 12 months (n = 176)				0.111***
0-2	74	42.1	51.3 (39.6-63.0)	
≥ 3	102	57.9	39.2 (29.5-48.8)	
Type of medical care (n = 163)				0.637**
SUS	72	44.1	40.2 (28.6-51.8)	
Private and Public-Private Partnership	91	55.9	43.9 (33.5-54.3)	
Diagnostic delay in months (n = 178)				0.982***
0-3	46	25.9	45.6 (30.6-60.6)	
≥ 4	132	74.1	45.4 (36.8-54.0)	
Disease time in months (n = 185)				0.681***
0-24	20	10.9	4.0 (16.4-63.5)	
≥ 25	165	89.1	44.8 (37.1-52.5)	
Current use of DMARDs (n = 168)				0.724**
No	46	27.3	45.6 (30.6-60.6)	
Yes	122	72.7	42.6 (33.7-51.5)	
Current use of biologicals (anti-TNF) (n = 172)				0.162**
No	116	67.4	42.2 (33.1-51.3)	

Table 1 Description of the sample and of the prevalence of working patients with rheumatoid arthritis in Blumenau, Santa Catarina state, Brazil, according to the independent variables, 2014 *(Continued)*

Variables	Sample		Working Patients	
	n^*	%	Prevalence (%) 95% CI	p
Yes	56	32.6	53.5 (40.0-67.0)	
HAQ score (n = 110)				0.009[***]
0-1	45	41.0	62.2 (47.4-76.9)	
1.1-3	65	59.0	36.9 (24.8-48.9)	
Rheumatoid factor (n = 160)				0.873[**]
0-60 (normal or low titer)	90	56.2	45.4 (35.0-56.0)	
≥ 61 (high titers)	70	43.8	44.2 (32.3-56.2)	
Radiography of hands with joint erosion (n = 151)				0.375[**]
No	62	41.0	50.0 (37.1-62.8)	
Yes	89	59.0	42.6 (32.2-53.1)	

95% CI 95% confidence interval
[*]Number of working patients with rheumatoid arthritis who were on sick leave or were disability retirees
[**]Chi-squared test
[***]Wald test

high functional disability, assessed using the HAQ (Table 2).

Discussion

The present study showed that job retention among RA patients in the city of Blumenau was 44.3%. Higher percentages of working RA patients were identified among low-income adult RA patients with high functional disability. The first variable is directly related to individual characteristics, the second reflects the socioeconomic context of the patient and the third reveals the degree of disability caused by RA.

Studies conducted in Germany and the Netherlands found 41% and 40% working RA patients, respectively [12, 18]. Furthermore, a systematic review of North American data found rates of working RA patients ranging from 22% to 76% [19]. Regarding the Brazilian data, a study conducted in Sorocaba found a prevalence of 46% working RA patients, similar to that found in the present study [20]. However, another study conducted in São Paulo found a 31% prevalence of such working patients, possibly due to different inclusion criteria and sampling and to the use of secondary data from medical records [13].

Age is a non-modifiable predictive factor of work disability. Our study confirmed this finding because the prevalence of working RA patients among elderly individuals was almost twice as high as that among adults. Synergistically, two systematic reviews of cohort studies on disability also reported the existence of this relationship [21, 22].

A study with 878 patients, conducted in the Netherlands, showed that a low socioeconomic status was related to worsened disease activity, physical and mental health and quality of life [23]. Similarly, a Latin American cohort with 1093 patients from 14 countries, including Brazil, concluded that low and middle incomes were associated with increased disease activity and higher HAQ scores [24]. Notably however, this association has not been consistently reported [25].

In contrast to the aforementioned findings, our study found a prevalence of working RA patients among low-income individuals who was 132% higher than that among individuals with a higher income. This finding suggests social inequality because the prevalence of working RA patients was expected to be higher among individuals with a higher income considering that higher income is usually associated with easier access to information, medical consultations and pharmacological treatments. This finding may be due to circumstances directly related to the individual, such as a lack of access to information, lack of knowledge of the right to disability retirement, limited legal expenses, lack of payment to social security and the need to work to avoid income loss.

Regarding the HAQ, the results showed that the prevalence of working RA patients was 73% higher among individuals with high disability than among individuals with a low HAQ score. This finding may be related to low-income patients with increased inflammatory activity of the disease and, therefore, increased disability [24]. Although this variable had a lower sample number than the others, an association with outcome was observed. An English study of two cohorts, totaling 244 patients, described HAQ as the most important factor of work disability [26].

Regarding education, the prevalence of working RA patients among the group with more than 4 years of study was 64% higher in the crude analysis; however,

Table 2 Crude and adjusted Poisson regression analyses of the prevalence of working patients with rheumatoid arthritis as a function of independent variables in Blumenau, Santa Catarina state, Brazil, 2014

Variables	Crude analysis		Adjusted analysis	
	PRc (95% CI)	p	PRa (95% CI)	p
Sex (n = 185)		0.943[*]		NS
Male	0.98 (0.70-1.38)			
Female	1			
Age in years (n = 185)		0.023		0.001
20-59 (adults)	1.33 (1.04-1.71)		1.90 (1.31-2.75)	
≥ 60 (elderly)	1		1	
Income in minimum wages (n = 154)		0.007		0.008
0-2	1.87 (1.18-2.96)		2.32 (1.24-4.36)	
> 2	1		1	
Education in completed years (n = 176)		0.000		0.676[**]
0-4	1.64 (1.28-2.10)		1.08 (0.74-1.58)	
> 4	1		1	
Self-reported skin color (n = 178)		0.669[*]		NS
White	1			
Black + Brown	1.1 (0.70-1.73)			
Presence of comorbidities (n = 181)		0.019		0.464[**]
No	1		1	
Yes	1.37 (1.05-1.80)		1.08 (0.74-1.58)	
Consultation with another rheumatologist (n = 181)		0.900[*]		NS
No	1			
Yes	0.98 (0.73-1.31)			
Number of visits in the last 12 months (n = 176)		0.121		0.619[**]
0-2	1.03 (0.99-1.08)		0.91 (0.65-1.28)	
≥ 3	1		1	
Type of medical care (n = 163)		0.637[*]		NS
SUS	1.06 (0.81-1.38)			
Private + Public-Private Partnership	1			
Diagnostic delay in months (n = 178)		0.982[*]		NS
0-3	1			
≥ 4	1.01 (0.73-1.36)			
Disease time in months (n = 185)		0.667[*]		NS
0-24	1			
≥ 25	0.91 (0.62-1.35)			
Current use of DMARDs (n = 168)		0.729[*]		NS
No	0.94 (0.69-1.28)			
Yes	1			
Current use of biologicals (n = 172)		0.184		0.481[**]
No	1.24 (0.90-1.71)		1.17 (0.79-1.73)	

Table 2 Crude and adjusted Poisson regression analyses of the prevalence of working patients with rheumatoid arthritis as a function of independent variables in Blumenau, Santa Catarina state, Brazil, 2014 *(Continued)*

Variables	Crude analysis		Adjusted analysis	
	PRc (95% CI)	p	PRa (95% CI)	p
Yes	1		1	
HAQ (n = 110)		0.017		0.017
0-1	1		1	
1.1-3	1.66 (1.09-2.54)		1.73 (1.10-2.72)	
Rheumatoid factor (n = 160)		0.873[**]		NS
0-60 (normal or low titer)	1			
≥ 61 (high titers)	1.02 (0.77-1.35)			
Radiography of hands with joint erosion (n = 151)		0.385[**]		NS
No	1			
Yes	1.14 (0.84-1.55)			

95% CI 95% confidence interval, *NS* non-significant p value, *PRc* crude prevalence ratio, *PRa* adjusted prevalence ratio
[*]Excluded from the adjusted analysis (p value > 0.20)
[**]Excluded from the final model (p value > 0.05)

when subjected to adjusted analysis, the variable lost significance. Despite this result, a systematic review of studies on RA found a significant association between higher levels of education and the prevalence of working patients [21]. The same result was found regarding the presence of comorbidities, which was initially 37% higher among working RA patients, although the lack of a significant association was subsequently assessed. A Saudi study also found no significant association between the prevalence of working patients and the presence of comorbidities, although comorbidities were found in 95% of the subjects [27]. Conversely, a longitudinal study conducted in the United States with patients from the National Data Bank for Rheumatic Diseases, a national database for rheumatologic diseases, found progression of work disability, particularly in individuals with cardiovascular disease and a high number of comorbidities [28].

Regarding the sociodemographic profile variables, although sex and self-reported skin color were not significantly associated with the outcome (possibly due to the predominance of white over brown and black individuals in the sample), studies describing significant associations between these variables and the prevalence of working patients have been reported in the literature. A study showed that women had a higher risk for being out of the labor force, whereas men were more likely to continue working and to report negative workplace experiences [29].

Regarding the care variables, a Brazilian study showed that diagnostic delay may increase the prevalence of loss of work capacity and found a mean diagnostic delay of 39 months [20]. Although a lower mean diagnostic delay was found in our study (27.6 months), the importance of this variable for early treatment is noteworthy.

Regarding the disease variables, disease time is directly related to decreased prevalence of working RA patients.

A cohort of Swedish patients with RA followed for 15 years showed that after 5, 10 and 15 years of disease, 65%, 61% and 56% of the individuals were actively working, respectively [30]. The lack of association and the decreased prevalence of outcome in our study may be related to the sample, which predominantly consisted of patients with established RA (> 2 years), to the mean disease time of approximately 10 years and to the fact that most subjects had higher levels of education.

Although the prevalence of working RA patients was not associated with the use of DMARDs or anti-TNF biologicals, several studies showing that these drugs may decrease the number of sick-leave days have been published [31–33]. The work capacity of patients may approximate that of healthy individuals during early treatment [34, 35].

The study limitations might include methodological differences caused by the lack of consistency in defining work disability [10], specific population characteristics, the very high HDI of the municipality of Blumenau (which differs from the rest of the country), the sample losses of some variables such as the HAQ score (which would likely be more significantly associated with the prevalence of working RA patients in a larger sample), possible memory biases of the respondents and reverse causation typical of cross-sectional studies.

The strengths of the study were the representative sample of the population of the municipality where the study was conducted (encompassing all social classes), the interviews conducted through pre-structured questionnaires by trained staff and the quality control of the interviews. The labor market context presumably had no effect on the results because the unemployment rate in Brazil in the study period ranged from 4.3% to 5.3%, in contrast to Blumenau, which had a 2% unemployment rate in 2014. Furthermore, the state of Santa Catarina had the lowest unemployment rate of all Brazilian states in 2015 (IBGE).

Conclusion

This study analyzed the prevalence of RA patients in the labor market in a southern region of Brazil. A higher prevalence of working RA patients was found among adult, low-income individuals with high functional disability. We suggest new population-based studies to improve the consistency of information on the employment status of patients with RA and to signal future budgetary impacts on social security.

Abbreviations

DMARDs: Disease-modifying antirheumatic drugs; FURB: Regional University of Blumenau; HAQ: Health assessment questionnaire; HDI: Human development index; MH: Ministry of Health; PR: Prevalence ratios; RA: Rheumatoid arthritis; SD : Standard deviation; SUS: Unified Health System; UBS: Primary care centers; UNPD: United Nations Development Program

Authors' contributions

RKSG and MRCN contributed to elaboration, literature review, statistical analysis and article writing. LCS, MOV and PHM contributed to writing and literature review. All approved final version for submission in journal.

Author details

[1]Specialty Center of the City of Blumenau, Blumenau, Santa Catarina State (SC), Brazil. [2]Specialty Center of the City of Brusque, Brusque, SC, Brazil. [3]School of Medicine, Regional University of Blumenau (Universidade Regional de Blumenau – FURB), Blumenau, Brazil. [4]Clinical Epidemiology Unit, Heart Institute, University Hospital, School of Medicine, University of São Paulo (Universidade de São Paulo – USP), São Paulo, SP, Brazil. [5]Centro de Referência Policlínica Lindolf Bell, Rua: Dois de Setembro, 1234 - Itoupava Norte, 3° andar, sala 1, Blumenau, SC CEP: 89052-003, Brazil.

References

1. Cheung PP, Dougados M, Andre V, Balandraud N, Chales G, Chary-Valckenaere I, et al. Improving agreement in assessment of synovitis in rheumatoid arthritis. Jt Bone Spine. 2013;80(2):155–9.
2. Mota LMH, Laurindo IMM, Neto LL dos S, FAC L, Viana SL, Mendlovitz PS, et al. Diagnóstico por imagem da artrite reumatoide inicial. Rev Bras Reumatol. 2012;52(5):761–6.
3. Hoy D, March L, Brooks P, Blyth F, Woolf A, Bain C, et al. The global burden of rheumatoid arthritis: estimates from the global burden of disease 2010 study. Ann Rheum Dis. 2014;73(6):968–74.
4. Gabriel SE. The epidemiology of rheumatoid arthritis. Rheum Dis Clin N Am. 2001;27:269–81.
5. Marques WV, Cruz VA, Rego J, da Silva NA. Influência das comorbidades na capacidade funcional de pacientes com artrite reumatoide. Rev Bras Reumatol. 2015;56(1):14–21.
6. Schoels M, Wong J, Scott DL, Zink A, Richards P, Landewé R, et al. Economic aspects of treatment options in rheumatoid arthritis: a systematic literature review informing the EULAR recommendations for the management of rheumatoid arthritis. Ann Rheum Dis. 2010;69(6):995–1003.
7. Kwoh CK, Simms RW, Anderson LG, Erlandson DM, Greene JM, Moncur C, et al. Guidelines for the management of rheumatoid arthritis: American College of Rheumatology ad hoc Committee on clinical guidelines. Arthritis Rheum. 1996;39(5):713–22.
8. Diretrizes P. Projeto Diretrizes Artrite Reumatóide : Diagnóstico e Tratamento Projeto Diretrizes; 2002. p. 1–15.
9. Han C, Smolen J, Kavanaugh A, St. Clair EW, Baker D, Bala M. Comparison of employability outcomes among patients with early or long-standing rheumatoid arthritis. Arthritis Care Res. 2008;59(4):510–4.
10. Verstappen SMM, Bijlsma JWJ, Verkleij H, Buskens E, Blaauw AAM, ter Borg EJ, et al. Overview of work disability in rheumatoid arthritis patients as observed in cross-sectional and longitudinal surveys. Arthritis Rheum 2004; 51(3):488–497.
11. Woolf AD, Pfleger B. Burden of major musculoskeletal conditions. Bull World Health Organ. 2003;81(9):646–56.
12. Merkesdal S, Ruof J, Schffski O, Bernitt K, Zeidler H, Mau W. Indirect medical costs in early rheumatoid arthritis: composition of and changes in indirect costs within the first three years of disease. Arthritis Rheum. 2001;44(3):528–34.
13. Louzada P, Souza BDB, Toledo RA, Ciconelli RM. Análise descritiva das caracteríticas demográficas e clínicas de pacientes com artrite reumatóide no estado de São Paulo. Brazil Rev Bras Reumatol. 2007;47(2):84–90.
14. Vilsteren van M, Boot CR, Knol DL, van Schaardenburg D, Voskuyl AE, Steenbeek R, et al. Productivity at work and quality of life in patients with rheumatoid arthritis. BMC Musculoskelet Disord. 2015;16(1):107.
15. De Abreu MM, Kowalski SC, Ciconelli RM, Ferraz MB. Avaliação do perfil sociodemográfico, clínico-laboratorial e terapêutico dos pacientes com artrite reumatóide que participaram de projetos de pesquisa na Escola Paulista de Medicina, nos últimos 25 anos. Rev Bras Reumatol. 2006;46(2):103–9.
16. Programa das Nações Unidas - PNUD. Atlas do Desenvolvimento Humano no Brasil 2003. Available from: http://www.pnud.org.br/atlas. [Accessed in 21 Feb 2016].
17. Instituto Brasileiro de Geografia e Estatística-IBGE. Sinopse do Censo Demográfico de 2010/2011. Available from: http://www.ibge.gov.br/home/estatistica/populacao/censo2010/. [Accessed in 21 Feb 2016].
18. Young A, Dixey J, Kulinskaya E, Cox N, Davies P, Devlin J, et al. Which patients stop working because of rheumatoid arthritis? Results of five years' follow up in 732 patients from the early RA study (ERAS). Ann Rheum Dis. 2002;61(4):335–40.
19. Cooper NJ. Economic burden of rheumatoid arthritis: a systematic review. Rheumatology (Oxford). 2000;39(1):28–33.
20. de Melo Jr VA, Aguiar FA, Baleroni TCG, Novaes GS. Análise temporal entre início dos sintomas, avaliação reumatológica e tratamento com drogas modificadoras de doença em pacientes com artrite reumatóide. Revista da Faculdade de Ciências Médicas de Sorocaba. 2008;10(2):12–5.
21. De Croon EM, Sluiter JK, Nijssen TF, Dijkmans BA, Lankhorst GJ, Frings-Dresen MH. Predictive factors of work disability in rheumatoid arthritis: a systematic literature review. Ann Rheum Dis. 2004;63:1362–7.
22. Detaille SI, Heerkens YF, Engels JA, van der Gulden JW, van Dijk FJ. Common prognostic factors of work disability among employees with a chronic somatic disease: a systematic review of cohort studies. Scand J Work Environ Health. 2009;35:261–81.
23. Jacobi CE, Mol GD, Boshuizen HC, Rupp I, Dinant HJ, Van Den Bos GAM. Impact of socioeconomic status on the course of rheumatoid arthritis and on related use of health care services. Arthritis Rheum. 2003;49(4):567–73.
24. Massardo L, Pons-Estel BA, Wojdyla D, Cardiel MH, Galarza-Maldonado CM, Sacnun MP, et al. Early rheumatoid arthritis in Latin America: low socioeconomic status related to high disease activity at baseline. Arthritis Care Res. 2012;64(8):1135–43.
25. Liao KP, Karlson EW. Classification and epidemiology of rheumatoid arthritis. Rheumatology. 2011;5:823–8.
26. Barrett EM, Scott DG, Wiles NJ, et al. The impact of rheumatoid arthritis on employment status in the early years of disease: a UK community-based study. Rheumatology. 2000;39:1403–9.
27. Janoudi N, Almoallim H, Husien W, Noorwali A, Ibrahim A. Work ability and work disability evaluation in Saudi patients with rheumatoid arthritis: special emphasis on work ability among housewives. Saudi Med J. 2013;34(11): 1167–72.
28. Michaud K, Wallenstein G, Wolfe F. Treatment and nontreatment predictors of health assessment questionnaire disability progression in rheumatoid arthritis: a longitudinal study of 18,485 patients. Arthritis Care Res (Hoboken). 2011;63(3):366–72.
29. Kaptein SA, Gignac MA, Badley EM. Differences in the workforce experiences of women and men with arthritis disability: a population health perspective. Arthritis Rheum. 2009;61:605–13.
30. Eberhardt K, Larsson BM, Nived K, Lindqvist E. Work disability in rheumatoid arthritis–development over 15 years and evaluation of predictive factors over time. J Rheumatol. 2007;34:481–7.

31. Augustsson J, Neovius M, Cullinane-Carli C, et al. Patients with rheumatoid arthritis treated with tumour necrosis factor antagonists increase their participation in the workforce: potential for significant long-term indirect cost gains (data from a population-based registry). Ann Rheum Dis. 2010;69: 126–31.

32. Sokka T. Work disability in early rheumatoid arthritis. Clin Exp Rheumatol. 2003;21:S71–4.

33. Puolakka K, Kautiainen H, Möttönen T, Hannonen P, Korpela M, Julkunen H, et al. Impact of initial aggressive drug treatment with a combination of disease-modifying antirheumatic drugs on the development of work disability in early rheumatoid arthritis: a five-year randomized followup trial. Arthritis Rheumatism. 2004;50:55–62.

34. Tiippana-Kinnunen T, Paimela L, Peltomaa R, Kautiainen H, Laasonen L, Leirisalo-Repo M. Work disability in Finnish patients with rheumatoid arthritis: a 15-year follow-up. Clin Exp Rheumatol. 2014;32:88–94.

35. Puolakka K, Kautiainen H, Mattonen T. Predictors of productivity loss in early rheumatoid arthritis: a year follow up study. Ann Rheum Dis. 2005;64:130–3.

11

Clinical and pathophysiologic relevance of autoantibodies in rheumatoid arthritis

Sara de Brito Rocha*, Danielle Cristiane Baldo and Luis Eduardo Coelho Andrade

Abstract

Rheumatoid arthritis (RA) is an autoimmune/inflammatory disease affecting 0.5 to 1% of adults worldwide and frequently leads to joint destruction and disability. Early diagnosis and early and effective therapy may prevent joint damage and lead to better long-term results. Therefore, reliable biomarkers and outcome measures are needed. Refinement of the understanding of molecular pathways involved in disease pathogenesis have been achieved by combining knowledge on RA-associated genes, environmental factors and the presence of serological elements. The presence of autoantibodies is a distinctive feature of RA. Rheumatoid Factor and Anti-Citrullinated Protein Antibodies are the two most remarkable autoantibodies in RA and provide different clinical and pathophysiological information. They precede the onset of disease symptoms and predict a more severe disease course, indicating a pathogenetic role in RA. Therefore, they promote a more accurate prognosis and contribute for a better disease management. Several RA-associated autoantibody systems have been identified: Anti-Carbamylated Antibodies, Anti-BRAF, Anti-Acetylated, Anti-PAD4 antibodies and others. Hopefully, the characterization of a comprehensive array of novel autoantibody systems in RA will provide unique pathogenic insights of relevance for the development of diagnostic and prognostic approaches compatible with an effective personalized medicine.

Keywords: Rheumatoid arthritis, Autoantibodies, ACPA, Anti-CarP, Rheumatoid factor, Personalized medicine

Introduction

Rheumatoid arthritis (RA) is an autoimmune/inflammatory disease affecting 0.5 to 1% of adults worldwide [1]. Women are three times more susceptible than men and the disease is more frequent at the age of 40–50 years [1]. RA frequently leads to joint destruction and disability [1]. Early diagnosis and early and effective therapy may prevent joint damage and lead to better long-term results [1]. Optimal management of RA is needed within 3 to 6 months after onset of disease, since substantial irreversible joint damage has been shown to occur within the first 2 years. Therefore, reliable biomarkers and outcome measures are needed in order to establish early diagnosis, assess prognosis, and achieve a better disease management [2, 3].

The etiology of rheumatoid arthritis (RA) is not known, although genetic, environmental factors and serological elements have been identified to play a role in disease initiation and progression [4]. Smoking is now a well-known environmental trigger [5]. Genetic contribution is estimated around 50 to 60% and therefore, genetic factors have an important impact on susceptibility to RA [4]. The strongest predisposing gene variants are found in the human leukocyte antigen (HLA) genes, accounting for 30 to 50% of overall genetic susceptibility to RA [6]. Multiple RA risk alleles within the HLA-DRB1 gene share a conserved amino acid sequence, leading to the "shared epitope" (SE) concept [6]. The presence of one HLA SE allele confers an odds ratio to develop RA around 4, and the presence of two SE copies increases the odds ratio to approximately 11 [7].

The presence of autoantibodies is a distinctive feature of RA. The two autoantibody systems most commonly used as an aid for diagnosing/classifying RA are rheumatoid factor (RF) and anti-citrullinated protein antibodies (ACPA). They precede the onset of disease symptoms and predict a more severe disease course, indicating a pathogenic role in RA. Therefore, they promote a more accurate prognosis and contribute for a better disease management. Their importance was recently emphasized by the inclusion of ACPA alongside the previously included RF on ACR/EULAR 2010 RA diagnostic criteria [8].

* Correspondence: sb.rocha@gmail.com
Rheumatology Division, Escola Paulista de Medicina, Universidade Federal de São Paulo, Disciplina de Reumatologia, Rua Botucatu 740, 3o andar, São Paulo, SP ZIP:04023-062, Brazil

The hypothesis that autoantibodies may play a pathophysiologic role has been fueled by the discovery of strong associations linking the HLA-DRB1 SE and PTPN22 alleles, smoking and the presence of autoantibodies, in particular ACPA [7]. Recently, other forms of post-translational modification have been associated with the generation of RA-relevant autoantigens and autoantibodies that can be used as useful biomarkers [9]. In predisposed subjects, failure in keeping self-tolerance might be elicited by post-translational modifications, since these processes might promote generation of neoepitopes and neo-(auto)antigens [9].

This article provides an update on the state of the art on autoantibodies in rheumatoid arthritis (RA).

Rheumatoid factor

Characteristics

The first autoantibody discovered in RA patients is the RF. It was first described in 1940 as an antibody directed against serum gamma-globulins and promoted the agglutination of sheep red blood cells sensitized by subagglutinating doses of rabbit antibodies [10]. In 1948, these antibodies were described in patients with RA, and in 1952 they were called RF due to their strong association with RA [10]. RF are autoantibodies that directly bind to the Fc portion of the aggregated IgG and are locally produced by B cells present in lymphoid follicles and germinal center-like structures that develop in inflamed RA synovium [10, 11].

RF testing in RA patients has a sensitivity ranging from 60 to 90% and a specificity ranging from 48 to 92%, according to different studies [10]. RF has limited specificity, since it can also be found in healthy controls and patients with other autoimmune diseases such as systemic lupus erythematosus and systemic sclerosis, and in non-autoimmune diseases, such as chronic infections and cancer [4, 10, 12] RF is found in multiple immunoglobulin isotypes (IgM, IgG and IgA) wherein IgM-RF is the one usually measured in most clinical laboratories, being detected in 60–80% of RA patients [12]. The simultaneous occurrence of IgM, IgA, and IgG RF is present in up to 52% of RA patients but in fewer than 5% of patients with other connective tissue diseases. The combined occurrence of IgM and IgA RF has high diagnostic specificity for rheumatoid arthritis, but the presence of IgA and IgG RF isotypes in absence of IgM-RF is less specific, since they are also prevalent in patients with diverse connective

tissue diseases [12, 13]. IgM-RF specificity increases considerably at high titres [4, 10, 12]. RF reactivity presents several differences in healthy and RA patients. Healthy subjects usually present poly-reactive, low affinity, low titer IgM class RF, whereas RA patients usually present more than one isotype RF at higher titer and with higher avidity [10]. It has been shown that high titer RF in healthy subjects is associated with increased risk of developing RA [14]. Finally, IgM RF has increased frequency in healthy elderly people, which suggests that they may be also related to the age-related immune deregulation [12, 14].

Role in pathogenesis

There is evidence supporting the concept that RF is a pathogenic autoantibody with a key role in the physiopathology of RA [15]. In normal conditions, transient production of low-affinity IgM RF is regularly induced by immune complexes [15] and polyclonal B-cell activators, such as bacterial lipopolysaccharides and Epstein-Barr virus [10]. The physiological role of RF under normal conditions includes promoting stability of IgG bound to solid surfaces, such as bacterial walls; enhancing immune complex clearance by increasing its stability and size; helping B cells uptake immune complexes, and thereby, efficiently present antigens to T cells; and facilitating complement fixation by binding to IgG containing immune complexes [15, 16]. High affinity and high-titer RF in RA synovial fluid are believed to exert such functions in a pathogenic manner and thus to potentiate inflammation and antigen trapping in the joints [16]. In RA, RF may induce the formation of immune complexes at the sites of synovial inflammation, ensuing the activation of complement and leukocyte infiltration (Fig. 1) [16]. B cells with RF specificity migrate into the synovium of RA patients, presenting a variety of antigens to T cells and this may contribute to the perpetuation of local inflammatory responses and amplification of RF production in the synovium. Thus, RF may prolong B cell survival and hence maintain its own production [11, 15, 16].

Clinical relevance

RF plays a pivotal role in the differential diagnosis and determination of prognosis of patients with arthritis [16]. It has been shown that RF is useful in predicting the development of RA, as the detection of IgM, IgA, and IgG RF

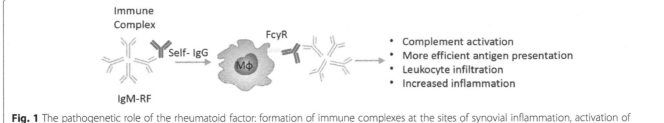

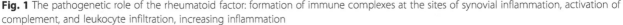

Fig. 1 The pathogenetic role of the rheumatoid factor: formation of immune complexes at the sites of synovial inflammation, activation of complement, and leukocyte infiltration, increasing inflammation

may predate disease onset by years [10]. The pre-clinical appearance of RF isotypes in serum follows a specific sequential evolution: first IgM RF, then IgA RF, and finally IgG RF [17]. High titers of RF have been associated with worse prognosis, more aggressive articular disease, increased disease activity, reduced rates of remission, higher prevalence of extra-articular manifestations, and increased morbidity and mortality, especially when in combination with ACPA [11, 17, 18].

Some studies have shown that immunosuppressive treatment can decrease RF serum levels, but the clinical usefulness of RF in monitoring disease activity and treatment response is limited [18]. Progressive decrease in RF levels parallels the decrease of disease activity in patients treated with conventional disease modifying anti-rheumatic drugs (DMARDs) or biologic agents such as infliximab, etanercept and adalimumab [4, 10]. The published data regarding the potential role of RF in predicting responses to antitumor necrosis factor alpha (TNF-α) in controversial, as one study suggests that the presence of RF predicts a negative response [19], whereas two other studies show that RF positivity before therapy is insufficient to predict the therapeutic response [20, 21]. It has been reported that high IgA RF pre-treatment levels are associated with a poor clinical response to TNF-α inhibitors [10]. Since high serum levels of RF are predictors of more severe disease forms, it is expected that B cell-depleting therapy can have a beneficial effect. Indeed, RF positivity seems to predict better response to rituximab [10, 15, 16] and to tocilizumab but not to abatacept [10, 22].

ACPA

Characteristics

The characterization of autoantibodies reacting with citrullinated peptides (ACPA) in RA was first reported in 1998 [9]. However, the history of ACPA starts in 1964 when fluorescence of anti-perinuclear factor (APF) was described in RA sera. Subsequently, anti-keratin antibodies (AKA) that had, as APF, a high specificity for RA, were reported. Over the years, other candidate citrullinated autoantigens have been identified, such as fibrinogen, vimentin, fibronectin and α-enolase [23]. The Sa antigen/autoantibody system was also reported as highly specific for RA. By 1998, van Venrooij's group was able to demonstrate that the common

denominator for several of these autoantibody systems was the reactivity against citrullinated peptides [23]. APF and AKA are related to the citrullinated protein filaggrin whereas Sa is related to citrullinated vimentin [23]. More recently, the term 'citrullinome' was used referring to the whole array of citrullinated proteins, 53 in all at this time, identified in sera and synovial fluid of RA patients [16, 23]. ACPA recognize peptides and proteins containing citrulline, a non-standard amino acid generated by the post-translational modification of arginine by peptidylarginine deiminase enzymes, in a calcium-dependent process known as citrullination (Fig. 2a) [11, 16]. Post-translationally modified proteins have been described to be particularly capable of inducing immunological tolerance breakdown and auto-antibody response. These modifications are critical for protein structure and biological function [24]. Citrullination occurs during many biologic processes, such as inflammation, apoptosis and keratinization. ACPA are produced by plasma cells in RA joints, and the citrullination of proteins during the inflammatory process seems to play a role in triggering cognate autoantibody production. Several citrullinated proteins can be found in RA synovium, however, fibrin is the major citrullinated protein in RA joint [11, 16].

ACPA are detected in approximately 2/3 of RA patients with a diagnostic specificity of 98% [16]. In the natural history of RA, ACPA immune response starts several years before diagnosis of the disease and the onset of symptoms, but in a restricted manner with low antibody titers and limited peptide reactivity. Fine specificity and epitope spreading, increase in titer, isotype switching and maturation of response gradually occur along the years towards the clinical onset of disease and tend to persist in the majority of patients. This evolution is associated with increase in the diversity of antibody structure that may result in the activation of more immune effector mechanisms [25].

Importantly, the rate of seroconversion of ACPA-negative early inflammatory arthritis (or early RA) to ACPA-positive disease is very low, thus suggesting that repeated testing during follow up may not have an added value [26]. In arthralgia patients, the development of arthritis is predicted not only by the presence of ACPA, but also by their levels [27]. High titer ACPA is also associated with the recognition of several citrullinated epitopes. Patients with arthralgia who

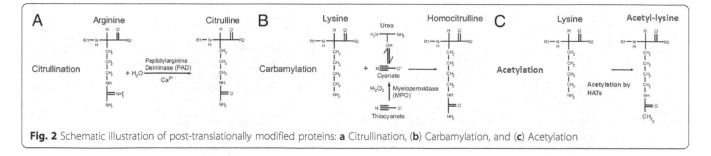

Fig. 2 Schematic illustration of post-translationally modified proteins: **a** Citrullination, (**b**) Carbamylation, and (**c**) Acetylation

have an extended ACPA repertoire are at higher risk of developing arthritis [27]. These findings are consistent with the notion that a broader ACPA recognition profile is associated with higher probability for the transition towards disease [25, 27].

ACPA can be present in different isotypes: IgG, IgA, IgM and IgE. In ACPA-positive patients with RA, IgG1 and IgG4 ACPA are usually present in almost 99% of patients, followed by IgG2 and IG3 in 80 and 60% of patients, respectively. IgM and IgA are present in around 60% of patients [12, 13, 25]. The fine specificity and isotype usage of ACPA in health and disease differs. Healthy family members of patients with RA have fewer ACPA isotypes than their relatives with the disease [10, 14]. The ACPA isotype distribution does not seem to significantly expand anymore during disease progression from undifferentiated arthritis to RA, indicating that most of the expansion of ACPA isotype happens before the onset of arthritis. Indeed, ACPA-positive patients with symptoms of RA for less than 12 weeks show no difference in the specificity and isotype repertoire of their ACPA response compared with patients with longer symptom duration [25]. Importantly, the number of isotypes used by ACPA also associate with RA prognosis, as the magnitude of the ACPA isotype profile at baseline reflects the risk of future radiographic damage, showing an odds ratio of 1.4-fold increase for every additional isotype [24, 28].

In patients with RA, ACPA do not show avidity maturation during longitudinal follow up. In fact, even in patients who displayed extensive isotype switching, ACPA avidity was relatively low. This data shows that there are intrinsic differences between the dynamics of development of RA-specific autoantibodies and protective antibodies against pathogens [25].

ACPA testing
The first enzyme-linked immunosorbent assay (ELISA) using citrullinated peptides (derived from filaggrin epitopes) was developed in 1988, which within 2 years was followed by the development of an ELISA based on artificial cyclic citrullinated peptides (CCP) [25]. The CCP2 assay, the first commercial version of this test, became available in 2002 and allowed the widespread routine testing for antibodies directed against citrullinated epitopes as a biomarker for RA [25]. The CCP2 peptides ensure the detection of a broad range of antibodies to citrullinated host proteins and proved to be extremely specific (98%) for RA, displaying a significantly higher specificity in comparison with the IgM RF [25]. The overall sensitivity of anti-CCP2 assays is similar to that of RF (60–80%), but anti-CCP2 antibody is positive in 20–30% of RF seronegative patients [29].

Other assays for detecting ACPA were subsequently developed, such as CCP3 and MCV (Mutated Citrullinated

Vimentin), with slight differences in terms of specificity and sensitivity [25]. CCP3 is based on ELISA using a collection of citrullinated peptides by a manufacturer distinct from the one that developed CCP2. Citrullinated vimentin has been identified as potential genuine autoantigen in the pathophysiology of RA, what has triggered the development of an ELISA assay for the detection of antibodies directed against mutated citrullinated vimentin (anti-MCV) [30]. Anti-MCV is a further development of the protocol for detecting antibodies to naturally citrullinated vimentin (Sa antigen) [31]. Studies show that anti-MCV assay does not appear to provide additional diagnostic performance over anti-CCP in RA patients [30]. However, when patients with early RA are compared with healthy controls, it has been reported that analysis of anti-MCV yields greater sensitivity and unchanged specificity as compared with anti-CCP2. Besides, anti-MCV appears to perform better than anti-CCP2 in identifying poor radiographic prognosis in patients with early RA [30].

There is still conflicting data regarding the diagnostic and monitoring value of anti-Sa antibodies. A recent study aiming to evaluate the prevalence and diagnostic significance of anti-Sa compared with anti-CCP2 did not demonstrate any additional diagnostic value of the anti-Sa autoantibody in comparison to the anti-CCP2 [31]. Despite high specificity (92–98%), anti-Sa antibodies showed a low diagnostic sensitivity (between 31 and 44%) [31]. However, it has also been suggested that the combined application of anti-CCP 2 and anti-Sa tests can improve the laboratory diagnosis of early RA, with a high specificity (99.4%), albeit with low sensitivity (50%) [32]. It has been shown that, the recently described anti-CarP antibody correlates with anti-Sa antibodies in RA. The association of anti-CarP with anti-Sa antibodies could not be explained by cross-reactivity and this finding is interesting since both autoantibodies are associated with radiographic progression. Therefore, co-expression of anti-CarP and anti-Sa may be confounding these reports. On the other hand, presence of both of them may be associated with improved ability to predict erosive RA [33]. The CCP3 was developed by a distinct company from anti-CCP2 and does not represent a traditional technical upgrade. Despite some controversy in the literature, there seems to be no argument for superiority of one over the other one. One study showed a significantly higher sensitivity for anti-CCP3 in testing RF-negative RA as well as the total RA population [29]. Recently, differences in the test performances accordingly to the moment of the natural history of RA were reported: in patients with established RA, CCP2 was more specific, whereas in subjects with undifferentiated inflammatory arthritis, CCP3 had a higher predictive value for development of RA [9].

Role in pathogenesis

The identification of ACPA has been a major breakthrough in the advancement of the understanding of the pathogenesis in RA. ACPA-positive and ACPA-negative disease have been shown to be associated with different genetic and environmental background, and therefore, different pathophysiological mechanisms should underlie these two separate disease subsets [25].

RA patients exhibit an abnormal humoral response to citrullinated proteins, which are expressed in any form of inflammation, in the synovium or elsewhere [25]. Normally, citrullinated proteins are regularly degraded and do not elicit any relevant humoral reaction of the immune system, therefore the presence of citrullinated proteins per se will not necessarily lead to chronic inflammation [3]. Citrullination has been reported to be a process present in a wide range of inflammatory tissues, suggesting that this is an inflammation-associated phenomenon that should be normally tolerated by the immune system. In fact, it has been widely demonstrated that the presence of citrullinated proteins is not specific for rheumatoid synovial tissue; rather, they can be observed in synovial tissue of patients with other arthropathies and in tonsils from patients with chronic tonsillitis, multiple sclerosis and type 1 diabetes [9].

Citrullination also seems to be implicated in several physiological processes, such as cell death pathways, in which intracellular calcium concentration raises to higher levels than in physiologic conditions, activating peptidylarginine deiminases (PAD) enzymes during apoptosis.

Immune cells infiltrating the inflamed tissue contain PAD enzymes. PAD activation due to high intracellular calcium concentration during cell death would promote citrullination of target antigens. Normally, the generated apoptotic bodies are rapidly removed by phagocytes, preventing inflammatory reactions. Any dysregulation of apoptosis or an ineffective clearance of apoptotic cell remnants may be involved in the breakdown of self-tolerance due to accumulation of dying cells and consequent accessibility of intra-cellular antigens. This scenario would promote the meeting of citrullinated proteins with the immune system leading to autoantibody generation in genetically predisposed individuals. This will ultimately result in immune complex formation, followed by upregulation of pro-inflammatory cytokines, which are regarded as the driving force of the chronic inflammation that is typical of RA (Fig. 3) [9].

Genetic factors, such as the HLA-DRB1 SE alleles, environmental factors, such as smoking and hormone levels, and the possible contribution of bacterial PAD enzymes might participate in this mechanism [5–7]. The development of an autoimmune response against citrullinated epitopes is facilitated by specific genetic predisposition. The presence of particular HLA-DRB1 alleles ("shared epitope"-SE) in RA patients contributes to the development of anti-CCP antibodies [3, 7, 8]. Carriage of SE alleles or the R620W allele of the general autoimmunity marker tyrosine phosphatase non-receptor type 22 (PTPN22) in smokers increases susceptibility to RA since SE related HLA binds citrullinated peptides more strongly and the R620W PTPN22 allele stimulates an exaggerated T cell response [5]. This T cell response may drive increased autoantibody production by B-cells, including ACPA [5, 7, 9]. Intriguingly, the strong association between SE-encoding HLA-DRB1 alleles and RA is only observed for ACPA-positive disease [6, 9].

Periodontitis is associated with increased risk for RA. The presence of periodontitis in patients with RA has been associated with seropositivity for RF and ACPA [34]. *Porphyromonas gingivalis*, a microbe that is the major causative agent for periodontitis, is the only prokaryotic organism expressing PAD, and can cause microbial and host protein citrullination [34]. Hypothetically, this may trigger an immunological response to citrullinated proteins in a subset of RA patients with periodontitis carrying SE alleles [9]. Just like chronic exposure to citrullinated proteins at periodontal sites could contribute to the breakdown of immune tolerance to citrullinated epitopes, chronic inflammation in the lungs from smokers may also predispose susceptible individuals to the development of ACPA and prime individuals to the development of RA [9]. The presence of ACPA before signs of inflammation in joints suggests that immunity against citrullinated proteins is initiated outside the joint [9]. Recent studies suggested that the lung is involved in the citrullination of proteins and may contribute for the generation of RA-related autoimmunity. Smoking has been shown to enhance PAD expression in bronchi-alveolar lavage cells with consequent generation of citrullinated proteins that may lead to citrulline autoimmunity in genetically susceptible RA subjects [7]. It was also shown that local production of ACPA can occur in lungs of patients with RA. Therefore, the lung might be a site of priming the immunity to citrullinated proteins (Fig. 4) [7].

Once generated, ACPA can induce damage as they activate the classical and alternative complement pathways. ACPA are also capable of triggering immune cell responses via Fc receptors (FcR). Immune complexes containing ACPA and citrullinated fibrinogen have been shown to induce TNFα secretion via engagement of FcR on macrophages [25]. ACPA bind to osteoclast surfaces, resulting in osteoclastogenesis and bone degradation [4]. Another mechanism by which ACPA mediate pro-inflammatory action may be through neutrophil extracellular traps (NET). ACPA can enhance the formation of NET, resulting in expel of immune-stimulatory molecules together with strongly immunogenic citrullinated

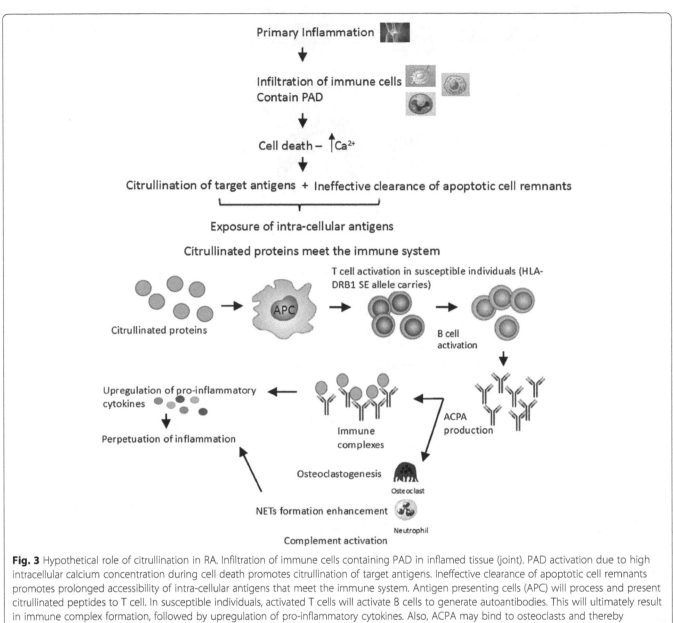

Fig. 3 Hypothetical role of citrullination in RA. Infiltration of immune cells containing PAD in inflamed tissue (joint). PAD activation due to high intracellular calcium concentration during cell death promotes citrullination of target antigens. Ineffective clearance of apoptotic cell remnants promotes prolonged accessibility of intra-cellular antigens that meet the immune system. Antigen presenting cells (APC) will process and present citrullinated peptides to T cell. In susceptible individuals, activated T cells will activate B cells to generate autoantibodies. This will ultimately result in immune complex formation, followed by upregulation of pro-inflammatory cytokines. Also, ACPA may bind to osteoclasts and thereby promote bone erosion, enhance NET formation by neutrophils and activate complement

autoantigens. These observations suggest a mechanism that may promote and perpetuate disease (Fig. 3) [24, 25].

The presence of both RF and ACPA is associated with increased systemic inflammation and disease activity in RA [4]. The combined presence of IgM-RF and ACPA mediates increased pro-inflammatory cytokine production in vitro [4]. RF seems to preferentially interact with hypoglycosylated IgG and ACPA IgG is hypoglycosylated as compared with total IgG. It is suggested that IgM-RF enhances the capacity of ACPA immune complexes to stimulate macrophage cytokine production, therefore providing a mechanistic link by which RF enhances the pathogenicity of ACPA immune complexes in RA [25].

Clinical relevance

ACPA are detected in serum samples up to 14 years before onset of the first symptoms of RA and IgM-RF up to 10 years [35]. The presence of ACPA is associated with more severe joint destruction and ACPA-positive patients develop erosions earlier and more abundantly than patients without ACPA [1, 9]. It is also associated with greater disease activity and poorer remission rates [9]. In addition, the extra-articular manifestations that often determine the severity and comorbidity of RA are also closely associated with ACPA positivity [25]. Both ACPA and RF have been found to associate with cardiovascular disease and mortality in RA patients [4]. Their presence predicts progression towards RA in patients

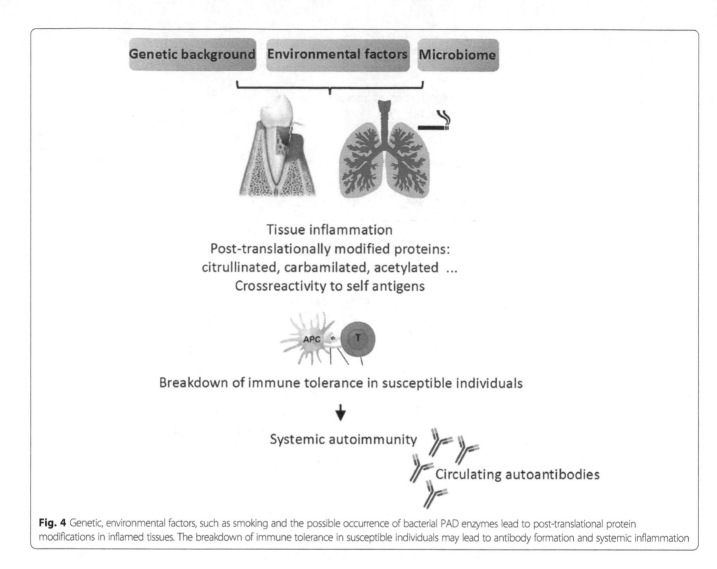

Fig. 4 Genetic, environmental factors, such as smoking and the possible occurrence of bacterial PAD enzymes lead to post-translational protein modifications in inflamed tissues. The breakdown of immune tolerance in susceptible individuals may lead to antibody formation and systemic inflammation

with undifferentiated arthritis and high levels are indicative for arthritis development in arthralgia patients [27]. ACPA positivity is also associated with the presence of RF and SE [29, 36]. Combination analysis showed independent additive effects of these three factors for high radiological risk [36]. It has been shown that anti-CCP2 has higher positive predictive value for erosive RA than RF, C-reactive protein (CRP), erythrocyte sedimentation rate (ESR) or matrix metalloproteinase-3 (MMP-3) serum levels [37]. ACPA-positive patients seem to respond better to treatment than ACPA-negative RA patients in an early phase of the disease, but achieve drug-free remission less frequently [4].

ACPA-positive patients with undifferentiated arthritis (UA) benefit from treatment with methotrexate being less likely to progress to RA, and doing so at a later time point, as compared with a placebo control group. In addition, fewer patients under methotrexate show radiographic progression over 18 months. In contrast, no effect of methotrexate therapy on progression to RA was observed in the ACPA-negative group [38]. ACPA-positive patients, with low and intermediate pre-treatment levels of ACPA respond better to methotrexate treatment in recent-onset cohorts, whereas high levels are associated with an insufficient response. Therefore, in patients with high ACPA levels, methotrexate monotherapy might be insufficient [39]. In the BeSt study, ACPA-positive patients initially treated with DMARD monotherapy had greater radiographic joint destruction after 2 years than ACPA-negative patients. However, when patients were treated initially with combination therapy (DMARD plus anti-TNF biologicals), no difference regarding joint destruction was observed between ACPA-positive and ACPA-negative patients. These observations suggest that ACPA-positive patients, especially those with high titer ACPA, require an aggressive initial approach in order to prevent radiographic progression [25].

ACPA titers can decrease over the course of disease when patients have a good response to therapy. DMARD induce a reduction of 25% or more in ACPA titers in half of the patients over the course of treatment [40].

Regarding response to TNF inhibitors, one study has shown that the presence of ACPA was associated with reduced response to those agents [41]. Other studies show that response to TNF inhibitors is associated with lower ACPA baseline titers and that there is around 30% reduction of serum ACPA titers after anti-TNF treatment [40]. However, several other reports showed little or no effect of anti-TNF therapy on ACPA titers [40]. Other immunobiologicals, such as abatacept, reduce CD20⁺ B cells in the synovial membrane of RA patients and the production of IL-2, IL-17, IL-22 in ACPA-positive but not in ACPA-negative RA patients [42, 43]. In these studies, anti-CCP2 positivity has been associated with EULAR response, suggesting that abatacept is more efficacious in ACPA-positive RA patients. Rituximab is associated with good to moderate EULAR response in ACPA-positive patients or in patients with high ACPA levels. Anti-CCP2 antibody levels after rituximab therapy present a more pronounced fall in responders relative to non-responders [44]. These data indicate that ACPA status may be relevant for treatment decisions in RA and support the hypothesis that RA can be classified into two different disease subsets: ACPA-positive and ACPA-negative RA [25].

Anti-carbamylated protein antibodies (anti-CarP)

Characteristics

Recently, a new autoantibody system has been described in RA, characterized by antibodies against carbamylated proteins, i.e., proteins that contain homocitrulline residues (anti-CarP antibodies). Antibodies in the serum of RA patients can discriminate citrullinated and carbamylated antigens and, therefore, this antibody system is independent from ACPA. In fact, anti-CarP antibodies may be detected in ACPA-negative patients and vice-versa [4, 45].

Carbamylation is defined as a post-translational modification in which a positively charged amino acid is replaced by a neutral amino acid. The most common carbamylation process refers to the conversion of lysine into homocitrulline. The chemical structure of homocitrulline resembles citrulline. Homocitrulline is one methylene group longer than citrulline (Fig. 2b) [40, 45, 46]. In contrast to citrullination, carbamylation is a non-enzymatic chemical reaction involving cyanate in the conversion of lysine into homocitrulline. Cyanate is naturally present in the several body fluids and in equilibrium with urea [45]. Under physiological conditions, the cyanate concentration is too low to allow extensive carbamylation of proteins. However, several conditions such as renal disease, inflammation and smoking can shift the balance towards predominance of cyanate over urea. In renal failure, the urea concentration increases, resulting in extensive carbamylation of proteins [47]. Smoking also increases the cyanate concentration and can enhance carbamylation. However, most carbamylation is believed to take place under

inflammatory conditions, when myeloperoxidase (MPO) is released from neutrophils, converting thiocyanate to cyanate, an essential driver for carbamylation [45]. As a consequence of excess carbamylation, protein and cellular dysfunction may occur, leading to systemic effects [45]. Decreased functional activity upon carbamylation has been reported for several enzymes and hormones. In susceptible individuals, extensive carbamylation will provide the trigger for the development an autoimmune response directed against carbamylated proteins (Fig. 5) [45].

Pathogenesis

In animal model, it has been shown that carbamylated proteins can trigger primary immune responses, inducing chemotaxis, T cell activation and antibody production, and subsequently, the production of IFN-γ, IL-10 and IL-17. The activation of T cells added to a strong antibody response will enable the recognition of carbamylated and citrullinated peptides within the joints, which may contribute to the development of erosive arthritis. Carbamylated and citrullinated peptides complement each other in the generation of the autoimmune response. The immune-activating effects of carbamylation enhance the arthritogenic properties of citrullinated peptides, therefore providing a novel mechanism for the pathogenesis of autoimmune arthritis [46].

Clinical relevance

Anti-CarP antibodies are detected in up to 45% of RA patients (45% IgG and 43% IgA anti-CarP). Notably, anti-CarP antibodies may occur in 16–30% of ACPA-negative patients (16% IgG and 30% IgA anti-CarP) [48]. Anti-CarP IgG antibodies seem to be associated with a more severe radiological progression in ACPA-negative RA, indicating that anti-CarP antibodies are a unique and relevant serological marker for ACPA-negative patients [48]. Recently, the presence of anti-CarP antibodies was associated also with higher disease activity and significantly more disability over time in patients with rheumatoid arthritis. Statistically significant associations were seen not only in ACPA-positive but also in ACPA-negative patients [45].

These autoantibodies can be detected more than 10 years before disease onset, at the same time of ACPA and before IgM-RF [4, 49]. The presence of anti-CarP antibodies of patients with arthralgia predicts the development of RA independently of ACPA [49]. Therefore, anti-CarP antibodies might be a useful biomarker to identify ACPA-negative "pre-RA" patients and newly diagnosed RA patients who require early and aggressive clinical intervention [45, 49].

The high specificity of anti-CarP antibodies for RA was suggested as these antibodies were not found in patients with other inflammatory rheumatic conditions or in normal healthy individuals [50]. However, one study

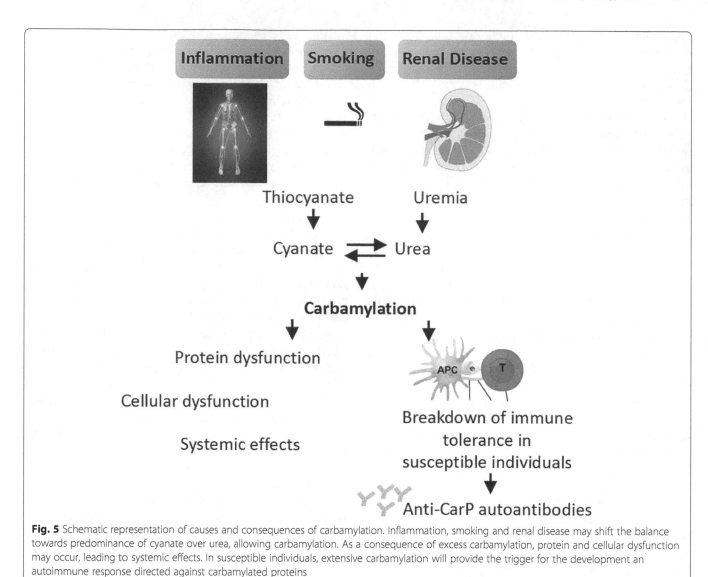

Fig. 5 Schematic representation of causes and consequences of carbamylation. Inflammation, smoking and renal disease may shift the balance towards predominance of cyanate over urea, allowing carbamylation. As a consequence of excess carbamylation, protein and cellular dysfunction may occur, leading to systemic effects. In susceptible individuals, extensive carbamylation will provide the trigger for the development an autoimmune response directed against carbamylated proteins

showed that anti-CarP antibodies are detectable in the serum of patients with active PsA and correlations between anti-CarP levels and disease activity were observed in polyarthritis patients that were negative for ACPA and RF. If confirmed, anti-CarP may be considered as the first evidence of the presence of autoantibodies in PsA [51]. Anti-CarP antibodies can also be found in juvenile idiopathic arthritis (JIA) patients. It has been shown that 16.7% of JIA patients are positive for anti-CarP, whereas only 6.4% are positive for ACPA and 8.1% for IgM-RF [52]. Genetic and environmental associations have not yet been investigated thoroughly, but one study showed that there were no significant associations between anti-CarP antibodies and smoking, PTPN22 alleles or HLA-DRB1, with the exception of the association identified for HLA-DRB1*03.. The lack of association with SE-HLA alleles may indicate a different biological mechanism for the formation of anti-CarP antibodies in comparison with the development of

ACPA and may represent an opportunity to identify additional molecular pathways involved in RA pathophysiology [53].

Anti-PAD4 antibodies
Characteristics and pathogenesis
PAD4 is a calcium dependent peptidylarginine deiminidase, one of the proteins that are responsible for the conversion of arginine into citrulline [4]. It has been recently demonstrated that PAD4 may undergo auto-citrullination, a process that might inactivate the enzyme as a mechanism of control. PAD4 citrullination modifies the structure of the enzyme, increasing its recognition by human autoantibodies [9, 54]. In fact, autoantibodies directed against PAD4 have indeed been identified in RA patients [4]. These antibodies not only target but also activate PAD, increasing the catalytic efficiency of the enzyme by decreasing its requirement for calcium [55]. Anti-PAD4 antibodies have

been reported to have predictive and prognostic value in RA patients [9].

PAD is found also in *Porphyromonas Gingivalis* (PPAD) However, recent data showed that PPAD expressed by *P gingivalis* is not citrullinated and PPAD citrullination is not recognized by anti-PAD antibodies in RA. Besides, anti-PPAD antibodies were not associated with ACPA levels and disease activity in RA and seem to have a protective role for periodontitis development in RA patients [9].

Clinical relevance

Anti-PAD4 antibodies are present in 22–45% of RA patients and can also be detected in 14% of SLE patients, but spondyloarthritis patients do not seem to have these auto-antibodies [4]. It has low specificity for RA diagnosis (< 50%) [4]. Anti-PAD4 antibodies are almost exclusively found in people with established RA and have been associated with severe disease in these patients [4]. These antibodies are associated with the presence of ACPA and are usually detected after ACPA appearance [56].

A specific group of anti-PAD4 antibodies cross-reacts with anti-PAD3 antibodies. This subset increases the catalytic capacity of PAD4 by decreasing its calcium requirement for citrullination. These antibodies are present in 12 to 18% of RA patients and its reactivity has been found only in anti-PAD4 positive RA patients. Importantly, these cross-reactive antibodies were associated with radiographic damage severity [55]. In addition, the prevalence and extent of interstitial lung disease was found to be higher among RA patients with anti-PAD3/4 cross-reactive antibodies [57]. Therefore, anti-PAD3/4 antibodies may serve as biomarker for disease prognosis, despite being detected at low frequency in RA patients [4].

Anti-BRAF antibodies
Characteristics and pathogenesis

BRAF (v raf murine sarcoma viral oncogene homolog B1) catalytic domain is a serine-threonine kinase that regulates the mitogen-activated protein kinase (MAPK) signaling pathway implicated in the production of pro-inflammatory cytokines. Anti-BRAF autoantibodies activate BRAF kinase activity, which may lead to production of pro-inflammatory cytokines and joint inflammation [54]. Anti-BRAF antibodies are present in 21–32% of RA patients.

Clinical relevance

These autoantibodies are present also in SLE and primary Sjögren's syndrome in a similar frequency to RA, and also in 4% of ankylosing spondylitis patients and 6% of healthy individuals [4, 54]. Although not specific for RA, anti-BRAF may be an interesting new autoantibody to identify ACPA-negative RA patients since 30% of anti-CCP2 negative RA patients were positive for anti-BRAF antibodies [54].

Other autoantibodies
Anti-RA-33 or anti-hnRNP A2 antibodies

RA-33 is an intracellular molecule that binds to the heterogeneous nuclear protein (hnRNP) A2, a part of the *splicosome*. Anti-RA-33 antinuclear antibodies are present in one third of RA patients. The reported frequency of anti-RA-33 antibodies is 13% in ACPA/RF-negative patients and 9% in non-RA patients. Anti-RA33 antibodies may not be useful as a clinical biomarker for diagnosing RA, however anti-RA33-positive patients seem to show a less severe disease so that these antibodies might serve as a prognostic marker for less aggressive disease [4].

Anti-malondialdehyde and anti-malondialdehyde acetaldehyde antibodies

Post-translational modifications due to lipid peroxidation can result in the presence of malondialdehyde (MDA) and malondialdehyde-acetaldehyde (MAA)–adducts. It was found that both MAA adducts and antibodies directed against these adducts were increased in the serum of RA patients, and a positive correlation between the presence of ACPA and anti-MAA antibodies was observed [58]. However, anti-MAA antibodies have also been detected in chronic liver diseases and in type 2 diabetes [59]. Antibodies against MDA-adducts, especially MDA-LDL, were found to associate with cardiovascular problems in RA patients.

Anti-acetylated peptide antibodies

Acetylation is a reversible enzymatic process where acetyl groups are added to free amines of lysine residues by Lys acetyltransferases (KAT) [60]. Acetylated lysine resembles homocitrulline, but the side chain terminal amine is replaced by a methyl moiety in acetylate lysine (Fig. 2c) [61].

Protein lysine acetylation is a key post-translational modification in cellular regulation, especially in histones and nuclear transcription regulators. Acetylation of cytoplasmic proteins regulates metabolic pathways and enzymatic functions [62]. IgG and IgA antibodies against acetylated vimentin peptides were detected in 35% of patients with early arthritis. However, data showed that anti-acetylated vimentin antibodies are relatively poor for predicting the development of anti-ACPA-negative RA. Their presence and frequency in established RA and their role in predicting disease severity and other clinically relevant outcomes in patients with RA remain to be established [61].

Anti-oxidized protein antibodies in RA

Several data suggest a role for oxidative stress in the pathogenesis of RA. Reactive oxygen species (ROS have been identified in the synovial fluid of 90% of RA patients [40]. Studies show that type II collagen (CII) post-translationally modified by ROS (ROS-CII) is present in the inflamed joints [63]. High titer anti-ROS-CII reactivity was observed in early RA regardless of ACPA status (93.8% in ACPA-positive patients and 91.6% in ACPA-negative patients). The sensitivity and specificity of anti-ROS-CII antibodies in early RA was 92 and 98%, respectively [40]. Anti-ROS-CII activity has not been detected in the serum of patients with other inflammatory diseases [40]. ROS-CII reactivity was lower in RA patients after their first DMARD treatment and this was associated with good response: 7.6% in serum samples of responders and 58.3% of serum samples in non-responders.[191]

Other less well-studied autoantibodies have been reported in RA. Autoantibodies against transthyretin, a hormone carrier, were found to be increased in RA patients when compared to healthy controls [4]. Antibodies against the hinge region of immunoglobulins, anti-hinge antibodies (AHA), have been reported in approximately 15–20% of RA patients. Despite low sensitivity, they seem to have high specificity for RA. ACPA antibodies may be fragmented by inflammation-associated proteases in the hinge region, creating novel epitopes that can be recognized by the immune system, resulting in AHA. These autoantibodies could modulate arthritis by binding to fragmented autoantibodies in the inflamed joint, which may lead to exacerbation of disease [64].

Conclusion

Several RA-associated autoantibody systems have been identified and many of these autoantibodies recognize post translationally modified proteins, indicating the immunogenicity of such proteins for human B cells.

RF and ACPA are the two most remarkable autoantibodies in RA and provide different clinical and pathophysiological information. ACPA exhibit high sensitivity with the highest predictive value for RA development and severity. These autoantibodies enabled the stratification of RA in ACPA-positive and ACPA-negative disease phenotype, with different genetic and environmental contribution factors. In addition, ACPA status predicts response to therapy. However, despite the diagnostic value of RF and ACPA, more serological markers are needed in order to improve early diagnosis and treatment of the patients as well as to lead to a better understanding of the molecular pathways involved in RA.

Recently, the identification of anti-CarP antibodies, also present in the serum of RF-negative/ACPA-negative RA patients filled another gap in the seronegative RA spectrum, and indicated further heterogeneity among RA patients. Hopefully, the progressive characterization of a comprehensive array of novel autoantibody systems in RA will provide unique pathogenic insights of relevance for the development of diagnostic and prognostic approaches compatible with an effective personalized medicine.

Acknowledgements
Not aplicable

Authors' contributions
All authors read and approved the final manuscript.

References

1. Moeez S, John P, Bhatti A. Anti-citrullinated protein antibodies: role in pathogenesis of RA and potential as a diagnostic tool. Rheumatol Int. 2013;33(7):1669–73.
2. Szodoray P, Szabó Z, Kapitány A, Gyetvai A, Lakos G, Szántó S, et al. Anti-citrullinated protein/peptide autoantibodies in association with genetic and environmental factors as indicators of disease outcome in rheumatoid arthritis. Autoimmun Rev. 2010;9(3):140–3.
3. Farid SS, Azizi G, Mirshafiey A. Anti-citrullinated protein antibodies and their clinical utility in rheumatoid arthritis. Inter J Rheum Dis. 2013;16(4):379–86.
4. Verheul MK, Fearon U, Trouw LA, Veale DJ. Biomarkers for rheumatoid and psoriatic arthritis. Clin Immunol. 2015;161(1):2–10.
5. Klareskog L, Malmström V, Lundberg K, Padyukov L, Alfredsson L. Smoking, citrullination and genetic variability in the immunopathogenesis of rheumatoid arthritis. Semin Immunol. 2011;23(2):92–8.
6. Imboden JB. The immunopathogenesis of rheumatoid arthritis. Annu Rev Pathol. 2009;4:417–34.
7. Kallberg H, Padyukov L, Plenge RM, Ronnelid J, Gregersen PK, van der Helm-van Mil AH, et al. Gene-gene and gene-environment interactions involving HLA-DRB1, PTPN22, and smoking in two subsets of rheumatoid arthritis. Am J Hum Genet. 2007;80(5):867–75.
8. Aletaha D, Neogi T, Silman AJ, Funovits J, Felson DT, Bingham CO 3rd, et al. Rheumatoid arthritis classification criteria: an American College of Rheumatology/European league against rheumatism collaborative initiative. Arthritis Rheum. 2010;62(9):2569–81.
9. Valesini G, Gerardi MC, Iannuccelli C, Pacucci VA, Pendolino M, Shoenfeld Y. Citrullination and autoimmunity. Autoimmun Rev. 2015;14(6):490–7.
10. Ingegnoli F, Castelli R, Gualtierotti R. Rheumatoid factors: clinical applications. Dis Markers. 2013;35(6):727–34.
11. Moura RA, Graca L, Fonseca JE. To B or not to B the conductor of rheumatoid arthritis orchestra. Clin Rev Allergy Immunol. 2012;43(3):281–91.
12. Nishimura K, Sugiyama D, Kogata Y, Tsuji G, Nakazawa T, Kawano S, et al. Meta-analysis: diagnostic accuracy of anti-cyclic citrullinated peptide antibody and rheumatoid factor for rheumatoid arthritis. Ann Intern Med. 2007;146(11):797–808.
13. Jónsson T, Steinsson K, Jónsson H, Geirsson AJ, Thorsteinsson J, Valdimarsson H. Combined elevation of IgM and IgA rheumatoid factor has high diagnostic specificity for rheumatoid arthritis. Rheumatol Int. 1998; 18(3):119–22.
14. Nielsen SF, Bojesen SE, Schnohr P, Nordestgaard BG. Elevated rheumatoid factor and long term risk of rheumatoid arthritis: a prospective cohort study. BMJ. 2012;345:e5244.
15. Edwards JC, Cambridge G. Rheumatoid arthritis: the predictable effect of small immune complexes in which antibody is also antigen. Br J Rheumatol. 1998;37(2):126–30.
16. Song YW, Kang EH. Autoantibodies in rheumatoid arthritis: rheumatoid factors and anticitrullinated protein antibodies. QJM. 2010;103(3):139–46.
17. Jónsson T, Arinbjarnarson S, Thorsteinsson J, Steinsson K, Geirsson AJ, Jónsson H, et al. Raised IgA rheumatoid factor (RF) but not IgM RF or IgG RF is associated with extra-articular manifestations in rheumatoid arthritis. Scand J Rheumatol. 1995;24(6):372–5.
18. Sokolove J, Johnson DS, Lahey LJ, Wagner CA, Cheng D, Thiele GM, et al. Rheumatoid factor as a potentiator of anti-citrullinated protein antibody-mediated inflammation in rheumatoid arthritis. Arthritis Rheumatol. 2014; 66(4):813–21.
19. Bos WH, Bartelds GM, Wolbink GJ, de Koning MH, van de Stadt RJ, van Schaardenburg D, et al. Differential response of the rheumatoid factor and anticitrullinated protein antibodies during adalimumab treatment in patients with rheumatoid arthritis. J Rheumatol. 2008;35(10):1972–7.
20. Bobbio-Pallavicini F, Caporali R, Alpini C, Moratti R, Montecucco C. Predictive value of antibodies to citrullinated peptides and rheumatoid factors in anti-TNF-alpha treated patients. Ann N Y Acad Sci. 2007;1109:287–95.
21. Klaasen R, Cantaert T, Wijbrandts CA, Teitsma C, Gerlag DM, Out TA, et al. The value of rheumatoid factor and anti-citrullinated protein antibodies as

predictors of response to infliximab in rheumatoid arthritis: an exploratory study. Rheumatology (Oxford). 2011;50(8):1487–93.

22. Maneiro RJ, Salgado E, Carmona L, Gomez-Reino JJ. Rheumatoid factor as predictor of response to abatacept, rituximab and tocilizumab in rheumatoid arthritis: systematic review and meta-analysis. Semin Arthritis Rheum. 2013;43(1):9–17.

23. van Beers JJ, Schwarte CM, Stammen-Vogelzangs J, Oosterink E, Božič B, Pruijn GJ. The rheumatoid arthritis synovial fluid citrullinome reveals novel citrullinated epitopes in apolipoprotein E, myeloid nuclear differentiation antigen, and β-actin. Arthritis Rheum. 2013;65(1):69–80.

24. Bax M, Huizinga TW, Toes RE. The pathogenic potential of autoreactive antibodies in rheumatoid arthritis. Semin Immunopathol. 2014;36(3):313–25.

25. Willemze A, Trouw LA, Toes RE, Huizinga TW. The influence of ACPA status and characteristics on the course of RA. Nat Rev Rheumatol. 2012;8(3):144–52.

26. Barra L, Pope J, Bessette L, Haraoui B, Bykerk V. Lack of seroconversion of rheumatoid factor and anti-cyclic citrullinated peptide in patients with early inflammatory arthritis: a systematic literature review. Rheumatology (Oxford). 2011;50(2):311–6.

27. van de Stadt LA, van der Horst AR, de Koning MH, Bos WH, Wolbink GJ, van de Stadt RJ, et al. The extent of the anti-citrullinated protein antibody repertoire is associated with arthritis development in patients with seropositive arthralgia. Ann Rheum Dis. 2011;70(1):128–33.

28. van der Woude D, Syversen SW, van der Voort EI, Verpoort KN, Goll GL, van der Linden MP, et al. The ACPA isotype profile reflects long-term radiographic progression in rheumatoid arthritis. Ann Rheum Dis. 2010;69(6):1110–6.

29. Szekanecz Z, Szabó Z, Zeher M, Soós L, Dankó K, Horváth I, et al. Superior performance of the CCP3.1 test compared to CCP2 and MCV in the rheumatoid factor-negative RA population. Immunol Res. 2013;56(2–3):439–43.

30. Bartoloni E, Alunno A, Bistoni O, Bizzaro N, Migliorini P, Morozzi G, et al. Diagnostic value of anti-mutated citrullinated vimentin in comparison to anti-cyclic citrullinated peptide and anti-viral citrullinated peptide 2 antibodies in rheumatoid arthritis: an Italian multicentric study and review of the literature. Autoimmun Rev. 2012;11(11):815–20.

31. Iwaszkiewicz C, Puszczewicz M, Białkowska-Puszczewicz G. Diagnostic value of the anti-Sa antibody compared with the anti-cyclic citrullinated peptide antibody in rheumatoid arthritis. Int J Rheum Dis. 2015;18(1):46–51.

32. Hou YF, Sun GZ, Sun HS, Pan WP, Liu WB, Zhang CQ. Diagnostic value of anti-Sa and anticitrullinated protein antibodies in rheumatoid arthritis. J Rheumatol. 2012;39(8):1506–8.

33. Challener GJ, Jones JD, Pelzek AJ, Hamilton BJ, Boire G, de Brum-Fernandes AJ, et al. Anti-carbamylated protein antibody levels correlate with anti-Sa (citrullinated vimentin) antibody levels in rheumatoid arthritis. J Rheumatol. 2016;43(2):273–81.

34. Dissick A, Redman RS, Jones M, Rangan BV, Reimold A, Griffiths GR, et al. Association of periodontitis with rheumatoid arthritis: a pilot study. J Periodontol. 2010;81(2):223–30.

35. Nielen MM, van Schaardenburg D, Reesink HW, van de Stadt RJ, van der Horst-Bruinsma IE, de Koning MH, et al. Specific autoantibodies precede the symptoms of rheumatoid arthritis: a study of serial measurements in blood donors. Arthritis Rheum. 2004;50(2):380–6.

36. De Rycke L, Peene I, Hoffman IE, Kruithof E, Union A, Meheus L, et al. Rheumatoid factor and anticitrullinated protein antibodies in rheumatoid arthritis: diagnostic value, associations with radiological progression rate, and extra-articular manifestations. Ann Rheum Dis. 2004;63(12):1587–93.

37. Shovman O, Gilburd B, Zandman-Goddard G, Sherer Y, Orbach H, Gerli R, et al. The diagnostic utility of anti-cyclic citrullinated peptide antibodies, matrix metalloproteinase-3, rheumatoid factor, erythrocyte sedimentation rate, and C-reactive protein in patients with erosive and non-erosive rheumatoid arthritis. Clin Dev Immunol. 2005;12(3):197–202.

38. van Dongen H, van Aken J, Lard LR, Visser K, Ronday HK, Hulsmans HM, et al. Efficacy of methotrexate treatment in patients with probable rheumatoid arthritis: a double-blind, randomized, placebo-controlled trial. Arthritis Rheum. 2007;56(5):1424–32.

39. Visser K, Goekoop-Ruiterman YP, de Vries-Bouwstra JK, Ronday HK, Seys PE, Kerstens PJ, et al. A matrix risk model for the prediction of rapid radiographic progression in patients with rheumatoid arthritis receiving different dynamic treatment strategies: post hoc analyses from the BeSt study. Ann Rheum Dis. 2010;69(7):1333–7.

40. Burska AN, Hunt L, Boissinot M, Strollo R, Ryan BJ, Vital E, et al. Autoantibodies to posttranslational modifications in rheumatoid arthritis. Mediat Inflamm. 2014;2014:492873.

41. Potter C, Hyrich KL, Tracey A, Lunt M, Plant D, Symmons DP, et al. Association of rheumatoid factor and anti-cyclic citrullinated peptide positivity, but not carriage of shared epitope or PTPN22 susceptibility variants, with anti-tumour necrosis factor response in rheumatoid arthritis. Ann Rheum Dis. 2009;68(1):69–74.

42. Kanbe K, Chiba J, Nakamura A. Immunohistological analysis of synovium treated with abatacept in rheumatoid arthritis. Rheumatol Int. 2013;33(7):1883–7.

43. Pieper J, Herrath J, Raghavan S, Muhammad K, Rv V, Malmström V. CTLA4-Ig (abatacept) therapy modulates T cell effector functions in autoantibody-positive rheumatoid arthritis patients. BMC Immunol. 2013;14:34.

44. Gardette A, Ottaviani S, Tubach F, Roy C, Nicaise-Roland P, Palazzo E, et al. High anti-CCP antibody titres predict good response to rituximab in patients with active rheumatoid arthritis. Joint Bone Spine. 2014;81(5):416–20.

45. Shi J, van Veelen PA, Mahler M, Janssen GM, Drijfhout JW, Huizinga TW, et al. Carbamylation and antibodies against carbamylated proteins in autoimmunity and other pathologies. Autoimmun Rev. 2014;13(3):225–30.

46. Mydel P, Wang Z, Brisslert M, Hellvard A, Dahlberg LE, Hazen SL, et al. Carbamylation-dependent activation of T cells: a novel mechanism in the pathogenesis of autoimmune arthritis. J Immunol. 2010;184(12):6882–90.

47. Wynckel A, Randoux C, Millart H, Desroches C, Gillery P, Canivet E, et al. Kinetics of carbamylated haemoglobin in acute renal failure. Nephrol Dial Transplant. 2000;15(8):1183–8.

48. Shi J, Knevel R, Suwannalai P, van der Linden MP, Janssen GM, van Veelen PA, et al. Autoantibodies recognizing carbamylated proteins are present in sera of patients with rheumatoid arthritis and predict joint damage. Proc Natl Acad Sci U S A. 2011;108(42):17372–7.

49. Shi J, van de Stadt LA, Levarht EWN, Huizinga TWJ, Toes REM, Trouw LA, et al. Anti carbamylated protein antibodies (anti-CarP) are present in arthralgia patients and predict the development of rheumatoid arthritis. Ann Rheum Dis. 2013;72:A31.

50. Scinocca M, Bell DA, Racapé M, Joseph R, Shaw G, McCormick JK, et al. Antihomocitrullinated fibrinogen antibodies are specific to rheumatoid arthritis and frequently bind citrullinated proteins/peptides. J Rheumatol. 2014;41(2):270–9.

51. Chimenti MS, Triggianese P, Nuccetelli M, Terracciano C, Crisanti A, Guarino MD, et al. Auto-reactions, autoimmunity and psoriatic arthritis. Autoimmun Rev. 2015;14(12):1142–6.

52. Muller PC, Anink J, Shi J, Levarht EW, Reinards TH, Otten MH, et al. Anticarbamylated protein (anti-CarP) antibodies are present in sera of juvenile idiopathic arthritis (JIA) patients. Ann Rheum Dis. 2013;72(12):2053–5.

53. Jiang X, Trouw LA, van Wesemael TJ, Shi J, Bengtsson C, Källberg H, et al. Anti-CarP antibodies in two large cohorts of patients with rheumatoid arthritis and their relationship to genetic risk factors, cigarette smoking and other autoantibodies. Ann Rheum Dis. 2014;73(10):1761–8.

54. Auger I, Charpin C, Balandraud N, Martin M, Roudier J. Autoantibodies to PAD4 and BRAF in rheumatoid arthritis. Autoimmun Rev. 2012;11(11):801–3.

55. Darrah E, Giles JT, Ols ML, Bull HG, Andrade F, Rosen A. Erosive rheumatoid arthritis is associated with antibodies that activate PAD4 by increasing calcium sensitivity. Sci Transl Med. 2013;5(186):186ra65.

56. Umeda N, Matsumoto I, Kawaguchi H, Kurashima Y, Kondo Y, Tsuboi H, et al. Prevalence of soluble peptidylarginine deiminase 4 (PAD4) and anti-PAD4 antibodies in autoimmune diseases. Clin Rheumatol. 2016;35(5):1181–8.

57. Giles JT, Darrah E, Danoff S, Johnson C, Andrade F, Rosen A, Bathon JM. Association of cross-reactive antibodies targeting peptidyl-arginine deiminase 3 and 4 with rheumatoid arthritis-associated interstitial lung disease. PLoS One. 2014;9(6):e98794.

58. Thiele GM, Duryee MJ, Anderson DR, Klassen LW, Mohring SM, Young KA, et al. Malondialdehyde-acetaldehyde adducts and anti-malondialdehyde-acetaldehyde antibodies in rheumatoid arthritis. Arthritis Rheumatol. 2015;67(3):645–55.

59. Vehkala L, Ukkola O, Kesäniemi YA, Kähönen M, Nieminen MS, Salomaa V, et al. Plasma IgA antibody levels to malondialdehyde acetaldehyde-adducts are associated with inflammatory mediators, obesity and type 2 diabetes. Ann Med. 2013;45(8):501–10.

60. Yang XJ, Seto E. Lysine acetylation: codified crosstalk with other posttranslational modifications. Mol Cell. 2008;31(4):449–61.

61. Juarez M, Bang H, Hammar F, Reimer U, Dyke B, Sahbudin I, et al. Identification of novel antiacetylated vimentin antibodies in patients with early inflammatory arthritis. Ann Rheum Dis. 2016;75(6):1099–107.

62. Zhao S, Xu W, Jiang W, Yu W, Lin Y, Zhang T, et al. Regulation of cellular metabolism by protein lysine acetylation. Science. 2010;327(5968):1000–4.

63. Winyard PG, Ryan B, Eggleton P, Nissim A, Taylor E, Lo Faro ML, et al. Measurement and meaning of markers of reactive species of oxygen, nitrogen and sulfur in healthy human subjects and patients with inflammatory joint disease. Biochem Soc Trans. 2011;39(5):1226–32.

12

High prevalence of obesity in rheumatoid arthritis patients: Association with disease activity, hypertension, dyslipidemia and diabetes

Maria Fernanda Brandão de Resende Guimarães[1]* (iD), Carlos Ewerton Maia Rodrigues[2], Kirla Wagner Poti Gomes[3], Carla Jorge Machado[4], Claiton Viegas Brenol[5], Susana Ferreira Krampe[5], Nicole Pamplona Bueno de Andrade[5] and Adriana Maria Kakehasi[4]

Abstract

Introduction: Rheumatoid arthritis (RA) is a well-documented independent risk factor for cardiovascular disease. Obesity may provide an additional link between inflammation and accelerated atherosclerosis in RA.

Objective: To evaluate the association between obesity and disease parameters and cardiovascular risk factors in RA patients.

Method: Cross-sectional study of a cohort of RA patients from three Brazilian teaching hospitals. Information on demographics, clinical parameters and the presence of cardiovascular risk factors was collected. Blood pressure, weight, height and waist circumference (WC) were measured during the first consultation. Laboratory data were retrieved from medical records. Obesity was defined according to the NCEP/ATPIII and IDF guidelines. The prevalence of obesity was determined cross-sectionally. Disease activity was evaluated using the DAS28 system (remission < 2.6; low 2.6–3.1; moderate 3.2–5.0; high > 5.1).

Results: The sample consisted of 791 RA patients aged 54.7 ± 12.0 years, of whom 86.9% were women and 59.9% were Caucasian. The mean disease duration was 12.8 ± 8.9 years. Three quarters were rheumatoid factor-positive, the mean body mass index (BMI) was 27.1 ± 4.9, and the mean WC was 93.5 ± 12.5 cm. The observed risk factors included dyslipidemia (34.3%), type-2 diabetes (15%), hypertension (49.2%) and family history of premature cardiovascular disease (16.5%). BMI-defined obesity was highly prevalent (26.9%) and associated with age, hypertension and dyslipidemia. Increased WC was associated with diabetes, hypertension, dyslipidemia and disease activity. Conclusion: Obesity was highly prevalent in RA patients and associated with disease activity.

Introduction

Obesity is caused by an imbalance between the ingestion and expenditure of food energy in previously healthy individuals, with sedentary lifestyle and excessive caloric intake as the main determinants. Genetic predisposition can also affect the risk of developing obesity, depending on lifestyle [1, 2]. Along with the accumulation of abdominal fat, obesity increases the risk of type 2 diabetes mellitus (DM II), dyslipidemia, systemic arterial hypertension (SAH), cardiovascular disease and hepatic steatosis [3, 4].

A growing body of evidence suggests that adipose tissue is not merely an inert energy store but an endocrine organ which communicates with the central nervous system, with a range of important functions, such as the production of hormones and proteins involved in physiological and pathological processes, including immunity and inflammation [5].

Biologically active substances released by the adipose tissue may contribute to a chronic condition of low-

* Correspondence: mfbresende@yahoo.com.br
[1]Serviço de Reumatologia, Hospital das Clínicas, Universidade Federal de Minas Gerais (UFMG), Rua Adolfo Pereira, 262, apto 901, Belo Horizonte, MG 30310-350, Brazil
Full list of author information is available at the end of the article

grade inflammation. High levels of these adipokines such as leptin, resistin and visfastine and low levels of adiponectin, which is an anti-inflammatory adipokine, may influence inflammation and increase disease activity in obese patients with rheumatoid arthritis (RA). Adipokines influence both the innate immune system (increasing cytokines such as interleukin 6 and 12 and tumor necrosis factor alpha) and the adaptive immune system by increasing T-helper 1 lymphocytes and decreasing regulatory T cells [6, 7].

Obese individuals often have elevated levels of circulating inflammatory markers such as C-reactive protein (CRP), tumor necrosis factor alpha, interleukin 6, and plasminogen activator inhibitor-1 [8, 9].

The documented association among obesity, increased cardiovascular risk (CVR) and inflammation, as well as the changes in body composition in patients with RA justify investigating the influence of obesity on these disease. The accumulation of body fat to the extent that it has a negative impact on health is usually diagnosed using anthropometric indicators such as the body mass index (BMI) and waist circumference (WC). Body weight is routinely registered in the clinical practice of rheumatologists, but in most studies on RA, this parameter is used only for demographic cohort characterization. More research is needed to evaluate the possible long-term effect of obesity on the course of RA [10]. High BMI values are believed to increase the risk of developing RA and compromise quality of life and treatment response [11–13], although some authors have found a negative correlation between BMI and radiographic progression in RA [14–16].

Obesity, especially the pathological fat mass dysfunction caused by inadequate secretion of pro-inflammatory adipokines, could be the link between increased CVR and rheumatic diseases [17–19].

The aim of the present study was to determine the prevalence of obesity (evaluated by both BMI and WC) in RA patients and to study the relationship between obesity and clinical parameters, cardiovascular risk factors and disease activity in RA patients.

Patients and methods

Patients over 18 years of both sexes diagnosed with RA according to the 1987 criteria of the American College of Rheumatology (ACR) [20] or the 2010 ACR/EULAR criteria [21] and with over 6 months of symptoms were invited to participate in the study during routine consultations at three Brazilian teaching hospitals (Ceará, Minas Gerais, and Rio Grande do Sul). Patients diagnosed with other connective tissue diseases (overlap syndromes), with the exception of secondary Sjögren syndrome were excluded.

Research ethics committee of each hospital approved the study and all participants gave their informed written consent.

Patients were submitted to clinical examination and swollen/tender joint assessment, and disease activity was scored using the DAS28 erythrocyte sedimentation rate (ESR) system. Scores was interpreted as follows: < 2.6 (clinical remission), 2.6–3.1 (low), 3.2–5.0 (moderate), and ≥ 5.1 (high) [22].

Information on RA (diagnostic criteria, duration), clinical manifestations, laboratory findings, extra-joint manifestations, comorbidities, previous and current treatments, and family history of cardiovascular disease (first-degree relatives, women < 65 years, men < 55 years) was collected during consultation or retrieved from medical records. Anthropometric measures were taken during the first encounter. The patients were weighed wearing light clothes and no shoes, height was measured with a single stadiometer, and BMI was calculated by dividing the weight (kg) by the height squared (m^2). Obesity was determined based on BMI and WC. The adopted BMI ranges were: normal (18.5–24.9), overweight (25–29.9) and obese (≥30) [23]. With the patient standing upright, WC was measured with a flexible tape in the horizontal plane midway between the lowest rib and the iliac crest [24].

Dyslipidemia was considered present when the level of high-density lipoproteins (HDL-c) was < 50 mg/dL and/or the level of triglycerides was ≥150 mg/dL and/or the patient was treated with lipid-lowering drugs. Positivity for metabolic syndrome (MetS) was based on the revised criteria of the National Cholesterol Education Program (NCEP) Adult Treatment Panel III and the criteria of the International Diabetes Federation (IDF) [24–26].

Statistical analysis

The findings were expressed as absolute values and percentages (continuous variables), central tendency (mean), dispersion (standard deviation) and range (minimum and maximum).

Univariate analysis with stratification of increased WC according to both IDF and NCEP (categories: increased vs. non-increased) and weight according to BMI (categories: low weight/eutrophic vs. overweight vs. obese) was performed. Student's t test was used to compare means for both IDF and NCEP, while the proportion of increased WC was analyzed for each level with Pearson's chi-square test or Fisher's test. Mean obesity values were compared using analysis of variance (ANOVA).

The level of statistical significance was set at 5% ($p < 0.05$). Variables with significance at the level of

25% or lower ($p < 0.25$) in the univariate analysis were further submitted to multivariate analysis.

A multivariate binomial logistic model was used for the dependent WC variables (IDF and NCEP), while BMI was analyzed with a multivariate multinomial logit model, considering the three categories ≤24.9 (reference), 25–29.9, and ≥ 30. Based on the assumption that similarities are greater within the same center than between centers (the three participating centers are in different geographical regions), we used Huber-White Sandwich variance estimators.

Because the variables DAS28 ESR and age were not normally distributed given Shapiro Wilk test for normality ($p < 0.05$), they were categorized in the multivariate models. In the larger and more complete model, the least significant variables by the Wald test were eliminated one by one. Only variables at the 5% level of significance ($p < 0.05$) remained in the final model.

Results
Patients
The sample consisted of 791 RA patients aged 54.7 ± 12.0 years, of whom 86.9% were women and 59.9% were Caucasian. The mean disease duration was 12.8 ± 8.9 years, and 75% were rheumatoid factor-positive. The mean BMI was 27.1 ± 4.9. WC was increased in 37.8% (IDF) or 32.6% (NCEP). Most patients (64.8%) were classified as overweight. CVR factors were observed in the following proportions: DM II 15%, SAH 49.2%, dyslipidemia 34.3%, obesity by BMI 26.9%. Prednisone, methotrexate and leflunomide were used by 62.6, 67.3 and 34.5% of patients, respectively. The mean DAS28 ESR score was 4.1 ± 1.5. Disease activity was moderate in 42.6% and high in 25.7%. CRP was 20.2 ± 81.6 mg/L and mean ESR was 28.2 ± 22.1 mm/h (Table 1).

Comparison of RA patients with regard to WC
In the univariate analysis, increased WC (IDF and NCEP) was associated with older age ($p < 0.001$) and with the presence of DM II, SAH and dyslipidemia ($p < 0.001$). Mean DAS28 ESR scores were also significantly higher among patients with increased WC (IDF and NCEP) ($p < 0.05$) (Tables 2 and 3).

Comparison of RA patients with regard to BMI
Average age was positively associated with BMI category (low weight/eutrophic, overweight, obesity) ($p = 0.037$). SAH was most prevalent among obese patients (66.5%), followed by overweight (43.4%) and low weight/eutrophic (42.7%) patients ($p < 0.001$). Dyslipidemia was considerably less prevalent among low weight/eutrophic patients than among overweight and obese patients ($p < 0.001$) (Table 4).

Variables independently associated with obesity in RA patients
In the final multivariate models (Table 5 and Fig. 1) non-white race/color was positively associated with increased WC (NCEP) (OR = 1.4; $p < 0.001$). Age between 50 and 59 years was positively associated with increased WC (NCEP) and obesity (OR = 2.9; $p < 0.05$) when compared to age < 40 years, while age between 60 and 69 years was positively associated with obesity (OR = 1.6; $p = 0.005$). SAH and dyslipidemia were positively associated with increased WC (IDF and NCEP) and obesity (OR > 2.0; $p < 0.001$). DM II was positively associated with increased WC (IDF and NCEP) and negatively associated with obesity (OR = 0.8; $p = 0.003$). Generally speaking, DAS28 ESR scores above 2.6 were positively associated with increased WC (IDF) (OR > 1.2; $p < 0.01$) (except for scores ≥5.1) and with overweight and obesity (OR > 1.7; $p < 0.01$) (except for scores between 3.2 and 5.1).

Discussion
To our knowledge, this is the first Brazilian multi-center study evaluating the prevalence of obesity (evaluated by both BMI and WC) in RA patients and its association with disease variables and other cardiovascular risk (CVR) factors. Obesity was highly prevalent, whether defined by BMI (26.9%) or WC (IDF = 37.8%; NCEP = 32.6%). Moreover, obesity was found to be associated with disease activity.

The inclusion of three centers in geographically diverse regions allowed us to draw a comprehensive profile of Brazilian RA patients and their regional peculiarities. Another strong point of our study was the simultaneous evaluation of several CVR factors, laboratory parameters and disease variables through multivariate analyses with the purpose of identifying obesity determinants in RA patients.

The increase in CVR in RA has been well documented. A meta-analysis of 24 mortality studies with more than 111,000 RA patients revealed that the standard mortality rate from cardiovascular disease was 1.59 (95% CI 1.46 to 1.73), with an increased risk of death from disease ischemic heart disease (and stroke). *Fransen* et al. also reported in a meta-analysis of 13 studies that compared to the general population, the relative risk of a cardiovascular event is 2.59 (95% CI 1.77 to 3.79) and 1.27 (95% CI 1.16 to 1.38) in patients with RA < 50 years compared to those above 50 years [27, 28].

Traditional CVR factors play an important role in RA patients and this was recently demonstrated by an article that studied the impact of each CVR factor and the risk that could be attributed to factors directly related to RA. The conclusion was that 30% of the risk of cardiovascular events was attributed to factors characteristic of RA

Table 1 Characteristics of 791 patients with rheumatoid arthritis from three Brazilian referral centers

Variable	N = 791 (100.0%)
Female sex (n; %)	687 (86.9)
Non-white race/color (n; %)	313 (40.1)
Age	
Mean ± SD	54.7 ± 12.0
Minimum; maximum	21; 85
Age group (n; %)	
< 40 years	89 (11.5)
40–49 years	159 (20.5)
50–59 years	257 (33.1)
60–69 years	190 (24.4)
≥ 70 years	82 (10.5)
Disease duration (years)	
Mean ± SD	12.8 ± 8.9
Minimum; maximum	0; 56
Disease duration (categories)	
< 5 years	135 (17.2)
5–9 years	193 (24.6)
10–14 years	183 (23.4)
15–19 years	115 (14.7)
20–24 years	78 (10.0)
≥ 25 years	79 (10.1)
Increased WC (IDF) (n; %)	288 (37.8)
Increased WC (NCEP) (n; %)	250 (32.6)
BMI	
Mean ± SD	27.1 ± 4.9
Minimum; maximum	17.0; 47.0
Overweight (BMI > 24.99 & < 30)	514 (64.8)
Obesity (BMI > 29.99)	209 (26.9)
Diabetes mellitus (n; %)	119 (15.0)
Systemic arterial hypertension (n; %)	389 (49.2)
Dyslipidemia (n; %)	265 (34.3)
Family history of CVD (n; %)	129 (16.5)
Smoking (n; %)	93 (13.0)
Use of methotrexate (n; %)	531 (67.3)
Use of prednisone (n; %)	492 (62.6)
Use of leflunomide (n; %)	273 (34.5)
Use of methotrexate + prednisone (n; %)	226 (29.0)
Use of methotrexate + leflunomide (n; %)	44 (5.7)
Use of prednisone + leflunomide (n; %)	70 (9.0)
C-reactive protein	
Mean ± SD	20.2 ± 81.6
Minimum; maximum	0; 1730
C-reactive protein > 5 (n; %)	395 (61.1)

Table 1 Characteristics of 791 patients with rheumatoid arthritis from three Brazilian referral centers (*Continued*)

Variable	N = 791 (100.0%)
Rheumatoid factor (n; %)	530 (75.0)
DAS28	
Mean ± SD	4.07 ± 1.54
Minimum; maximum	0.0; 8.64
DAS28 (categories) (n; %)	
Remission	123 (17.3)
Low activity	102 (14.4)
Moderate activity	302 (42.6)
High activity	182 (25.7)
ESR	
Mean ± SD	28.2 ± 22.1
Minimum; maximum	0; 150
Metabolic syndrome	
NCEP (n;%)	250 (32.6)
IDF (n;%)	288 (37.8)

SD standard deviation, *IQI* interquartile interval, *WC* waist circumference, *CVD* cardiovascular disease, *ESR* erythrocyte sedimentation rate, *BMI* body mass index, *DAS28* disease activity score in 28 joints, *IDF* International Diabetes Federation, *NCEP* National Cholesterol Education Program Adult Treatment Panel III

and the remainder of CVR was attributed to the traditional ones. Each of these risk factors worsens the cardiovascular clinical outcome of RA patients in different proportions: SAH = OR: 1.62 (1.31–2), DM II = OR: 1.49 (1.0–2, 06), dyslipidemia (LDL). = OR: 1.15 (1.04–1.27)) [29]. In our series, we found a high prevalence of CVR factors: hypertension (49.2%), DM II (15%) and dyslipidemia (34.3%).

Most of our patients were overweight or obese women with long-standing RA and moderate disease activity, indicating a relatively serious condition with high risk of cardiovascular disease. Relevantly, in a recent study based on a cohort of 338 RA patients, MetS was highly prevalent (51.3%, one of the highest prevalences reported in the literature) and associated with disease activity [30].

Our results show that RA patients with increased WC have more CVR factors (such as DM II, SAH and dyslipidemia) than RA patients with normal WC, and that these variables have an independent influence on the prevalence of obesity. Other authors have reported higher WC values in RA patients than in controls [31, 32]; in our study, despite the absence of a control group, the prevalence of increased WC may be considered very high. This is supported by a recent meta-analysis on MetS in RA patients which revealed increased WC to be the most frequent component of the syndrome, matching the results of several others [33–35]. These findings point to the

Table 2 Comparison of rheumatoid arthritis patients with regard to waist circumference (IDF)

Variable	Normal WC $n = 474$ (100.0%)	Increased WC $n = 288$ (100.0%)	Total $n = 762$ (100%)	p-value
Female sex (n; %)	408 (86.1)	225 (78.1)	663 (87.0)	0.326
Non-white race/color (n; %)	189 (39.8)	113 (39.2)	302 (39.6)	0.902
Age (mean ± SD)	52.6 ± 12.6	58.0 ± 10.0	54.6 ± 12.0	< 0.001
Disease duration (mean ± SD)	12.9 ± 9.3	12.7 ± 8.1	12.8 ± 8.9	0.798
Diabetes mellitus (n; %)	27 (5.6)	90 (31.2)	117 (15.3)	< 0.001
Systemic arterial hypertension (n; %)	150 (31.6)	231 (80.2)	381 (50.0)	< 0.001
Dyslipidemia (n; %)	112 (23.6)	144 (50.0)	256 (33.5)	< 0.001
Family history of CVD (n; %)	75 (15.8)	53 (18.4)	128 (16.7)	0.360
Smoking (n; %)	62 (13)	31 (10.7)	93 (12.2)	0.293
Use of methotrexate (n; %)	320 (67.5)	192 (66.6)	512 (67.1)	0.989
Use of prednisone (n; %)	304 (64.1)	169 (58.6)	473 (62.0)	0.090
Use of leflunomide (n; %)	154 (32.4)	110 (38.1)	264 (34.6)	0.109
C-reactive protein (mean ± SD)	16.6 ± 44.0	26.7 ± 123.2	20.3 ± 82.6	0.136
Rheumatoid factor (n; %)	320 (67.5)	197 (68.4)	517 (67.8)	0.456
DAS28 (mean ± SD)	3.99 ± 1.56	4.23 ± 1.48	4.08 ± 1.53	0.047

SD standard deviation, *WC* waist circumference, *CVD* cardiovascular disease, *DAS28* disease activity score in 28 joints, *IDF* International Diabetes Federation

need for better control of modifiable CVR factors and the adoption of more aggressive treatment strategies in this patient population, including adequate diet and pressure control associated with regular physical activity [30].

The finding of BMI-defined obesity in 26.9% of our patients is compatible with the literature. Obesity is associated with CVR factors in the general population and, more strongly, in RA patients. Thus, in a recent study involving over fifteen thousand RA patients, BMI-defined obesity was more prevalent among patients (20%) than among healthy controls, and even higher figures have been reported (31.6%) [34, 36]. The association between obesity and RA disease activity has also been reported before [37]. However, the use of BMI as a measure of obesity may be confounded by variations in body composition (fat vs. lean mass), compromising the accuracy of the method in this patient population. Our group and other researchers have therefore proposed alternative cut-off values for obesity in RA patients [38, 39]. Another strategy, adopted in the present study, is to employ WC in addition to BMI as an indicator of obesity.

Another important finding of this study was the positive association between DAS28 ESR scores and increased WC (IDF). Similar results were obtained by *Abourazzak* et al. who observed an association between IDF-defined MetS (thus, increased WC) and disease activity [31]. This is supported by a Finnish study showing a high prevalence of abdominal obesity in RA patients (52%) in association with greater disease activity,

physical incapacity and sedentary lifestyle [40]. In another study based on a sample of 1696 RA patients, abdominal and BMI-defined obesity were both associated with higher DAS28 ESR scores, limited physical functioning and smaller likelihood of sustained remission [41]. However, although the association between obesity and RA disease activity is well documented, little is known about the effect of diet and lifestyle changes on clinical improvement and/or sustained remission.

DAS28 ESR scores above 2.6 were correlated with IDF-defined obesity, overweight (BMI 25–29.9) and obesity (BMI ≥30). However, high DAS28 ESR scores were not associated with IDF-defined obesity, and BMI-defined overweight and obesity were not associated with moderate disease activity. One possible explanation for this is that the sample may not have provided sufficient statistical power to perform multivariate analyses and estimate disease activity in all categories. Moreover, many authors have criticized the interpretation of results based solely on *p*-values, insisting on the need to view results from the epidemiological perspective and include odds ratios and confidence intervals in the analysis [42]. In the present study, the confidence intervals for all the DAS28 ESR categories were greater than 1 (absence of association), indicating a positive association between disease activity and obesity. In addition, all the estimated odds ratios were greater than 1 (except for moderate activity in patients with BMI ≥30).

Our study has several limitations, one of which is the cross-sectional study design, making it impossible

Table 3 Comparison of rheumatoid arthritis patients with regard to waist circumference (NCEP)

Variable	Normal WC n = 488 (100.0%)	Increased WC n = 250 (100.0%)	Total n = 767 (100%)	p-value
Female sex (n; %)	442 (93.2)	225 (78.1)	667 (86.9)	0.082
Non-white race/color (n; %)	195 (41.1)	109 (37.8)	304 (39.6)	0.111
Age (mean ± SD)	52.8 ± 12.6	58.4 ± 12.0)	57 ± 12.0	< 0.001
Disease duration (mean ± SD)	12.9 ± 9.2	12.7 ± 8.2	12.8 ± 8.9	0.866
Diabetes mellitus (n; %)	27 (5.6)	89 (30.9)	116 (15.1)	< 0.001
Systemic arterial hypertension (n; %)	172 (36.2)	209 (72.5)	381 (49.6)	< 0.001
Dyslipidemia (n; %)	122 (25.7)	134 (46.5)	256 (33.3)	< 0.001
Family history of CVD (n; %)	81 (17.1)	47 (16.3)	128 (16.7)	0.290
Smoking (n; %)	66 (13.9)	27 (9.3)	93 (12.1)	0.371
Use of methotrexate (n; %)	350 (73.8)	165 (57.3)	515 (67.1)	0.866
Use of prednisone (n; %)	329 (69.4)	149 (51.7)	478 (62.3)	0.212
Use of leflunomide (n; %)	169 (34.6)	99 (39.6)	268 (34.9)	0.060
C-reactive protein (mean ± SD)	16.4 ± 42.7	28.3 ± 131.9	20.1 ± 82.1	0.087
Rheumatoid factor (n; %)	353 (74.5)	168 (58.3)	521 (67.9)	0.655
DAS28 (mean ± SD)	3.98 ± 1.54	4.29 ± 1.50	4.08 ± 1.53	0.012

SD standard deviation, WC waist circumference, CVD cardiovascular disease, DAS28 disease activity score in 28 joints, NCEP National Cholesterol Education Program Adult Treatment Panel III

to identify cause and effect. Another is the lack of a control group for comparisons with healthy individuals. Moreover, considering the impact of physical exercise on BMI, WC and disease activity, our failure to control for sedentary lifestyle may have limited the study. Another issue that should be emphasized is that we did not analyze the effect of the genetic background among RA patients, especially the HLA-DRB1 locus, which has been associated with disease susceptibility, and has also been associated with disease activity, radiological severity, mortality and response to treatment. Finally, by restricting recruitment to

Table 4 Clinical characteristics according to category of body mass index (BMI)

Variable	Low weight or eutrophic n = 274 (100%)	Overweight n = 295 (100%)	Obese n = 209 (100%)	Total n = 788 (100%)	p-value
Female sex (n; %)	236 (86.1)	254 (86.1)	185 (88.5)	675 (85.6)	0.467
Non-white race/color (n; %)	103 (37.6)	120 (40.7)	83 (39.7)	462 (58.6)	0.554
Age (mean ± SD)	53.5 ± 13.3	54.6 ± 12.1	56.6 ± 9.9	57.0 ± 12.0	0.037
Disease duration (mean ± SD)	13.4 ± 9.6	12.9 ± 8.6	12.3 ± 8.3	12.9 ± 8.9	0.389
Diabetes mellitus (n; %)	36 (13.1)	44 (14.9)	37 (17.7)	117 (14.8)	0.168
Systemic arterial hypertension (n; %)	117 (42.7)	128 (43.4)	139 (66.5)	384 (48.7)	< 0.001
Dyslipidemia (n; %)	70 (25.5)	98 (33.2)	92 (44.0)	260 (32.9)	< 0.001
Family history of CVD (n; %)	41 (14.9)	50 (16.9)	37 (17.7)	128 (16.2)	0.379
Smoking (n; %)	35 (12.8)	36 (12.2)	21 (10.0)	92 (11.7)	0.319
Use of methotrexate (n; %)	189 (68.9)	196 (66.4)	137 (65.5)	522 (66.2)	0.558
Use of prednisone (n; %)	162 (59.1)	188 (63.7)	131 (62.7)	481 (61.0)	0.342
Use of leflunomide (n; %)	94 (34.3)	104 (35.2)	73 (34.9)	271 (34.3)	0.972
C-reactive protein (mean ± SD)	18.7 ± 59.0	14.7 ± 36.2	31.0 ± 138.9	20.4 ± 82.3	0.137
Rheumatoid factor (n; %)	187 (68.2)	192 (65.1)	144 (68.9)	523 (66.4)	0.762
DAS28 (mean ± SD)	3.97 ± 1.58	4.06 ± 1.49	4.21 ± 1.52	4.07 ± 1.53	0.298

SD standard deviation, CVD cardiovascular disease, DAS28 disease activity score in 28 joint

Table 5 Final multivariate models: Odds Ratios and 95% confidence intervals for four different outcomes

Variable	Increased vs. non-increased WC (IDF) OR (95% CI)		Increased vs. non-increased WC (NCEP) OR (95% CI)		Overweight vs. low weight/eutrophic OR (95% CI)		Obese vs. low weight/eutrophic OR (95% CI)	
Non-white race/color (ref: white)	–	–	1.4***	1.2; 1.7	–	–	–	–
Age (ref: ≤39 years)								
40–49 years	–	–	1.2	0.9; 1.6	0.9	0.4; 2.4	2.5***	1.7; 3.7
50–59 years	–	–	1.9***	1.4; 2.4	1.2	0.5; 2.7	2.9*	1.3; 6.5
60–69 years	–	–	0.9	0.5; 1.6	1.3	0.9; 1.8	1.6**	1.2; 2.3
≥70 years	–	–	1.0	0.4; 2.2	0.9	0.7; 1.2	1.5	0.6; 3.7
Diabetes mellitus (ref: no DM)	4.5***	3.5; 5.7	7.4***	3.7; 15.0	1.1	0.6; 1.9	0.8**	0.7; 0.9
SAH (ref: no SAH)	6.4***	4.9; 8.2	8.9***	4.5; 17.9	0.9	0.6; 1.6	2.5***	2.1; 3.0
Dyslipidemia (ref: no dyslipidemia)	2.1***	1.8; 2.5	2.2***	1.6; 2.9	1.4***	1.2; 2.6	2.2***	1.5; 3.1
DAS28 (ref: ≤2.59; remission)								
2.60–3.19 (low activity)	1.8**	1.3; 2.5	–	–	2.2***	1.6; 3.1	1.8***	1.3; 2.4
3.2–5.09 (moderate activity)	1.3***	1.2; 1.4	–	–	1.2	0.7; 1.9	1.0	0.6; 1.6
≥5.1 (high activity)	1.8	0.9; 3.3	–	–	1.8**	1.3; 2.6	1.9**	1.1; 3.2

*p <0.05; **p <0.01; ***p <0.001;
SAH = systemic arterial hypertension; DAS28 = disease activity score in 28 joints; Overweight = BMI >24.99 and <30;Obese = BMI>29.9; Low weight/eutrophic = BMI<25

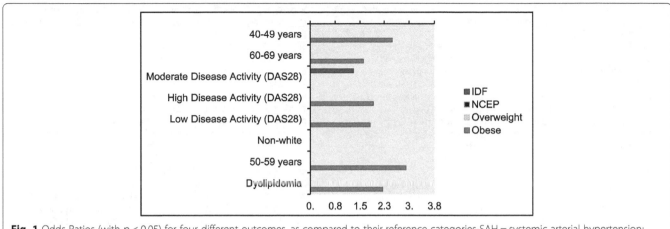

Fig. 1 Odds Ratios (with p < 0.05) for four different outcomes, as compared to their reference categories-SAH = systemic arterial hypertension; DAS28 = disease activity score in 28 joints; Overweight = BMI > 24.99 and < 30; Obese = BMI > 29.9; Low weight/eutrophic = BMI < 25. Reference categories for obese and overweight = low weight/eutrophic; for NCEP and for IDF = non-increased WCce.

patients from regional referral centers, a bias may have been introduced, increasing the proportion of severe cases and overestimating the prevalence of obesity.

Conclusion

Our study revealed a high frequency of abdominal obesity in RA patients and a positive association between obesity and CVR factors and disease activity, pointing to the need for better control of the disease and related risk factors. Larger prospective multi center studies are needed to evaluate the effect of WC reduction on RA disease activity.

Acknowledgements
None.

Authors' contributions
All authors were involved in drafting the article or revising it critically for important intellectual content, and all authors approved the final version to be submitted for publication. Dr. Guimaraes had full access to all study data and takes responsibility for the integrity of the data. Study conception and design: Guimaraes, Rodrigues, Gomes, Machado, Brenol, Krampe,de Andrade, Kakehasi. Acquisition of data: Guimaraes, Rodrigues. Poti, Brenol, Kakehasi. Analysis and interpretation of data: Guimaraes, Rodrigues, Kakehasi.

Author details
[1]Serviço de Reumatologia, Hospital das Clínicas, Universidade Federal de Minas Gerais (UFMG), Rua Adolfo Pereira, 262, apto 901, Belo Horizonte, MG 30310-350, Brazil. [2]Programa de Pós-graduacão em Ci ncias Médicas, Universidade de Fortaleza (UNIFOR), Fortaleza, Brazil. [3]Universidade de Fortalea e Hospital Geral de Fortaleza-HGF, Fortaleza, Brazil. [4]Faculdade de Medicina, Universidade Federal de Minas Gerais (UFMG), Belo Horizonte, Brazil. [5]Faculdade de Medicina, Universidade Federal do Rio Grande do Sul (UFRGS), Porto Alegre, Alegre, Brazil.

References
1. Jung RT. Obesity as a disease. Br Med Bull. 1997;53(2):307–21.
2. Hubert HB, Feinleib M, McNamara PM, Castelli WP. Obesity as an independent risk factor for cardiovascular disease: a 26-year follow-up of participants in the Framingham heart study. Circulation. 1983;67(5):968–77.
3. Blüher M. Adipose tissue dysfunction in obesity. Exp Clin Endocrinol Diabetes. 2009;117(6):241–50.
4. Van Gaal LF, Mertens IL, De Block CE. Mechanisms linking obesity with cardiovascular disease. Nature. 2006;444(7121):875–80.
5. Hotamisligil GS. Inflammation and metabolic disorders. Nature. 2006; 444(7121):860–7.
6. Ouchi N, Parker JL, Lugus JJ, Walsh K. Adipokines in inflammation and metabolic disease. Nat Rev Immunol. 2011;11(2):85–97.
7. Versini M, Jeandel PY, Rosenthal E, Shoenfeld Y. Obesity in autoimmune diseases: not a passive bystander. Autoimmun Rev. 2014;13(9):981–1000.
8. Whitlock G, Lewington S, Sherliker P, Clarke R, Emberson J, Halsey J, et al. Body-mass index and cause-specific mortality in 900 000 adults: collaborative analyses of 57 prospective studies. Lancet. 2009;373(9669): 1083–96.
9. Shimomura I, Funahashi T, Takahashi M, Maeda K, Kotani K, Nakamura T, et al. Enhanced expression of PAI-1 in visceral fat: possible contributor to vascular disease in obesity. Nat Med. 1996;2(7):800–3.
10. Stavropoulos-Kalinoglou A, Metsios GS, Koutedakis Y, Kitas GD. Obesity in rheumatoid arthritis. Rheumatology (Oxford). 2011;50(3):450–62.
11. García-Poma A, Segami MI, Mora CS, Ugarte MF, Terrazas HN, Rhor EA, et al. Obesity is independently associated with impaired quality of life in patients with rheumatoid arthritis. Clin Rheumatol. 2007;26(11):1831–5.
12. Klaasen R, Wijbrandts CA, Gerlag DM, Tak PP. Body mass index and clinical response to infliximab in rheumatoid arthritis. Arthritis Rheum. 2011;63(2): 359–64.
13. Symmons DP, Bankhead CR, Harrison BJ, Brennan P, Barrett EM, Scott DG, et al. Blood transfusion, smoking, and obesity as risk factors for the development of rheumatoid arthritis: results from a primary care-based incident case-control study in Norfolk, England. Arthritis Rheum. 1997;40(11): 1955–61.
14. Kaufmann J, Kielstein V, Kilian S, Stein G, Hein G. Relation between body mass index and radiological progression in patients with rheumatoid arthritis. J Rheumatol. 2003;30(11):2350–5.
15. Van der Helm-van Mil AH, van der Kooij SM, Allaart CF, Toes RE, Huizinga TW. A high body mass index has a protective effect on the amount of joint destruction in small joints in early rheumatoid arthritis. Ann Rheum Dis. 2008;67(6):769–74.
16. Westhoff G, Rau R, Zink A. Radiographic joint damage in early rheumatoid arthritis is highly dependent on body mass index. Arthritis Rheum. 2007; 56(11):3575–82.
17. Abella V, Scotece M, Conde J, López V, Lazzaro V, Pino J, et al. Adipokines, metabolic syndrome and rheumatic diseases. J Immunol Res. 2014;2014: 343746.
18. Lago F, Gómez R, Conde J, Scotece M, Gómez-Reino JJ, Gualillo O. Cardiometabolic comorbidities and rheumatic diseases: focus on the role of fat mass and adipokines. Arthritis Care Res (Hoboken). 2011;63(8):1083 90.
19. Gómez R, Conde J, Scotece M, Gómez-Reino JJ, Lago F, Gualillo O. What's new in our understanding of the role of adipokines in rheumatic diseases? Nat Rev Rheumatol. 2011;7(9):528–36.

20. Arnett FC, Edworthy SM, Bloch DAet al (1988) The American rheumatism association 1987 revised criteria for the classification of rheumatoid arthritis. Arthritis Rheum 31:315–324.

21. Aletaha D, Neogi T, Silman AJet al (2010) 2010 rheumatoid arthritis classification criteria: an American College of Rheumatology/European league against rheumatism collaborative initiative. Arthritis Rheum 62:2569–2581.

22. Aletaha D, Smolen J. The simplified disease activity index (SDAI) and the clinical disease activity index (CDAI): a review of their usefulness and validity in rheumatoid arthritis. Clin Exp Rheumatol. 2005;23:S100–8.

23. Physical status: the use and interpretation of anthropometry. Report of a WHO expert committee. World Health Organ Tech Rep Ser 1995; 854:1–452.

24. Alberti KG, Zimmet P, Shaw J. Metabolic syndrome--a new world-wide definition. A consensus statement from the international diabetes federation. Diabet Med. 2006;23:469–80.

25. Alberti KG, Eckel RH, Grundy SM, Zimmet PZ, Cleeman JI, Donato KA, Fruchart JC, James WP, Loria CM, Smith SC Jr (2009) International Diabetes Federation Task Force on Epidemiology and Prevention; Hational Heart, Lung, and Blood Institute; American Heart Association; World Heart Federation; International Atherosclerosis Society; International Association for the Study of Obesity. Harmonizing the metabolic syndrome: a joint interim statement of the International Diabetes Federation Task Force on Epidemiology and Prevention; National Heart, Lung, and Blood Institute; American Heart Association; World Heart Federation; International Atherosclerosis Society; and International Association for the Study of Obesity. Circulation 20;120(16):1640–1645.

26. Grundy SM, Cleeman JI, Daniels SR, Donato KA, Eckel RH, Franklin BA, Gordon DJ, Krauss RM, Savage PJ, Smith SC Jr, Spertus JA, Costa F (2005) American Heart Association; National Heart, Lung, and Blood Institute. Diagnosis and management of the metabolic syndrome: an American Heart Association/National Heart, Lung, and Blood Institute scientific statement. Circulation 25;112(17):2735–2752.

27. Avina-Zubeita JA, Choi HK, Sadatsafavi M, et al. Risk of cardiovascular mortality in patients with rheumatoid arthritis: a meta-analysis of observational studies. Arthitis Rheum. 2008;59(12):1690e7.

28. Fransen J, Kazema-Bajestani SM, Bredi SJ, et al. Rheumatoid arthritis disadvantages younger patients for cardiovascular diseases: a meta-analysis. PLoS One. 2016;11(6):e0157360.

29. Crowson CS, Rollefstad S, Ikdahl E, et al. Impact of risk factors associated with cardiovascular outcomes in patients with rheumatoid arthritis. Ann Rheum Dis. 2018;77(1):48–54.

30. Gomes KWP, Luz AJP, Felipe MRB, Beltrão LA, Sampaio AXC, Rodrigues CEM. Prevalence of metabolic syndrome in rheumatoid arthritis patients from northeastern Brazil: association with disease activity. Mod Rheumatol. 2017; 9:1–6 https://doi.org/10.1080/14397595.2017.1316813.

31. Abourazzak FE, Mansouri S, Najdi A, Tahiri L, Nejjari C, Harzy T. Prevalence of metabolic syndrome in patients with rheumatoid arthritis in Morocco: a cross-sectional study of 179 cases. Clin Rheumatol. 2014;33(11):1549–55.

32. Rajput R, Dangi A, Singh H. Prevalence of glucose intolerance in rheumatoid arthritis patients at a tertiary care centre in Haryana. Diabetes Metab Syndr. 2017;20 https://doi.org/10.1016/j.dsx.2017.07.032.

33. Zafar ZA, Mahmud TH, Rasheed A, Wagan AA. Frequency of metabolic syndrome in Pakistani cohort of patients with rheumatoid arthritis. J Pak Med Assoc. 2016;66(6):671–6.

34. Galarza-Delgado DA, Azpiri-Lopez JR, Colunga-Pedraza IJ, Cárdenas-de la Garza JA, Vera-Pineda R, Wah-Suárez M, Arvizu-Rivera RI, Martínez-Moreno A, Ramos-Cázares RE, Torres-Quintanilla FJ, Valdovinos-Bañuelos A, Esquivel-Valerio JA, Garza-Elizondo MA. Prevalence of comorbidities in Mexican mestizo patients with rheumatoid arthritis. Rheumatol. 2017;5 https://doi.org/10.1007/s00296-017-3769-3.

35. Hallajzadeh J, Safiri S, Mansournia MA, Khoramdad M, Izadi N, Almasi-Hashiani A, Pakzad R, Ayubi E, Sullman MJ, Karamzad N (2017) Metabolic syndrome and its components among rheumatoid arthritis patients: a comprehensive updated systematic review and meta-analysis. PLoS one 23; 12(3):e0170361. https://doi.org/10.1371/journal.pone.0170361.

36. Albrecht K, Richter A, Callhoff J, et al. Body mass index distribution in rheumatoid arthritis: a collaborative analysis from three large German rheumatoid arthritis databases. Arthritis Res Ther. 2016;18:149 https://doi.org/10.1186/s13075-016-1043-9.

37. Jawaheer D, Olsen J, Lahiff M, Forsberg S, Lähteenmäki J, da Silveira IG, Rocha FA, Magalhães Laurindo IM, Henrique da Mota LM, Drosos AA, Murphy E, Sheehy C, Quirke E, Cutolo M, Rexhepi S, Dadoniene J,

Verstappen SM, Sokka T. QUEST-RA. Gender, body mass index and rheumatoid arthritis disease activity: results from the QUEST-RA study. Clin Exp Rheumatol. 2010;28(4):454–61.

38. Stavropoulos-Kalinoglou A, Metsios GS, Koutedakis Y, Nevill AM, Douglas KM, Jamurtas A, van Zanten JJ, Labib M, Kitas GD. Redefining overweight and obesity in rheumatoid arthritis patients. Ann Rheum Dis. 2007;66(10): 1316–21.

39. Guimarães MFBR, Pinto MRDC, Raid RGSC, Andrade MVM, Kakehasi AM. Which is the best cutoff of body mass index to identify obesity in female patients with rheumatoid arthritis? A study using dual energy X-ray absorptiometry body composition. Rev Bras Reumatol. 2017;57(4):279–85.

40. Uutela T, Kautiainen H, Järvenpää S, Salomaa S, Hakala M, Häkkinen A. Waist circumference based abdominal obesity may be helpful as a marker for unmet needs in patients with RA. Scand J Rheumatol. 2014;43(4):279–85 https://doi.org/10.3109/03009742.2013.858769.

41. Ajeganova S, Andersson ML, Hafström I. BARFOT study group. Association of obesity with worse disease severity in rheumatoid arthritis as well as with comorbidities: a long-term followup from disease onset. Arthritis Care Res (Hoboken). 2013;65(1):78–87. https://doi.org/. https://doi.org/10.1002/acr.21710.

42. Susarla SM, Hopper RA (2018) Discussion: why the p value alone is not enough: the need for confidence intervals in plastic surgery research. Plast Reconstr Surg 141(1):163e-164e. https://doi.org/10.1097/PRS. 0000000000003965.

13

Rheumatoid artrhitis treatment in Brazil: Data from a large real-life multicenter study

Ana Paula Monteiro Gomides[1][*] [iD], Cleandro Pires de Albuquerque[1], Ana Beatriz Vargas Santos[2], Manoel Barros Bértolo[3], Paulo Louzada Júnior[4], Rina Dalva Neubarth Giorgi[5], Sebastião Cezar Radominski[6], Maria Fernanda B. Resende Guimarães[7], Karina Rossi Bonfiglioli[8], Maria de Fátima Lobato da Cunha Sauma[9], Ivânio Alves Pereira[10], Claiton Viegas Brenol[11], Licia Maria Henrique da Mota[1] and Geraldo da Rocha Castelar Pinheiro[2]

Abstract

Background: Last decades witnessed great technological advances in rheumatoid arthritis (RA) management, but their implementation in clinical practice might prove difficult. Despite the efficacy demonstrated in controlled trials this information needs to be confirmed by real life data. This study assessed real-life treatment among RA patients.

Methods: REAL study included Brazilian RA patients from eleven centers. Interview and medical records were performed. Continuous variables were compared using Student's t or Mann-Whitney and categorical variables were assessed with chi-square or Fisher's exact tests.

Results: 1115 patients were included, women 89.5%. Median age 56.6 years, disease duration 152.5 months; 78.7% were rheumatoid fator positive; 55.2% had erosive disease; DAS28 (disease activity index-28 joints) = 3.5, HAQ (health assessment questionnaire) =0.875. The median duration of symptoms until the start of first DMARD was 12 months. A total of 529 (47.2%) patients used corticosteroids; 1022 (90.8%) were on conventional synthetic (cs) DMARDs and 406 (36.1%) on biological (b) DMARDs. Methotrexate (MTX) was the most frequent csDMARD: 748 (66.5%) patients, followed by leflunomide (LFN), used by 381 (33.9%) of patients. MTX was associated to LFN in 142 (12.6%) patients. Only five (0.4%) patients used triple therapy (MTX + hydroxychloroquine + sulfasalazine) or sulfasalazine in monotherapy.

Conclusions: Despite advances in therapeutic resources, roughly half RA patients failed achieve T2T goals and 55.2% developed erosive disease. The frequent use of corticosteroids and delay in initiating DMARDs were demonstrated. Issues concerning timely access to medical care are crucial for effective management.

Keywords: Rheumatoid arthritis, Drug therapy, Observational study, Latin America

Background

Rheumatoid arthritis (RA) is a chronic systemic auto-immune disease characterized by inflammatory involvement of the peripheral synovial joints [1]. Delays in diagnosis and initiation of disease-modifying anti-rheumatic drugs (DMARDs) can lead to joint destruction, deformities, and impairment of the patient's functional capacity and quality of life [2, 3].

In recent decades, there have been great advances in the management of RA, including new effective drugs and the advent of the "treat to target" (T2T) concept, based on frequent clinical assessment and adjustments as needed to attain sustained remission or low disease activity. Another important incorporated concept was that of a window of opportunity for most effective treatment. It is believed that early diagnosis and treatment with strict control of disease activity are associated with better outcomes and prognosis [4].

Current standards of care in RA incorporate these concepts and postulate a rational stepwise approach to the pharmacological treatment of the disease [5–7]. Although widely accepted by rheumatologists, T2T implementation and its actual benefits in day-to-day clinical

* Correspondence: anapmgomides@gmail.com
[1]Universidade de Brasília- UnB, Brasília, DF, Brazil
Full list of author information is available at the end of the article

practice are still not well established [8]. Unlike research settings, in real-life scenarios, constraints in access to healthcare resources, especially in less developed countries, might hinder the achievement of treatment goals and produce deviations from the expected standards of care [8].

The extent to which the recent advances in RA management are effectively being translated into better disease control in day-to-day practice can only be assessed through real-life epidemiological data. This study was aimed to assess the real-life patterns of treatment and their end results in terms of disease control, among RA patients in Brazil.

Methods

The REAL study assembled a cohort of RA patients attending eleven public health centers, from different regions of the country. From August, 2015 to April, 2016, each center enrolled approximately 100 consecutive patients [9]. Subjects should be 18 years of age or older, meet the American Rheumatism Association (1987) or American College of Rheumatology/European League Against Rheumatism (2010) classification criteria [10, 11], and have been followed up at their respective center for at least six months. Patients with comorbidities that could pose obstacle the planned assessment were excluded. Subjects were submitted to structured clinical interview with physical exam and thorough review of medical records, including laboratorial and imaging aspects. Data reported herein are cross-sectional, corresponding to the baseline assessment of participants, who would then be followed up for 12 months.

Disease activity was assessed using the Disease Activity Index-28 Joints (DAS28) and the Clinical Disease Activity Index (CDAI) [12]. Functional capacity (disability) was determined using the Health Assessment Questionnaire (HAQ) [13]. Health-related quality of life was assessed by the 12-Item Short-Form Health Survey (SF-12) [14]. Erosive disease was characterized by the finding of erosions (breaking of the cortical bone) in at least three separate joints at any of the following sites: proximal interphalangeal, metacarpophalangeal, wrist, and metatarsophalangeal joints [15]. Rheumatoid factor and anti-cyclic citrullinated peptide antibody (anti-CCP) were defined as positive "low titer", when exceeding by less than 3 times the upper limit of normality, and as "high titer" when reaching 3 times the upper limit of normality or above.

Continuous variables were compared using Student's t test or Mann-Whitney test, based on whether or not normality requirements were fulfilled. Categorical variables were compared using the chi-square test or Fisher's exact test [16]. A p value < 0.05 was deemed significant. Statistical analysis was performed using SAS 9.4 (SAS Institute Inc., Cary, North Carolina) and SPSS 20.0 (IBM Corp. Armok, NY). The study was approved by the local ethics committee and all participants granted informed consent.

Results

A total of 1115 patients (89,5% female, median age of 56.6 years and median disease duration of 152.5 months) were included. An extended description of demographic characteristics of the REAL cohort has already been published [9] and are shown in Table 1. The Table 2 summarizes the patients' clinical characteristics.

By the time of assessment, 15 (1.3%) patients were in clinical remission without any medication. Five hundred twenty-nine patients (47.2%) were on corticosteroids, and 21 (1.9%) took corticosteroids as their sole DMARD. The median (equivalent) dose of prednisone was 5 mg/day (interquartile range, IQR = 1). Among patients who were not on corticosteroids, 367 (61.6%) reported their previous use. Corticosteroid users, compared to non-users, showed higher mean scores (standard deviation, SD) on DAS28-ESR 3.9 (1.6) vs. 3.4 (1.4), DAS28-CRP 3.6 (1.5) vs. 3.1 (1.3), and HAQ 1.1 (0.8) vs. 0.8 (0.7), $p < 0.001$ for all comparisons. Some features indicative of aggressive or refractory disease were associated with corticosteroid use (Table 3). There was no association between gender and corticosteroid use ($p = 0.43$).

Overall, 1022 patients (90.8%) used conventional synthetic DMARDs (in monotherapy or combination); 406 (36.1%) used a biological DMARD; 23 (5.7%) of the biological DMARD users had it in monotherapy. Tofacitinib was then the only target-specific synthetic DMARD available in Brazil, taken by 9 (0.8%) of cohort's patients

Table 1 Demographic data of patients with rheumatoid arthritis in the REAL study [9]

Demographic data	Absolute value or%	n
Years of study – median (min-max)	8 (0–20)	1081
Ethnicity		1115
White	56.8%	
Black	10.9%	
Pardo	31.3%	
Others	1.0%	
Social Class[a]		1115
A	1.4%	
B1	3.5%	
B2	18.4%	
C1	27.4%	
C2	31.3%	
D-E	18.0%	

[a] Social classes based on average household income (Brazil criterion) A1: R $ 20,888 B1: R $ 9254 B2: R $ 4852 C1 R $ 2705 C2 R $ 1625 D- E: R $ 768

Table 2 RA patients' clinical characteristics in the REAL cohort

Clinical Variable	Results	N[a]
Disease duration[b], median (min-max)	152.5 (8–683)	1115
Positive rheumatoid factor (%)	78.7	1105
Positive ACPA (%)	76.8	477
Time to first DMARD[c], median (min-max)	12 (0–624)	995
Erosive disease (%)	55.2	1105
DAS28-ESR, median (min-max)	3.5 (0.3–8.2)	932
DAS28-CRP, median (min-max)	3.7 (1.0–8.1)	944
CDAI, median (min-max)	9 (0–70)	1122
HAQ, median (min-max)	0.875 (0–3)	1121
SF-12 physical component, median (min-max)	36.1 (17.5–55.9)	1035
SF-12 mental component, median (min-max)	46.9 (14.3–72.0)	1035
Remission (DAS28-ESR)	26.2%	
Low disease activity (DAS28-ESR)	15.1%	
Moderate disease activity (DAS28-ESR)	41.8%	
High disease activity (DAS28-ESR)	16.9%	

[a] Numbers of patients assessed for each clinical variable. [b] Total disease duration in months. [c] Time-interval from first symptoms to first prescribed DMARD (in months). *ACPA* anti-citrullinated peptide antibody. *DAS28* Disease Activity Score – 28 joints. *ESR* erythrocyte sedimentation rate. *CDAI* Clinical Disease Activity Index. *HAQ* Health Assessment Questionnaire. *SF-12* 12-Item Short-Form Health Survey

at that moment. The most prescribed therapeutic regimens of conventional synthetic DMARDs are presented in Table 4. The triple therapy with methotrexate (MTX) + sulfasalazine (SSZ) + hydroxichloroquine (HCQN) was used in only 5 patients (0.4%); a similar figure was observed for sulfasalazine monotherapy (5 patients, 0.4%). Table 5 reports the total frequencies of use for each synthetic and biological DMARDs (whether in combination or monotherapy).

Patients on methotrexate (MTX), whether in combination or not, compared to those not using the drug, had lower DAS28-CRP: mean (SD) score of 3.2 (1.3) for the MTX group and 3.4 (1.4) for the non-MTX group ($p = 0.0043$). There was also a trend toward lower DAS28-ESR in MTX users [3.6 (1.5) vs. 3.7 (1.5), $p = 0.056$].

MTX was less prescribed to patients with interstitial pneumonia, compared to those without this feature (OR 0.44; 95%CI: 0.24–0.82; $p = 0.008$). Leflunomide was less prescribed to individuals with subcutaneous nodules (OR 0.52; 95%CI: 0.31–0.87; $p = 0.011$). Patients on biological DMARDs, compared to those with only conventional synthetic drugs, showed higher scores on HAQ, mean (SD): 1.03 (0.76) vs. 0.90 (0.77), $p = 0.007$. Some features of aggressive or refractory disease were also associated with biological DMARD prescription (Table 6).

Discussion

The Brazilian Ministry of Health provides free access to nearly all currently approved synthetic and biological DMARDs for the treatment of RA, and new technologies are continuously assessed for possible incorporation. To grant access to such costly drugs, the Ministry requires a medical prescription along with founded explanation of clinical motives, including data on disease activity scores. Moreover, the continuity of treatment depends on medical reports, which should account for current disease status on a regular 3-month basis. In other words, the Brazilian protocol for the management of RA does incorporate all relevant concepts and resources with proven efficacy in clinical trials. Nonetheless, concerns about extrapolating findings from controlled trials to larger uncontrolled scenarios, especially in less-favored economic backgrounds, are warranted [17, 18]. The actual patterns of disease management in these population settings and their end results must be assessed through real-life data. The REAL study applied to that task.

The cohort was composed mainly of patients with long-term established RA (median of 152.5 months), with white race predominance (56.8%) and a high prevalence of females (89.5%). The female prevalence herein was similar to that in GLADAR, a multicenter study conducted in 14 Latin American countries, but higher than expected in North American and European populations [19]. The white race predominance followed a characteristic of the Brazilian population [20].

Table 3 Rheumatoid arthritis features associated with corticosteroid use

Clinical feature[a]	N(%)[b]	Odds ratio for corticosteroid use (95% CI)
Moderate or high disease activity[c] (DAS28-ESR)	543 (58.7)	1.50 (1.15–1.96)
Moderate or high disease activity[c] (DAS28-CRP)	437 (57.3)	1.59 (1.23–2.06)
High-titer rheumatoid factor[d]	616 (56.1)	1.64 (1.29–2.08)
Positive anti-CCP	368 (76.8)	2.27 (1.48–3.51)
Erosive disease[e]	602 (54.9)	1.56 (1.23–1.98)
Anemia	78 (7.03)	2.37 (1.46–3.85)
Subcutaneous nodules	92 (8,3)	1.82 (1.18–2.82)

[a] Groups of patients with and without each feature were compared (binary logistic regression); $p < 0.05$ for all comparisons. [b] Total numbers and percentage of patients with the clinical feature among all those assessed for that variable. [c] Defined as DAS28 score > 3.2 [d] Defined as at least 3 times the upper limit of normality [e] Defined as at least 3 erosions in some specified joints (see methodology)

Table 4 Preferred therapeutic regimens of conventional synthetic disease-modifying antirheumatic drugs (DMARDs) in Brazil

Synthetic DMARD Regimen[a]	N (%)
Methotrexate monotherapy	154 (13.7)
Methotrexate + corticosteroid	135 (12.0)
Methotrexate + leflunomide	95 (8.4)
Methotrexate + leflunomide + corticosteroid	55 (4.9)
Leflunomide monotherapy	52 (4.6)
Methotrexate + antimalarial (hydroxichloroquine or chloroquine)	31 (2.8)
Leflunomide + corticosteroid	30 (2.7)
Antimalarial (hydroxichloroquine or chloroquine monotherapy)	17 (1.5)
Other[b]	140 (12.4)

[a] NSAIDs allowed for pain relief on an as-needed basis. [b] All other regimens of conventional synthetic DMARD whether in monotherapy or combination (none exceeding 1.5% of prescriptions individually)

A high prevalence of rheumatoid factor was observed (78.7%), similar to that in other Latin American and Brazilian studies. This feature has been associated with more aggressive disease, worse prognosis and possibly extra-articular manifestations [19, 21]. A high positivity rate for anti-CCP (76.8%) was also found. Roughly, half of the patients failed to achieve the T2T goals of remission or low disease activity (as assessed by DAS28-ESR), exhibiting moderate or high disease activity instead. A similar proportion of patients had developed erosive disease. HAQ and SF-12 scores evidenced a noticeable impairment of health status and health-related quality of life in the cohort [22].

A high use of corticosteroids was identified (47.2%), associated with some features of more aggressive disease, that is, higher disability (HAQ) and disease activity (DAS28) scores, high-titer rheumatoid factor, positivity to anti-CCP, erosive disease, anemia, and subcutaneous nodules. Even greater corticosteroid use (up to 66%) was shown in Latin America by the GLADAR study [19].

Table 5 Total frequencies of conventional synthetic and biological DMARDs in the REAL cohort

DMARD	N (%)
Methotrexate	748 (66.5)
Leflunomide	381 (33.9)
Hydroxychloroquine	120 (10.7)
Sulfasalazine	55 (4.9)
Abatacept	73 (6.5)
Etanercept	66 (5.9)
Tocilizumab	60 (5.3)
Adalimumab	54 (4.8)
Infliximab	50 (4.4)
Rituximab	49 (4.4)
Golimumab	37 (3.3)
Certolizumab	17 (1.5)

However, GLADAR assessed patients with early RA, when corticosteroids are most used, while our cohort was composed mainly of established RA, when corticosteroids should be used only transiently for control of flares.

A selection bias toward more aggressive or refractory disease in tertiary healthcare centers might partially account for this high corticosteroid use, as well as for the high proportions of patients not achieving T2T goals and developing erosive disease. Nonetheless, issues related to timely access to medical care might also be playing a role in this scenario, ultimately determining delays in proper diagnosis and treatment and consequent loss of the window of opportunity for best results. In fact, the median delay from first symptoms to first prescribed DMARD in the cohort was 12 months, noticeably above the generally accepted width of (the first) 3 to 6 months of disease for initiating treatment, in order to attain the best possible results [23].

Methotrexate was the most widely used DMARD in Brazil (in 66.5% of patients), whether in monotherapy or in combinations. The MTX-containing regimens described herein are similar to those reported in other studies [15, 24]. MTX users showed lower clinical disease activity (as assessed by DAS28-ESR) than nonusers. Rheumatologists were less prone to prescribe MTX to patients with interstitial pneumonia, possibly because of concerns about interstitial lung disease progression or MTX-associated pneumonitis, even though this issue is still controversial [25].

Leflunomide was the second most commonly used DMARD (33.9% of patients) in our cohort, a much larger number than in GLADAR (4%) [19]. Brazilian rheumatologists plainly prefered leflunomide to sulfasalazine (used in only 4.9% of patients), two drugs deemed as comparable in efficacy [26]. It's our clinical impression, and based on these numbers, it might also be the case with other Brazilian rheumatologists, that leflunomide seems advantageous over sulfasalazine in

Table 6 Clinical features associated with biological DMARD use

Clinical feature[a]	N(%)[b]	Odds ratio for bDMARD use (95% CI)
High-titer rheumatoid factor[c]	616 (56.1)	1.45 (1.12–1.86)
Interstitial pneumonia[d]	42 (3.8)	1.84 (0.99–3.42)
Erosive disease[e]	602 (54.9)	1.47 (1.14–1.89)
Cutaneous vasculitis	13 (1.2)	4.12 (1.26–13.47)
Subcutaneous nodules	92 (8.3)	1.73 (1.13–2.66)

[a] Groups of patients with and without each feature were compared (binary logistic regression); $p < 0.05$ for all comparisons. [b] Total numbers and percentage of patients with the clinical feature among all those assessed for that condition. [c] Defined as at least 3 times the upper limit of normality [d] Defined by findings suggestive of interstitial X-ray disease: ground-glass opacities, fibrosis compatible lesions (honeycombing, traction bronchiectasis / bronchiolectasis, irregular interlobular septal thickening, and irregular interfaces) [e] Defined as at least 3 erosions in some specified joints (see methodology)

our population (yet to be verified in a clinical trial). Even hydroxychloroquine (10.7%), currently recommended for RA treatment in only special situations, was favored in comparison to sulfasalazine. The reasons underlying this relative disregard for sulfasalazine and clear preference for leflunomide among Brazilian rheumatologists might be worth studying, from a pharmacogenetic point of view.

Moreover, a significant proportion of patients (13.3%) were using the MTX + leflunomide combination, with or without corticosteroids. Although the efficacy of this regimen has been demonstrated, it is rarely used in other countries due to concerns about adverse effects, especially hepatotoxicity [27–29]. Nonetheless, the SMILE study ($n = 2975$) found the combination of MTX + leflunomide to be well tolerated, with adverse events comparable to those of monotherapy with each drug [30]. Given its relative low cost, it is an alternative to be considered before starting a biological therapy, especially in locations with scarce resources.

The use of triple therapy with MTX + hydroxychloroquine + sulfasalazine was extremely low (0.4% of patients) in our cohort. Infrequent use of this combination therapy was also reported in the USA [31]. However, this is a low-cost regimen, with efficacy comparable to biological DMARDs in some scenarios. In low-income countries, this option should be considered, before starting a biological DMARD, particularly for patients without poor prognostic factors [32, 33]. Brazilian rheumatologists should probably be heeding this therapeutic regimen more carefully.

Biological DMARD use (36.1%) in our cohort was more frequent than in studies of early RA conducted in Brazil and Latin America [17, 19, 21]. Patients treated early in the course of disease are supposed to respond better and to require less of the more advanced resources, such as biological DMARDs, in the stepwise approach to RA management [23]. Biological DMARD use was associated with some features of disease aggressiveness, i.e., higher disability (HAQ) scores, high-titer rheumatoid factor, erosive disease, pulmonary fibrosis, subcutaneous nodules and cutaneous vasculitis.

The nature of the data gathered by the REAL study, i.e., reflecting real-life clinical patterns of RA management in Brazil, warrants caution in extrapolating these findings to other population settings. Nevertheless, the study describes for the first time with such a scale the dynamics of real-life treatment of RA in this region, and might serve as a proxy to a better understanding of RA treatment specificities in developing countries, especially in Latin America.

Conclusions

In summary, we demonstrated herein that, in real-life, despite granted access to all advanced pharmacological resources for RA management in Brazil, roughly half of the patients did not achieve T2T goals and developed erosive disease. A high use of corticosteroids was observed in association with signs of aggressive or refractory disease. There was a clear preference for leflunomide over sulfasalazine among Brazilian rheumatologists for the treatment of RA. Triple therapy with MTX + sulfasalazine + hydroxichloroquine was seldom used. Methotrexate plus leflunomide combined therapy was common. Issues concerning timely access to healthcare resources, thus avoiding delays in initiating a DMARD within the first months of disease, might be crucial to effective RA management.

Abbreviations
Anti-CCP: Anti-cyclic citrullinated peptide antibody; CDAI: Clinical Disease Activity Index; DAS28: Disease Activity Index-28 Joints; DMARD: Disease-modifying anti-rheumatic drugs; HAQ: Health Assessment Questionnaire; SF 12: 12-Item Short-Form Health Survey

Acknowledgments
We thank the Brazilian Society of Rheumatology and the Rheumatology team of the University Hospital of Brasília - HUB-UnB for support of this project.

Authors' contributions
All authors made substantial contributions to the acquisition of data, have been involved in drafting the manuscript or revising it critically for important intellectual content, gave final approval of the version to be published and have participated sufficiently in the work to take public responsibility for appropriate portions of the content; and agreed to be accountable for all aspects of the work in ensuring that questions related to the accuracy or integrity of any part of the work are appropriately investigated and resolved. In addition, GRCP, ABVS and LMHM also made substantial contributions to

conception and design of the study. The authors read and approved the final manuscript.

Competing interests

APMG: Has received personal support and consulting fees from Pfizer. GRCP: Has received consulting fees from AbbVie, Bristol-Myers Squibb, Eli Lilly, Glaxosmithkline, Janssen, Pfizer, Sanofi Genzyme and Roche; ABVS: Has received supporting for international medical events from AbbVie and Janssen; CPA: Has received personal fees and/or non-financial support from Pfizer, AbbVie, AstraZeneca, Janssen, Bristol-Myers Squibb, Roche, Novartis and UCB, outside the submitted work; MBB: Has participated in clinical and/or experimental studies related to this work and sponsored by Roche; has delivered speeches at events related to this work and sponsored by AbbVie and Pfizer; PLJ: Has received supporting for internationals congresses from Bristol-Myers Squibb, UCB and consulting fees from Pfizer; RDNG: Has received consulting fees, speaking fees and supporting for internationals congresses from Roche, Pfizer, Bristol-Myers Squibb, UCB, Eli-Lilly, AbbVie, Abbott and EMS; SCR: Has received consulting and speaking fees from Abbvie, Janssen, Pfizer, Roche and UCB; MFBRG: Has received speaking fees and supporting for congresses from AbbVie, Bristol-Myers Squibb, Janssen, Novartis, Pfizer, Roche and UCB; KRB: Has received speaking fees and supporting for international congresses from Roche, Pfizer, Bristol-Myers Squibb, Abbvie and Janssen; MFLCS: No financial disclosures; CVB: Has participated in clinical and/or experimental studies related to this work and sponsored by AbbVie, BMS, Janssen, Pfizer and Roche; has received personal or institutional support from AbbVie, BMS, Janssen, Pfizer and Roche; has delivered speeches at events related to this work and sponsored by AbbVie, Janssen, Pfizer and Roche; IAP: Has received consulting fees, speaking fees and supporting for internationals congresses from Roche, Pfizer, UCB Pharma, Eli-Lilly, Abbvie and Janssen; ESFC: No financial disclosures; LMHM: Has received personal or institutional support from AbbVie, Janssen, Pfizer and Roche; has delivered speeches at events related to this work and sponsored by AbbVie, Janssen, Pfizer, Roche and UCB.

Author details

[1]Universidade de Brasília- UnB, Brasília, DF, Brazil. [2]Universidade do Estado do Rio de Janeiro, Rio de Janeiro, RJ, Brazil. [3]Universidade Estadual de Campinas, Campinas, SP, Brazil. [4]Faculdade de Medicina da Universidade de Ribeirao Preto, Universidade de Sao Paulo, Ribeirão Preto, SP, Brazil. [5]Instituto de Assistência Médica ao Servidor Público Estadual, Hospital do Servidor Público Estadual de São Paulo, São Paulo, SP, Brazil. [6]Universidade Federal do Paraná, Curitiba, PR, Brazil. [7]Universidade Federal de Minas Gerais, Belo Horizonte, MG, Brazil. [8]Universidade de São Paulo, São Paulo, SP, Brazil. [9]Universidade Federal do Pará, Belém, PA, Brazil. [10]Universidade Federal de Santa Catarina, Florianópolis, SC, Brazil. [11]Universidade Federal do Rio Grande do Sul, Porto Alegre, RS, Brazil.

References

1. Majithia V, Geraci SA. Rheumatoid arthritis: diagnosis and management. Am J Med. 2007;120:936–9.
2. Van der Horst-Bruinsma IE, Speyer I, Visser H, Breedvelt FC, Hazes GM. Diagnosis and course of early-onset arthritis: results of a special early arthritis clinic compared to routine patient care. Br J Rheumatol. 1998;37:1084–8.
3. Nell VPK, Machold KP, Eberl G, Stamm TA, Uffmann M, Smolen JS. Benefit of very early referral and very early therapy with disease-modifying anti-rheumatic drugs in patients with early rheumatoid arthritis. Rheumatol. 2004;43:906–14.
4. Smolen JS, Aletaha D, Bijlsma JW, Breedveld FC, Boumpas D, Burmester G. Treating rheumatoid arthritis to target: recommendations of an international task force. Ann Rheum Dis. 2010;69:631–7.
5. Mota LMH, Kakehasi AM, Gomides APM, Duarte ALBP, Cruz BA, Brenol CV et al. 2017 recommendations of the Brazilian Society of Rheumatology for the pharmacological treatment of rheumatoid arthritis. Adv Rheumatol 2018; 58:2. https://doi.org/https://doi.org/10.1186/s42358-018-0005-0.
6. Smolen JS, Landewé R, Bijlsma J, Burmester G, Chatzidionysiou K, Dougados M, et al. EULAR recommendations for the management of rheumatoid arthritis with synthetic and biological disease-modifying antirheumatic drugs: 2016 update. Ann Rheum Dis. 2017;76:960–77.
7. Singh JA, Saag KG, Bridges SL, Akl EA, Bannuru RR, Sullivan MC, et al. 2015 American College of Rheumatology Guideline for the treatment of rheumatoid arthritis. Arthritis Care Res. 2016;68:1–25.
8. Solomon DH, Bitton A, Katz JN, Radner H, Brown E, Fraenkel L. Treat to target in rheumatoid arthritis: fact, fiction or hypothesis? Arthritis Rheumatol. 2014;66:775–82.
9. Castelar-Pinheiro GR, Vargas-Santos AB, Albuquerque CP, Bértolo MB, Júnior PL, Giorgi RDN et al The REAL study: a nationwide prospective study of rheumatoid arthritis in Brazil. Adv Rheumatol 2018. https://doi.org/https://doi.org/10.1186/s42358-018-0017-9.
10. Arnett FC, Edworthy SM, Bloch DA, McShane DJ, Fries JF, Cooper NS, et al. The American rheumatism association 1987 revised criteria for the classification of rheumatoid arthritis. ArthritisRheum. 1998;31:315–24.
11. Aletaha D, Neogi T, Silman AJ, Funovits J, Felson DT, Bingham CO 3rd, et al. 2010 rheumatoid arthritis classification criteria: an American College of Rheumatology/European league against rheumatism collaborative initiative. Arthritis Rheum. 2010;62:2569–81.
12. Gaujoux-Viala C, Mouterde G, Baillet A, Claudepierre P, Fautrel B, Le Loët X, et al. Evaluating disease activity in rheumatoid arthritis: which composite index is best? A systematic literature analysis of studies comparing the psychometric properties of the DAS, DAS28, SDAI and CDAI. Joint Bone Spine. 2012;79:149–55.
13. Fries JF, Spitz P, Kraines RG, Holman HR. Measurement of patient outcome in arthritis. Arthritis Rheum. 1980;23:137–45.
14. Ware J Jr, Kosinski M, Keller SD. A 12-item short-form health survey: construction of scales and preliminary tests of reliability and validity. Med Care. 1996 Mar;34(3):220–33.
15. Van der Heijde D, Van der Helm-van MAH, Aletaha D, Bingham CO, Burmester GR, et al. EULAR definition of erosive disease in light of the 2010 ACR/EULAR rheumatoid arthritis classification criteria. Ann Rheum Dis. 2013; 72(4):479–81.
16. Agresti A. An introduction to categorical data analysis. 2nd ed. New York: Wiley; 2007.
17. Mota LM, Brenol CV, Palominos P, Pinheiro GR. Rheumatoid arthritis in Latin America: the importance of an early diagnosis. Clin Rheumatol. 2015; 34(Suppl 1):S29–44.
18. Saturni S, Bellini F, Braido F, Paggiaro P, Sanduzzi A, Scichilone N, et al. Randomized Controlled Trials and real life studies. Approaches and methodologies: a clinical point of view. Pulm Pharmacol Ther. 2014;27(2):129–38.
19. Cardiel MH, Pons-Estel BA, Sacnun MP, Wojdyla D, Saurit V, Marcos JC, et al. Treatment of early rheumatoid arthritis in a multinational inception cohort of Latin American patients: the GLADAR experience. J Clin Rheumatol. 2012; 18(7):327–35.
20. Instituto Brasileiro de Geografia e Estatistica - IBGE ; População; 2010. Available from: www.ibge.gov.br. Accessed 23 Mar 2018.
21. Mota LMH, Laurindo IMM, Neto LLS. Características demográficas e clínicas de uma coorte de pacientes com artrite reumatoide inicial. Rev Bras Reumatol. 2010;50(3):235–48.
22. Linde L, Sorensen J, Ostergaard M, Horslev-Petersen K, Rasmussen C, Jensen DV, et al. What factors influence the health status of patients with rheumatoid arthritis measured by the SF-12v2 health survey and the health assessment questionnaire? J Rheumatol. 2009;36(10):2183–9.
23. Raza K, Filer A. The therapeutic window of opportunity in rheumatoid arthritis: does it ever close? Ann Rheum Dis. 2015;74(5):793–4.
24. Swierkot J, Szechiński J. Methotrexate in rheumatoid arthritis. Pharmacol Rep. 2006;58(4):473–92.
25. Conway R, Low C, Coughlan RJ, O'Donnell MJ, Carey JJ. Methotrexate and lung disease in rheumatoid arthritis: a meta-analysis of randomized controlled trials. Arthritis Rheumatol. 2014;66(4):803–12.
26. Scott DL, Smolen JS, Kalden JR, van de Putte LB, Larsen A, Kvien TK, et al. Treatment of active rheumatoid arthritis with leflunomide: two year follow up of a double blind, placebo controlled trial versus sulfasalazine. Ann Rheum Dis. 2001;60(10):913–23.
27. Kremer JM, Genovese MC, Cannon GW, Caldwell JR, Cush JJ, Furst DE, et al. Concomitant leflunomide therapy in patients with active rheumatoid arthritis despite stable doses of methotrexate. A randomized, double-blind, placebo-controlled trial. Ann Intern Med. 2002;137(9):726–33.
28. Roon ENV, Tim LTA, Houtman NM, Spoelstra P, Brouwers JR. Leflunomide for the treatment of rheumatoid arthritis in clinical practice. Drug Saf. 2004; 27(5):345–52.

29. Administration USFDA. Drug Safety Communication: new boxed warning for severe liver injury with arthritis drug Arava (leflunomide). https://www.fda.gov/drugs/drug-safety-and-availability. Accessed 15 Mar 2018.

30. Bird P, Griffiths H, Tymms K, Nicholls D, Roberts L, Arnold M, et al. The SMILE study—safety of methotrexate in combination with leflunomide in rheumatoid arthritis. J Rheumatol. 2013;40(3):228–35.

31. O'Dell JR. Triple therapy with methotrexate, sulfasalazine, and hydroxychloroquine in patients with rheumatoid arthritis. Rheum Dis Clin North. 1998;24(3):465–77.

32. Bansback N, Phibbs CS, Sun H, O'Dell JR, Brophy M, Keystone EC, et al. Triple therapy versus biologic therapy for active rheumatoid arthritis: a cost-effectiveness analysis. Ann Intern Med. 2017;167(1):8–16.

33. Mary J, De Bandt M, Lukas C, Morel J, Combe B. Triple Oral therapy versus antitumor necrosis factor plus methotrexate (MTX) in patients with rheumatoid arthritis and inadequate response to MTX: a systematic literature review. JRheumatol. 2017;44(6):773–9.

14

High frequency of methotrexate intolerance in longstanding rheumatoid arthritis: Using the methotrexate intolerance severity score (MISS)

Jéssica Martins Amaral[1*] (iD), Maria José Menezes Brito[2] and Adriana Maria Kakehasi[3]

Abstract

Background: Methotrexate (MTX) intolerance is frequent, and its early identification may impact treatment, leading to timely changes in medication that may promote patient compliance and better control of rheumatoid arthritis (RA). The objective of this study was to identify the frequency of, and risk factors for, MTX intolerance using the Brazilian Portuguese version of the Methotrexate Intolerance Severity Score (MISS) questionnaire in patients with RA.

Methods: This cross-sectional study was performed between April 2018 and April 2019 and enrolled patients with RA in regular use of oral or subcutaneous MTX for at least 3 months. Patients were invited to answer the Brazilian Portuguese version of the MISS questionnaire, and MTX intolerance was defined by a score ≥ 6 points. Age, sex, disease duration, time of MTX use, dose, route of administration, concomitant medications, comorbidities, smoking, and Disease Activity Score for 28joint (DAS28) data were collected from institutional medical records.

Results: Among 120 patients, 103 (85.8%) were female, the mean age was 61 (±12.5) years, the mean duration of disease was 16 (±10.3) years, and the average duration of MTX use was 7 (±5.5) years. The frequency of MTX intolerance was 21.6%. The most frequent symptoms reported after the use of MTX were nausea (92.3%), abdominal pain (46.1%), and vomiting (30.7%). Behavioral symptoms occurred in 96.1% of patients with MTX intolerance, the most frequent being restlessness and irritability. Patients who used corticosteroids were more likely to develop MTX intolerance than those not using corticosteroids (odds ratio = 2.73; 95% confidence interval, 1.06 to 7.06; $p = 0.038$). Conversely, increasing age showed marginally significant association with decreased risk of MTX intolerance ($p = 0.059$).

Conclusions: The use of the MISS questionnaire disclosed high frequencies of anticipatory, associative, and behavioral symptoms in MTX-intolerant patients, and the use of corticosteroid increases the risk of MTX intolerance. We suggest that the MISS questionnaire be used routinely in clinical practice.

Keywords: Rheumatoid arthritis, Methotrexate, Questionnaire, Intolerance

* Correspondence: jessicamartinsmk@yahoo.com.br
[1]Post Graduate Program in Sciences Applied to Adult Health Care, Federal University of Minas Gerais, Avenida Alfredo Balena, 190 room 193 Santa Efigênia, Belo Horizonte, Minas Gerais ZIP 30130-100, Brazil
Full list of author information is available at the end of the article

Background

Rheumatoid arthritis (RA) is a systemic, autoimmune inflammatory disease whose manifestations occur in synovial joints and in different organs and systems, causing chronic pain, bone erosion and progressive disability [1]. Methotrexate (MTX) is the most important disease-modifying antirheumatic drug in the treatment of RA. Use of MTX is indicated for first-line therapy of RA and occupies a prominent position in many guidelines and recommendations for the treatment of rheumatic diseases [1–3]. In spite of its effectiveness and low cost, MTX can cause gastrointestinal side effects, such as abdominal pain, nausea, vomiting and diarrhea [4, 5]. Although folic acid supplementation during MTX treatment may reduce such effects, many patients discontinue treatment, something that negatively impacts disease control and quality of life [4]. In addition, patients may develop anticipatory symptoms, which occur prior to MTX intake, and associative symptoms, when patients think about the drug, as well as behavioral symptoms [6, 7]. These adverse effects arise as a response to previous symptoms experienced by patients on MTX and are not often clinically evident; therefore, they are often inadequately managed [7].

Given the lack of specific tools to assess the adverse effects associated with the use of MTX, the Methotrexate Intolerance Severity Score (MISS) was developed [7]. This is currently the only questionnaire that formally evaluates MTX intolerance taking into account the most frequent side effects as well as anticipatory, associative and behavioral symptoms – which are very important in the identification of intolerance. This tool was developed and validated in patients with juvenile idiopathic arthritis [7], and it has also been validated for use in patients with juvenile idiopathic arthritis in the French language [8]. Furthermore, the MISS questionnaire has also been used to determine the prevalence of MTX intolerance in patients with RA and psoriatic arthritis in several countries [4, 7–9]. More recently, the MISS questionnaire has also been validated in Brazilian Portuguese for use in adults with RA [10].

Early identification of MTX intolerance may impact treatment, so that changes in medications may occur at the right time, promoting patient compliance and, consequently, disease control [9].

Thus, the objective of this study was to identify the frequency of MTX intolerance using the Brazilian Portuguese version of the MISS questionnaire in patients with RA in a Brazilian rheumatology service, as well as factors that may be associated with MTX intolerance.

Methods

Study design and approval

This cross-sectional study was performed in a University rheumatology service in Brazil from April 2018 to April 2019. The study was approved by the institutional ethics committee, and all patients provided a signed informed consent form.

Patient eligibility and assessment

One hundred and 20 patients diagnosed with RA according to the American College of Rheumatology (ACR) 1987 criteria [11] or ACR/European League Against Rheumatism 2010 criteria [12], and in regular use of oral or subcutaneous MTX for at least 3 months, were invited to answer the MISS questionnaire; all patients had participated in the validation stage of the Brazilian Portuguese version of the MISS. Patients who had psychiatric illnesses or history of noncompliance with earlier treatments were excluded.

The MISS questionnaire contains twelve items divided into four dimensions: abdominal pain (three questions), nausea (three questions), vomiting (two questions), and behavioral complaints (four questions). The symptoms occurring after MTX intake, before MTX intake (anticipatory symptoms) and/or when thinking of taking MTX (associative symptoms). The possible answers (and corresponding score in points) for each item are no complaints (0), mild complaints (1), moderate complaints (2), and severe complaints (3). Points are summed to give a score that may range from 0 to 36. The definition of MTX intolerance is given by a score of 6 or more points, with at least 1 point in the anticipatory, associative, or behavioral symptoms [7]. Additional data, collected from institutional medical records, were age, sex, disease duration, time of MTX use, dose, route of administration, concomitant medications, other comorbidities, smoking, and disease activity as assessed by Disease Activity Score in 28 joints (DAS28) [13].

The Brazilian Portuguese version of the MISS questionnaire is shown in the Additional file 1.

Statistical analysis

The primary outcome of interest was MTX intolerance. Univariate analyses were performed to explore the association of demographic and clinical variables with MTX intolerance; categorical variables were assessed using Pearson's Chi-Square test or Fisher's exact test, depending on the number of cases and categories. Quantitative variables were assessed using t-test or the Mann-Whitney test, depending on their distribution; normality was assessed using the Shapiro-Wilk test, and homoscedasticity using the Levene test. Variables in the univariate analyses with a p-value < 0.25 were inserted in a multivariate logistic regression model to assess independent risk factors for MTX intolerance. Odds ratios (OR) from the multivariate model were computed in order to indicate an increased risk of MTX intolerance with values above 1.00. Model fit was assessed using the

Hosmer-Lemeshow test, and statistical significance was considered for two-sided p-values < 0.05.

Results

Demographic and clinical characteristics

Among the 120 patients who participated in the study, 103 (85.8%) were female, the mean age was 61 ($\pm$ 12.5) years, the mean duration of disease was 16 ($\pm$ 10.3) years, and the average duration of MTX use was 7 ($\pm$ 5.5) years. These and other patient characteristics are shown in Table 1.

Frequency and characteristics of MTX intolerance

Considering all 120 patients, 27 (22.5%) presented symptoms of anticipation, 36 (30%) presented symptoms of association, and 41 (34.2%) showed behavioral symptoms. Table 2 displays the prevalence of symptoms among patients with and without MTX intolerance. MTX intolerance was present in 26 of 120 patients (21.6%), of whom women. The most frequent symptom after MTX intake among patients with MTX intolerance was nausea, in 24 (92.3%) patients, followed by abdominal pain, in 12 (46.1%) patients, and vomiting, in eight (30.7%) patients. Among these same patients, the most frequent pre-treatment symptoms in the nausea domain were associative in 22 (84.6%) and anticipatory in 18 (69.2%) patients. Therefore, all 26 patients with MTX intolerance presented symptoms in the nausea domain either after taking MTX or as anticipatory or associative symptoms. In the abdominal pain domain, associative and anticipatory symptoms occurred in three (11.5%) and two (7.6%) patients with MTX intolerance, respectively. Anticipatory symptom related to vomiting occurred in two (7.6%) of those patients. Finally, behavioral symptoms occurred in 25 (96.1%) patients with MTX intolerance; among these symptoms, the most frequent were restlessness and irritability (Table 2).

Predictors of MTX intolerance

In univariate analyses, age as continuous variable ($p = 0.089$), female sex ($p = 0.022$), MTX dose above 17.5 mg/week ($p = 0.126$), and use of non-steroidal anti-inflammatory agents ($p = 0.203$), proton-pump inhibitor ($p = 0.164$), corticosteroids ($p = 0.054$), and antiemetics ($p = 0.217$), were deemed possibly associated with the presence of MTX intolerance, due to a p-value < 0.25, as pre-specified in Methods, and thus carried forward to the multivariate analysis. This study did not reveal association of MTX intolerance with other variables, such as subcutaneous or oral formulation, or folic acid dosing. Of these variables, only age and use of corticosteroids were retained in the final logistic regression model, presented in Table 3. In this multivariate analysis, use of corticosteroid was significantly associated with MTX

Table 1 Baseline characteristics of the patients at the time of completing the MISS questionnaire

Characteristics	$N = 120$
Qualitative	
Female (%)	103 (85.8)
MTX, subcutaneous (%)	66 (55)
MTX dose (mg/week)	
< 10 (%)	1 (0.8)
10.1–17.5 (%)	31 (25.8)
> 17.5 (%)	88 (73.4)
Leflunomide (%)	29 (24.2)
Nonsteroidal anti-inflammatory drugs (%)	9 (7.5)
Disease-modifying antirheumatic drugs – biological (%)	28 (23.3)
Corticosteroids (%)	63 (52.5)
Proton-pump inhibitors (%)	56 (46.7)
Antiemetics (%)	1 (0.8)
Folic acid	
No (%)	7 (5.8)
5 mg/week (%)	92 (76.7)
10 mg/week or more (%)	21 (17.5)
DAS 28 moderate and high disease activity (%)	51 (45.5)
Smoking	
No (%)	74 (62.2)
Current smoker (%)	15 (12.6)
Ex-smoker (%)	30 (25.2)
Seropositive RA (%)	92 (76.7)
Hypertension (%)	68 (56.7)
Diabetes mellitus (%)	29 (24.2)
Dyslipidemia (%)	36 (30.0)
Hypothyroidism (%)	15 (12.5)
Fibromyalgia (%)	10 (8.3)
Gastroesophageal reflux disease (%)	12 (10.3)
Antidepressant (%)	24 (20)
Quantitative	
Mean age, years (SD)	61 (12.5)
Mean disease duration, years (SD)	16 (10.3)
Mean MTX usage duration, years (SD)	7 (5.5)
Mean dose of MTX, mg/week (SD)	20 (5.1)
Mean DAS28 (SD)	3.25 (3.1)

DAS 28 Disease activity score in 28 joints; *MTX* Methotrexate; *SD* Standard deviation

intolerance (OR = 2.73; 95% confidence interval [CI], 1.06 to 7.06; $p = 0.038$). With regard to age, the association was not statistically significant, but the results indicate a trend for a 3% reduction in the risk of MTX intolerance for every increase of 1 year of age (OR = 0.97; 95% CI, 0.93 to 1.0; $p = 0.059$).

Table 2 Prevalence of MTX-related symptoms in MTX-tolerant and MTX-intolerant patients

Symptoms	MTX-intolerant **N** = 26 (%)	MTX-tolerant **N** = 94 (%)
Abdominal pain		
After taking MTX	12 (46.15)	3 (3.19)
Anticipatory	2 (7.69)	2 (2.12)
Associative	3 (11.53)	1 (1.06)
Nausea		
After taking MTX	24 (92.30)	44 (46.80)
Anticipatory	18 (69.23)	7 (7.44)
Associative	22 (84.61)	13 (13.82)
Vomiting		
After taking MTX	8 (30.76)	9 (9.57)
Anticipatory	2 (7.69)	1 (1.06)
Behavioral complaints		
Restlessness	20 (76.92)	10 (10.63)
Crying	11 (42.30)	1 (1.06)
Irritability	20 (76.92)	7 (7.44)
Refusal of MTX	16 (61.53)	4 (4.25)

MTX Methotrexate

Discussion

In the current study, we have found a frequency of 21.6% of MTX intolerance among RA patients. The most frequent symptoms reported after the use of MTX were nausea (92.3%), abdominal pain (46.1%), and vomiting (30.7%). Patients who used corticosteroids were nearly three times more likely to develop MTX intolerance than those not using corticosteroids. Conversely, increasing age was associated with a decreasing risk of MTX intolerance.

To our knowledge, this is the first study developed in Brazil using a validated questionnaire to assess MTX intolerance in patients with RA. The prevalence of MTX intolerance we found is within the range reported in studies using the MISS questionnaire reported elsewhere. For example, a study performed in Utrecht, in the Netherlands, found a prevalence of MTX intolerance of 11% among patients with RA and psoriatic arthritis [14]. In a study conducted in Pakistan, this frequency was 33.3% among RA patients [4]. Finally, a recent study from Saudi Arabia among RA patients who used MTX for at least 3 months found that 39.5% of them had a positive score for MTX intolerance using the MISS questionnaire [15]. The frequency of the most common symptoms reported by our patients after the use of MTX were similar to those from the Dutch study, in which 100% of the patients reported nausea, 46.9% abdominal pain, and 31.3% vomiting [14].

In addition to experiencing gastrointestinal symptoms after receiving the drug, patients in our study with MTX intolerance exhibited anticipatory, associative, and behavioral symptoms. The occurrence of these symptoms before the ingestion of MTX supports the idea that classical conditioning mechanisms play an important role in the development of MTX intolerance [7]. The presence of these symptoms has also been noted in studies among patients with juvenile idiopathic arthritis [7, 16]. The study that developed and applied the MISS questionnaire in children with juvenile idiopathic arthritis highlighted the most frequently conditioned stimuli reported at the outpatient clinic: the yellowish color of the medication and the fluids used to administer MTX, such as water or orange juice. Such stimuli may lead to the conditioned response of anticipatory and associative effects [7]. It is accepted that such symptoms occur due to stimulation of higher centers of the central nervous system [17]. In line with this hypothesis, cognitive-behavioral therapy may have benefits in the treatment of MTX-intolerant patients [7, 18]. A recent study in patients with juvenile idiopathic arthritis showed positive results using desensitization and pre-processing of ocular movements to treat MTX-intolerant patients, promoting more adherence to treatment and increasing patient's quality of life [18]. Other measures that can be taken to ameliorate symptoms include decreasing the dose of MTX [19], changing the route of administration from oral to parenteral, introduction of folic acid [5, 20], and introducing an antiemetic [21].

It is worth noting that often times the anticipatory, associative and behavioral symptoms are not clinically evident, hence not adequately monitored. This can affect the continuity of the treatment and lead to a decrease in the

Table 3 Multivariate analysis of risk factors for methotrexate intolerance

Variable	Coefficient	Standard error	*P*-value	OR	95% confidence interval	
					Lower limit	Upper limit
Corticosteroids						
Yes	1.00	0.48	0.038	2.73	1.06	7.06
No						
Age (years)	−0.03	0.02	0.059	0.97	0.93	1.00

OR Odds ratio

patient's quality of life [7]. In view of this, it is very important to monitor MTX intolerance in daily clinical practice, which makes the use of the MISS questionnaire advantageous, as it allows for early detection of symptoms. In our findings, no association of MTX intolerance with other variables was observed. Ensuring adequate tolerance and greater adherence to MTX can prevent therapeutic failures, minimize the high cost of treating rheumatic diseases, and ultimately promote better disease control.

Several studies have indicated that corticosteroid use increases the risk of gastrointestinal adverse events [22, 23]. Our findings suggest that patients who used corticosteroids were more likely to develop MTX intolerance. Glucocorticoids may have dual action on the gastric mucosa: physiological gastroprotective and pathological proulcerogenic one. The prolongation of the action, instead of the dose of exogenous glucocorticoids, can be a significant factor for the undesirable effects of glucocorticoids on the gastric mucosa [24]. Since previous studies using the MISS questionnaire have found no association between concomitant medications and MTX intolerance, further studies are needed to elucidate the association between corticosteroid use and MTX intolerance. Our study suggests a trend for decreasing risk of MTX intolerance with increasing age. Previous studies among patients with RA and psoriatic arthritis have also shown an association between age and MTX intolerance, with older patients (> 65 years) being less likely to have MTX intolerance than their younger counterparts [14]. With regard to other potential risk factors for MTX intolerance, further, large-sample studies are needed to better elucidate additional issues associated with MTX intolerance, given its large impact on non-compliance with drug treatment.

Conclusion

In conclusion, MTX intolerance is relatively frequent in RA patients, even those under treatment for prolonged periods of time. The use of the MISS questionnaire discloses high frequencies of anticipatory, associative, and behavioral symptoms in MTX-intolerant patients, and such symptoms potentially contribute to lower adherence to treatment. The use of corticosteroid seemingly increases the risk of MTX intolerance. The early identification of MTX intolerance may allow more adequate medical treatment, with timely changes in medication that may improve patient compliance, disease control, and well-being. Therefore, we strongly recommend that the evaluation of MTX intolerance be included in daily clinical practice, and for that purpose we suggest using the MISS questionnaire.

Study limitations

The relatively small number of participants is a limitation of this study. The data were collected from a single tertiary hospital, which might limit the generalization of our findings to the general population. Furthermore, other studies are needed to elucidate the association between age and corticosteroid use and MTX intolerance.

Abbreviations

ACR: American college of rheumatology; CI: Confidence interval; MISS: Methotrexate intolerance severity score; MTX: Methotrexate; OR: Odds ratio; RA: Rheumatoid arthritis

Acknowledgements

Authors acknowledges editorial assistance funded by AbbVie.

Authors' contributions

JMA collected, analyzed and interpreted the patient data regarding the identification of MTX intolerance, and was a major contributor in writing the manuscript. MJMB was an important contributor in writing the manuscript. AMK analyzed and interpreted the patient data and was a major contributor in writing the manuscript. The author (s) read and approved the final manuscript.

Author details

[1]Post Graduate Program in Sciences Applied to Adult Health Care, Federal University of Minas Gerais, Avenida Alfredo Balena, 190 room 193 Santa Efigênia, Belo Horizonte, Minas Gerais ZIP 30130-100, Brazil. [2]Applied Nursing Department, Nursing School Federal University of Minas Gerais, Belo Horizonte, Minas Gerais, Brazil. [3]Post Graduate Program in Sciences Applied to Adult Health Care, Federal University of Minas Gerais, Belo Horizonte, Minas Gerais State, Brazil.

References

1. Smolen JS, Aletaha D, McInnes IB. Rheumatoid arthritis. Lancet. 2016; 388(10055):2023–38.
2. Mota L, Kakehasi AM, Gomides APM, Duarte A, Cruz BA, Brenol CV, et al. 2017 recommendations of the Brazilian Society of Rheumatology for the pharmacological treatment of rheumatoid arthritis. Adv Rheumatol. 2018;58(1):2.
3. Singh JA, Saag KG, Bridges SL Jr, Akl EA, Bannuru RR, Sullivan MC, et al. 2015 American College of Rheumatology Guideline for the treatment of rheumatoid arthritis. Arthritis Rheumatol. 2016;68(1):1–26.
4. Fatimah N, Salim B, Nasim A, Hussain K, Gul H, Niazi S. Frequency of methotrexate intolerance in rheumatoid arthritis patients using methotrexate intolerance severity score (MISS questionnaire). Clin Rheumatol. 2016;35(5):1341–5.
5. Brunner HI, Johnson AL, Barron AC, Passo MH, Griffin TA, Graham TB, et al. Gastrointestinal symptoms and their association with health-related quality of life of children with juvenile rheumatoid arthritis: validation of a gastrointestinal symptom questionnaire. J Clin Rheumatol. 2005;11(4):194–204.
6. van der Meer A, Wulffraat NM, Prakken BJ, Gijsbers B, Rademaker CM, Sinnema G. Psychological side effects of MTX treatment in juvenile idiopathic arthritis: a pilot study. Clin Exp Rheumatol. 2007;25(3):480–5.
7. Bulatovic M, Heijstek MW, Verkaaik M, van Dijkhuizen EH, Armbrust W, Hoppenreijs EP, et al. High prevalence of methotrexate intolerance in juvenile idiopathic arthritis: development and validation of a methotrexate intolerance severity score. Arthritis Rheum. 2011;63(7):2007–13.
8. Chausset A, Fargeix T, Pereira B, Echaubard S, Duquesne A, Desjonqueres M, et al. MISS questionnaire in French version: a good tool for children and parents to assess methotrexate intolerance. Clin Rheumatol. 2017;36(6):1281–8.
9. Virdi P, Singh B, Singh R. Role of methotrexate intolerance severity score (miss) in rheumatoid arthritis to know methotrexate intolerance: a 2-year prospective study. Int J Adv Res. 2017;5:2542–8.
10. Amaral JM, Brito MJM, Kakehasi AM. Cultural adaptation and validation of the methotrexate intolerance severity score in Brazilian Portuguese for adults with rheumatoid arthritis. J Clin Rheumatol. 2019.
11. Arnett FC, Edworthy SM, Bloch DA, McShane DJ, Fries JF, Cooper NS, et al. The American rheumatism association 1987 revised criteria for the classification of rheumatoid arthritis. Arthritis Rheum. 1988;31(3):315–24.

12. Aletaha D, Neogi T, Silman AJ, Funovits J, Felson DT, Bingham CO 3rd, et al. 2010 rheumatoid arthritis classification criteria: an American College of Rheumatology/European league against rheumatism collaborative initiative. Arthritis Rheum. 2010;62(9):2569–81.

13. Prevoo MLL, van't Hof MA, Kuper HH, et al. Modified disease activity scores that include twenty-eight joint counts. Arthritis Rheum. 1995;38:44–48.14.

14. Calasan MB, van den Bosch OF, Creemers MC, Custers M, Heurkens AH, van Woerkom JM, et al. Prevalence of methotrexate intolerance in rheumatoid arthritis and psoriatic arthritis. Arthritis Res Ther. 2013;15(6):R217.

15. Albaqami J, Alshalhoub R, Almalag H, Dessougi M, Al Harthi A, Bedaiwi MK, et al. Prevalence of methotrexate intolerance among patients with rheumatoid arthritis using the Arabic version of the methotrexate intolerance severity score. Int J Rheum Dis. 2019;22(8):1572–7.

16. van Dijkhuizen EH, Pouw JN, Scheuern A, Hugle B, Hardt S, Ganser G, et al. Methotrexate intolerance in oral and subcutaneous administration in patients with juvenile idiopathic arthritis: a cross-sectional, observational study. Clin Exp Rheumatol. 2016;34(1):148–54.

17. Hornby PJ. Central neurocircuitry associated with emesis. Am J Med. 2001; 111(Suppl 8A):106S–12S.

18. Hofel L, Eppler D, Storf M, Schnobel-Muller E, Haas JP, Hugle B. Successful treatment of methotrexate intolerance in juvenile idiopathic arthritis using eye movement desensitization and reprocessing - treatment protocol and preliminary results. Pediatr Rheumatol Online J. 2018;16(1):11.

19. Murray KJ, Lovell DJ. Advanced therapy for juvenile arthritis. Best Pract Res Clin Rheumatol. 2002;16(3):361–78.

20. Alsufyani K, Ortiz-Alvarez O, Cabral DA, Tucker LB, Petty RE, Malleson PN. The role of subcutaneous administration of methotrexate in children with juvenile idiopathic arthritis who have failed oral methotrexate. J Rheumatol. 2004;31(1):179–82.

21. Ravelli A, Martini A. Methotrexate in juvenile idiopathic arthritis: answers and questions. J Rheumatol. 2000;27(8):1830–3.

22. Moghadam-Kia S, Werth VP. Prevention and treatment of systemic glucocorticoid side effects. Int J Dermatol. 2010;49(3):239–48.

23. Piper JM, Ray WA, Daugherty JR, Griffin MR. Corticosteroid use and peptic ulcer disease: role of nonsteroidal anti-inflammatory drugs. Ann Intern Med. 1991;114(9):735–40.

24. Filaretova L, Podvigina T, Yarushkina N. Physiological and pharmacological effects of glucocorticoids on the gastrointestinal tract. Curr Pharm Des. 2020;26(25):2962–70.

15

Characterization of falls in adults with established rheumatoid arthritis and associated factors

Mariana de Almeida Lourenço[*], Flávia Vilas Boas Ortiz Carli and Marcos Renato de Assis

Abstract

Background: Rheumatoid arthritis patients may have an increased risk of falls due to changes caused by the disease such as muscle weakness, joint impairment, reduced mobility and postural instability. The aim of this study was to prospectively analyze the occurrence of falls in RA patients and its risk factors.

Methods: A cohort of 86 RA patients were assessed over 1 year for disease activity using the Disease Activity Score (DAS-28), for functionality using the Health Assessment Questionnaire (HAQ), for the characterization of falls and for the use of medications, and they were subjected to the Berg Balance Scale (Berg), Timed Up and Go (TUG), 6-Minute Walk (6MWT) and Short Physical Performance Battery (SPPB) tests. The Kolmogorov-Smirnov, Spearman's correlation, Student's t, Mann-Whitney and chi-square tests were performed with a significance level of $P \leq 0.05$.

Results: A total of 86 patients were evaluated, of which 48.8% had at least one fall and 75.6% reported having a fear of falling. No association of falls with age, disease duration, functional capacity, disease activity or physical performance was found. Patients with poorer performance in the physical tests had more functional impairment, higher disease activity and more advanced age. No differences in physical or functional performance, disease activity, gender or fear of falling were found between fallers and non-fallers; only a greater amount of medications used was found in the group of fallers.

Conclusions: The occurrence of falls was high and associated with a previous history of falls and polypharmacy, with no association with disease activity or duration, functional capacity, physical performance, age or gender.

Keywords: Postural balance, Physical aptitude, Rheumatoid arthritis, Accidental falls

Background

Falls have a multifactorial etiology in the elderly, mainly due to intrinsic factors such as decreased muscle strength, balance deficits, and gait pattern changes. These age-related changes can also be observed in other diseases [1–3].

Rheumatoid arthritis (RA) is a chronic systemic inflammatory autoimmune disease of joint predominance, with a high prevalence of falls occurring in 14.3 to 54% of patients over a one-year period, which are high values compared to the general population [4–19]. This increased risk of falls may be due to pain, edema, deformities, loss of muscle strength or gait changes, and prospective studies have shown associations with altered balance, use of psychotropic medications, fear of falling and previous falls [4–8]. However, findings regarding several other risk factors, the characterization of falls and the consequences of falls in RA patients are still scarce or contradictory.

The aim of this study was to prospectively analyze the occurrence of falls in RA patients for 1 year and to investigate whether physical fitness and balance tests, medication use, previous history of falls, disease activity and functionality are associated with falls.

Methods
Sample
A prospective study based on the sample of a previous retrospective study composed of 99 patients diagnosed

* Correspondence: maalmeida1@terra.com.br
Marília School of Medicine, R. Pedro Martins, 209. Marília/SP – Brazil, Marília, São Paulo CEP 17519-430, Brazil

with RA was conducted at the Rheumatology outpatient clinic of the Marília School of Medicine [19, 20].

Adults with a diagnosis of RA according to the American College of Rheumatology (ACR) classification criteria of 1987 and/or the 2010 ACR/EULAR (European League Against Rheumatism) RA classification criteria were included [21]. Patients with cognitive impairments precluding them from answering the questionnaires, using a wheelchair or with other physical disabilities that impeded the execution of the tests were excluded.

The study was approved by the Research Ethics Committee of the Marília School of Medicine, protocol CAAE: 22845513.3.0000.5413. All participants signed the informed consent form.

Procedure

The rheumatologist confirmed the RA diagnosis and performed the measurements to assess disease activity, and the nurse collected the blood samples. Next, the anthropometric data were measured, and the functional questionnaires and physical tests were applied by the nurse and the physical therapist.

From the initial evaluation, the patients were followed up for 1 year by quarterly telephone contact to record the occurrence of falls and their characteristics. After 12 months, the disease activity and functionality assessments and physical tests were repeated.

Instruments

Patients were assessed for disease activity using the Disease Activity Score (DAS-28) [21], for functional capacity using the Health Assessment Questionnaire (HAQ) [22, 23] and for the occurrence of falls using a fall characterization questionnaire [19, 20].

The following physical tests were performed:

The Berg Balance Scale was used to determine risk factors for loss of independence and falls in the elderly. The scale has 14 items common to daily life, scored from 0 to 4, with a higher fall risk associated with lower scores. The predictive value of falls in the elderly ranges from 45 to 48 [24–27].

The Short Physical Performance Battery (SPPB) was used to assess standing balance, walking ability and sit-to-stand performance. The three items are scored from 0 to 4, with poorer physical function associated with lower scores. Standing balance is evaluated in three positions with progressive difficulty - feet together, with the hallux leaning against the medial edge of the opposite heel and with the hallux leaning against the posterior edge of the opposite heel. Walking is evaluated by measuring time, in seconds, for a distance of four meters. In the sit-to-stand evaluation using a chair, the action is performed five times with the arms crossed in front of the chest, and time is also recorded in seconds [28, 29].

The Timed Up and Go Test (TUG) was used to assess body balance and risk of falls, especially in the elderly. The test begins with the patient sitting on a chair, then getting up, walking a three-meter distance, making a 180° turn, returning and sitting on the same chair. The different lengths of time spent indicate the following: ≤10 s - elderly without balance alteration and with low risk of falls; between 10 and 20 s - elderly with no significant balance alteration but presenting some weakness and medium risk of falls; and ≥ 20 s - elderly with a high risk of falls [30]. Other studies consider a higher risk of falls between 10 and 14 s [24, 31, 32].

The 6-Minute Walk Test (6MWT) was used to assess functional capacity and exercise tolerance through the distance an individual is able to walk on a hard, flat surface for 6 min. In healthy adults, the reference values are 580 m for men and 500 m for women [33, 34].

Statistical analysis

The Kolmogorov-Smirnov (KS) test was used to evaluate the normality of the data distribution. Values were expressed as the mean and standard deviation (SD) for variables with normal distribution and as the median and percentages for the others. Correlations were analyzed using Spearman's test, and other analyses were conducted using Student's t-test, the Mann-Whitney U-test and chi-square tests with a significance level of $p < 0.05$. The statistical program used was SPSS v.21 (IBM Armonk, NY, USA, 2012).

Results

A total of 99 patients were included in the study, but 13 were lost – three died, three had medical follow-up unit changes, three were not found, two were bedridden, one refused to participate, and one suffered an ankle sprain – leaving 86 patients. The majority of the sample consisted of white married women with a mean age of 55 ± 11.8 years (Table 1).

There were 67 fall episodes in the one-year follow-up period; 48.8% of these patients fell at least once, and 75.6% reported the fear of experiencing a fall episode. Falls occurred most often at home (58.2%), in the morning (41.8%), while the patients walked (65.7%) and due to tripping and slipping (65.5%), and fracture occurred in three falls (4.4% of the total).

No association was found between the number of falls and age, disease duration, functional capacity, disease activity or physical performance. Patients with poorer performance on the physical tests had more functional impairment, higher disease activity and advanced age. The higher disease activity was associated with poorer

Table 1 Characteristics of the sample of patients with rheumatoid arthritis

Participants, n		86
Women, n (%)		76 (88.4)
Age (years), mean ± SD (min-max)		55 ± 11.8 (23–88)
BMI (kg/m^2), mean ± SD (min-max)		27.7 ± 5.3 (15.35–40.04)
Self-reported ethnicity, n (%)	White	54 (62.8)
	Mixed	20 (23.3)
	Black	12 (14)
Marital status, n (%)	Married	52 (62.8)
	Single	14 (16.3)
	Divorced	10 (11.6)
	Widowed	8 (9.3)
Duration of disease (years), median (P25–75) (min-max)		10 (5–16.5); (2–40)
Self-reported associated diseases (%)	HBP	53.5
	Osteoporosis	17.4
	DM	12.6
	Labyrinthitis	11.6
	HF	8.1
	Fibromyalgia	7.0
	Hypothyroidism	7.0
	Depression	3.4
Falls in the previous year (%)		37.4
Walking aids (%)		9.3

n: number; %: percentage; SD: standard deviation; min: minimum; max: maximum; BMI: body mass index; kg: kilogram; m^2: square meter; P25–75: 25th percentile and 75th percentile; HBP: high blood pressure; DM: diabetes mellitus; HF: heart failure

physical performance, poorer functional capacity and longer disease duration (Table 2).

There was no significant difference in functional capacity or disease activity in the initial evaluation and after 1 year. However, in the physical tests, better performance was observed in the final evaluation when compared to the initial evaluation (Table 3).

When divided into groups according to the occurrence of falls, considering fallers as patients with at least one fall episode during the follow-up period, no significant differences were found between fallers and non-fallers

regarding physical or functional performance, disease activity, gender or fear of falling (Tables 4 and 5). The number of medications used and history of falls differed significantly between fallers and non-fallers (Table 5).

Discussion

The incidence of falls in this sample of RA patients was high (48.8%) compared to that found in the literature, which shows ranges from 14.3 to 54% in retrospective studies and from 18.8 to 50% in prospective studies [4–9, 11–19]. The incidence of falls

Table 2 Correlations between the number of falls with clinical variables and functional tests

	Number of falls, r (P)	Age, r (P)	HAQ, r (P)	DAS28, r (P)
Age	0.059 (0.592)	–	−0.109 (0.317)	0.034 (0.755)
RA duration	−0.077 (0.483)	0.187 (0.087)	0.066 (0.550)	0.224 (0.039)*
HAQ	0.151 (0.165)	−0.109 (0.317)	–	0.468 (0.000)*
DAS28	0.004 (0.973)	0.034 (0.755)	0.468 (0.000)*	–
Berg	−0.127 (0.244)	−0.367 (0.001)*	−0.541 (0.000)*	−0.422 (0.000)*
6MWT	−0.124 (0.260)	−0.244 (0.024)*	−0.495 (0.000)*	−0.294 (0.006)*
TUG	0.064 (0.558)	0.243 (0.025)*	0.557 (0.000)*	0.363 (0.001)*
SPPB	−0.121 (0.266)	−0.291 (0.007)*	−0.658 (0.000)*	−0.404 (0.000)*

RA: rheumatoid arthritis; HAQ: Health Assessment Questionnaire; DAS28: Disease Activity Score 28; Berg: Berg Balance Scale; 6MWT: 6-min walk test; TUG: Timed Up and Go; SPPB: Short Physical Performance Battery; r: Spearman's correlation; P: significance level

Table 3 Initial and final scores on physical, functional and disease activity tests

	Initial	Final	P
HAQ, median (P25–75)	0.62 (0.12–1.25)	0.62 (0.12–1.37)	0.318
DAS28, mean (±SD)	3.40 (±1.17)	3.58 (±1.32)	0.215
6MWT (meters), mean (±SD)	391.27 (±103.78)	429.52 (±129.01)	0.001
Berg, median (P25–75)	53 (49.75–56)	55 (50.75–56)	0.019
TUG (seconds), median (P25–75)	8.89 (7.59–11.69)	8.75 (7.14–11.28)	0.071
SPPB, median (P25–75)	10 (8–12)	11 (9–12)	0.001

HAQ: Health Assessment Questionnaire; DAS28: Disease Activity Score 28; 6MWT: 6-min walk test; Berg: Berg Balance Scale; TUG: Timed Up and Go; SPPB: Short Physical Performance Battery; P25–75: 25th percentile and 75th percentile; SD: standard deviation; P: t test significance level

observed was also high compared to that of non-institutionalized elderly individuals, which ranges from 15.9 to 56.3% [2]. Although age is an important risk factor for falls, the association between falls and advanced age was not observed in this sample, which is in agreement with previous RA studies [4–6, 12, 15, 35].

Comparing fallers with non-fallers, there was again agreement with other RA studies but a difference from what occurs in the elderly - there was no predominance of falls among females. It is possible that no difference was observed between men and women because both genders have decreased muscle mass and similar patterns of medication consumption [5–7, 15, 35].

The use of several medications may increase the occurrence of falls due to interactions between medications or their side effects. In the present study, we found a significant difference between fallers and non-fallers in relation to polypharmacy. Armstrong et al. [15] reported an association between a higher number of medications and a higher risk of falling, while Stanmore et al. [36] found that using four or more medications more than doubles the risk of falling in RA patients. An association has also been found between falls and the use of medications such as antihypertensives, diuretics, sedatives, antidepressants and antipsychotics [6, 8, 15, 36–39].

The history of falls was associated with the occurrence of new falls, which indicates the need for special attention in the evaluation of RA patients who have already fallen [4, 6, 7, 36].

Most of the sample presented moderate disease activity, which, similar to the study by Bohler et al. [12], was associated with poorer performance in most physical tests, but not the occurrence of falls. Koerich et al. [40] argued that the level of disease activity may influence physical performance (Berg and TUG), suggesting an increased risk of falling or dependence in performing activities of daily life. The lack of association between poor physical performance and disease activity with the presence of falls may be related to the time of evaluation, which usually occurs at the beginning or end of the study and not at the time of the falls. Another reasonable explanation is that the increased disease activity results in restriction of activities and therefore reduces the individuals' exposure to situations with a risk of falls.

Other studies have indicated functional disability as a risk factor for falls, but in our study, although it was associated with poorer performance in physical tests, it was not correlated with falls [4, 9, 12, 13, 19, 20, 35]. In a prospective study with 80 patients in Japan, Hayashibara et al. [6] found no relationship between functional disability and the presence of falls and explained that the

Table 4 Differences between disease activity and physical and functional performance in fallers and non-fallers

	Fallers (n = 42)	Non-fallers (n = 44)	Test	P
HAQ	0.81 (0.22–1.75)	0.50 (0.12–1.34)	U = 763.5	0.164
DAS28	3.70 (±1.49)	3.47 (±1.16)	t = −0.798	0.427
6MWT	376.31 (±100.74)	405.88 (±105.79)	t = 1.320	0.190
Berg	53 (47.75–55.25)	54.5 (50–56)	U = 787	0.229
TUG	9.27 (7.89–11.62)	8.73 (7.35–12.08)	U = 852	0.660
SPPB	10 (7.75–11)	10.5 (9–12)	U = 784.5	0.219

HAQ: Health Assessment Questionnaire; DAS28: Disease Activity Score 28; 6MWT: 6-min walk test; Berg: Berg Balance Scale; TUG: Timed Up and Go; SPPB: Short Physical Performance Battery; P: significance level; t: t test; U: Mann-Whitney U-test
Values are expressed as the mean (± standard deviation) or median (25th - 75th percentile)

Table 5 Differences between number of medications, history of falls, gender and fear of falling between fallers and non-fallers

		Occurrence of falls (n)		χ^2	P
		No	Yes		
Polypharmacy	Up to three medications	20	9	5.55	0.018
	Four or more	24	33		
History of falls	Yes	10	22	8.087	0.004
	No	34	20		
Gender	Female	38	38	0.354	0.552
	Male	6	4		
Fear of falling	Present	31	31	0.120	0.729
	Absent	13	11		

χ^2: chi-square; P: significance level

findings were due to the fact that five of the eight HAQ categories assess the function of the upper limbs.

Although the physical tests used in the present study are aimed at the elderly population, RA patients may present an early decrease in muscle strength, physical activity and balance in a pattern similar to that of elderly individuals, anticipating the risks resulting from the aging process. This may explain the finding that performance on physical tests was correlated with age: the older the patient, the poorer the physical performance. Although the four physical tests were significantly correlated among themselves, no significant association was found between any of the tests and the occurrence of falls. While some studies found an association between poorer performance on physical tests and a greater occurrence of falls or risk of falling, others found no such association [6, 11, 12, 16, 19, 36, 37]. The lack of standardization in the choice of tests for the RA population may be an important factor to be considered when analyzing these results, a gap that was observed by Santana et al. [41].

Several studies suggest that prospective studies be conducted to minimize memory bias [13–15, 19]. Cummings et al. [42], in a prospective, 12-month study of the elderly, found that 13–32% of the participants who fell did not report the episode at the end of the evaluation period. The follow-up strategies used were calendars, journals, fall log cards and self-reports to the researcher at the time of the fall. The present study has a methodological advantage, as it obtained the information quarterly by telephone, which improved the reliability of the report of falls and facilitated detailed clarification regarding the characteristics [4–8, 36].

Conclusions

The occurrence of falls in RA patients is high and is associated with a previous history of falls and polypharmacy, showing no association with disease activity or duration, functional capacity, physical performance, age or gender. In addition, the performances in the physical tests were associated with each other, and a poorer physical condition was related to greater disease activity, poorer functional capacity and older age.

Authors' contributions
The rheumatologist (MRA) confirmed the RA diagnosis and performed the measurements to assess disease activity, and the nurse (FVBOC) collected the blood samples. Next, the anthropometric data were measured, and the functional questionnaires and physical tests were applied by the nurse and the physical therapist (MAL). All authors read and approved the final manuscript.

References

1. Pinho TAM, Silva AO, Tura LFR, Moreira MASP, Gurgel SN, Smith AAF, et al. Avaliação do risco de quedas em idosos atendidos em Unidade Básica de Saúde. Rev Esc Enferm USP. 2012;46(2):320–7.

2. Sandoval RA, Sá ACAM, Menezes RL, Nakatani AYK, Bachion MM. Ocorrência de quedas em idosos não institucionalizados : revisão sistemática da literatura. Rev Bras Geriatr Gerontol. 2013;16(4):855–63.

3. Oliveira AS, Trevizan PF, Bestetti MLT, Melo RC. Fatores ambientais e risco de quedas em idosos: revisão sistemática. Rev Bras Geriatr Gerontol. 2014;17(3): 637–45.

4. Smulders E, Schreven C, Weerdesteyn V, van den Hoogen FHJ, Laan R, Van Lankveld W. Fall incidence and fall risk factors in people with rheumatoid arthritis. Ann Rheum Dis. 2009 [cited 2013 may 23];68(11):1795–1796. Available from: http://www.ncbi.nlm.nih.gov/pubmed/19822719.

5. Stanmore EK, Oldham J, Skelton DA, O'Neill T, Pilling M, Campbell AJ, et al. Fall incidence and outcomes of falls in a prospective study of adults with rheumatoid arthritis. Arthritis Care Res (Hoboken). 2013;65(5):737–44.

6. Hayashibara M, Hagino H, Katagiri H, Okano T, Okada J, Teshima R. Incidence and risk factors of falling in ambulatory patients with rheumatoid arthritis: a prospective 1-year study. Osteoporos Int. 2010 [cited 2013 may 23];21(11):1825–33. Available from: http://www.ncbi.nlm.nih.gov/pubmed/20119662.

7. Bugdayci D, Paker N, Rezvani A, Kesiktas N, Yilmaz O, Sahin M, et al. Frequency and predictors for falls in the ambulatory patients with rheumatoid arthritis: a longitudinal prospective study. Rheumatol Int. 2013 Apr;33(10):2523–7.

8. Brenton-Rule A, Dalbeth N, Bassett S, Menz HB, Rome K. The incidence and risk factors for falls in adults with rheumatoid arthritis: a systematic review. Semin Arthritis Rheum. 2015;44:389–98.

9. Kaz Kaz H, Johnson D, Kerry S, Chinappen U, Tweed K, Patel S. Fall-related risk factors and osteoporosis in women with rheumatoid arthritis. Rheumatology (Oxford). 2004;43(10):1267–71. Available from: https://academic.oup.com/rheumatology/article-lookup/doi/10.1093/rheumatology/keh304

10. Pereira IA, Mota LMH, Cruz BA, Brenol CV, Fronza LSR, Bertolo MB, et al. Consenso 2012 da Sociedade Brasileira de Reumatologia sobre o manejo de comorbidades em pacientes com artrite reumatoide. Rev Bras Reum. 2012; 52(4):474–95.

11. Duyurçakit B, Nacir B, Erdem HR, Karagoz A, Saraçoglu M. Fear of falling, fall risk and disability in patients with rheumatoid arthritis. Turk J Rheumatol. 2011;26(3):217–25.

12. Böhler C, Radner H, Ernst M, Binder A, Stamm T, Aletaha D, et al. Rheumatoid arthritis and falls: the influence of disease activity. Rheumatology (Oxford). 2012 [cited 2013 may 23];51(11):2051–2057. Available from: http://www.ncbi.nlm.nih.gov/pubmed/22879462.

13. Marques WV, Cruz VA, Rêgo J, Silva NA. Influência da capacidade funcional no risco de quedas em adultos com artrite reumatoide. Rev Bras Reum. 2014;54(5):404–8.

14. Fessel KD, Nevitt MC. Correlates of fear of falling and activity limitation among persons with rheumatoid arthritis. Arthritis Care Res. 1997;10(4): 222–8.

15. Armstrong C, Swarbrick CM, Pye SR, O'Neill TW. Occurrence and risk factors for falls in rheumatoid arthritis. Ann Rheum Dis. 2005;64(11):1602–4.

16. Jamison M, Neuberger GB, Miller PA. Correlates of falls and fear of falling among adults with rheumatoid arthritis. Arthritis Care Res (Hoboken). 2003; 49(5):673–80.

17. Schober HC, Maass K, Maass C, Reisinger EC, Schröder G, Kneitz C. Value of fall-risk tests for patients with rheumatoid arthritis. Z Rheumatol. 2011;70(7): 609–14.

18. Sugioka Y, Koike T. Fall risk and fracture. Associated factors for falls in patients with inflammatory polyarthritis. Clin Calcium. 2013;23(5):701–5.

19. Lourenço MA, Roma I, Assis MR. Ocorrência de quedas e sua associação com testes físicos, capacidade funcional e aspectos clínicos e demográficos em pacientes com artrite reumatoide. Rev Bras Reum. 2017;57(3):217–23.

20. Lourenço MA, Roma I, Assis MR. Correlação entre instrumentos de avaliação da funcionalidade e equilíbrio em pacientes com artrite reumatoide. Rev Bras Educ Fís Esporte. 2015;29(3):345–53.

21. Da Mota LMH, Cruz BA, Brenol CV, Pereira IA, Fronza LSR, Bertolo MB, et al. Consenso da Sociedade Brasileira de Reumatologia 2011 para o diagnóstico e avaliação inicial da artrite reumatoide. Rev Bras Reumatol. 2011;51(3):207–19.

22. Bruce B, Fries JF. The Health Assessment Questionnaire (HAQ). Clin Exp Rheumatol. 2005;23(5 SUPPL. 39):S14–8.

23. Ferraz MB, Oliveira LM, Araujo PMP, Atra E, Tugwell P. Crosscultural reliability of the physical ability dimension of the health assessment questionnaire. J Rheumatol. 1990 Jun;17(6):813–7.

24. Figueiredo KMOB, Lima KC, Guerra RO. Instrumentos de avaliação do equilíbrio corporal em idosos. Rev Bras Cineantropom Desempenho Hum. 2007;9(4):408–13.

25. Pimentel RM, Scheicher ME. Comparação do risco de queda em idosos sedentários e ativos por meio da escala de equilíbrio de Berg. Fisioter Pesq. 2009;16(1):6–10.

26. Miyamoto ST, Lombardi Junior I, Berg KO, Ramos LR, Natour J. Brazilian version of the Berg balance scale. Braz J Med Biol Res. 2004 Sep;37(9):1411–21. Available from: https://www.ncbi.nlm.nih.gov/pubmed/15334208.

27. Berg KO, Maki BE, Williams JI, Holliday PJ, Wood-Dauphinee SL. Clinical and laboratory measures of postural balance in an elderly population. Arch Phys Med Rehabil. 1992;73(11):1073–80.

28. Nakano MM, Diogo MJDe, Jacob Filho W. Versão brasileira da Short Physical Performance Battery - SPPB: adaptação cultural e estudo da confiabilidade. UNICAMP; 2007.

29. Sayers SP, Jette AM, Haley SM, Heeren TC, Guralnick JM, Fielding RA. Validation of thelate-life function and disability instrument. J Am Geriatr Soc. 2004;52(9):1554–9.

30. Guimarães LHCT, Galdino DCA, Martins FLM, Vitorino DFM, Pereira KL, Carvalho EM. Comparação da propensão de quedas entre idosos que praticam atividade física e idosos sedentários. Rev Neurociências. 2004;12(2): 68–72.

31. Shumway-Cook A, Brauer S, Woollacott M. Predicting the probability for falls in community-dwelling older adults using the timed up & go test. Phys Ther. 2000;80(9):896–903.

32. Podsiadlo D, Richardson S. The timed "Up & Go": a test of basic functional mobility for frail elderly persons. J Am Geriatr Soc [Internet]. 1991 Feb;39(2): 142–8. Available from: http://www.ncbi.nlm.nih.gov/pubmed/1991946.

33. Cipriano Junior G, Yuri D, Bernardelli GF, Mair V, Buffolo E, Branco JNR. Avaliação da Segurança do Teste de Caminhada dos 6 Minutos em Pacientes no Pré-Transplante Cardíaco. Arq Bras Cardiol. 2009;92(4):312–9.

34. Rondelli R, Oliveira A, Corso SD, Malaguti C. Uma atualização e proposta de padronização do teste de caminhada de seis minutos. Fisioter Mov. 2009; 22(2):249–59.

35. Oswald AE, Pye SR, O'Neill TW, Bunn D, Gaffney K, Marshall T, et al. Prevalence and associated factors for falls in women with established inflammatory polyarthritis. J Rheumatol. 2006 Apr;33(4):690–4. Available from: http://www.ncbi.nlm.nih.gov/pubmed/16482644.

36. Stanmore EK, Oldham J, Skelton D a, O'Neill T, Pilling M, Campbell a J, et al. Risk factors for falls in adults with rheumatoid arthritis: A prospective study. Arthritis Care Res (Hoboken). 2013 Feb;

37. Metlı NB, Kurtaran A, Akyüz M. Impaired balance and fall risk in rheumatoid arthritis patients. Turk J Phys Med Rehab. 2015;61:344–51.

38. Robbins AS, Rubenstein LZ, Josephson KR, Schulman BL, Osterweil D, Fine G. Predictors of falls among elderly people. Results of two population-based studies. Arch Intern Med. 1989;149:1628–33.

39. Furuya T, Yamagiwa K, Ikai T, Inoue E, Taniguchi A, Momohara S, et al. Associated factors for falls and fear of falling in Japanese patients with rheumatoid arthritis. Clin Rheumatol. 2009 Nov [cited 2013 may 23];28(11): 1325–30. Available from: http://www.ncbi.nlm.nih.gov/pubmed/19618097.

40. Koerich J, Armanini KK, Iop RR, Borges Júnior NG, Domenech SC, Gevaerd MS. Avaliação do equilíbrio corporal de pacientes com artrite reumatoide. Fisioter e Pesq. 2013;20(4):336–42.

41. De Santana FS, Nascimento DDC, De Freitas JPM, Miranda RF, Muniz LF, Santos Neto L, et al. Avaliação da capacidade funcional em pacientes com artrite reumatoide: implicações para a recomendação de exercícios físicos. Rev Bras Reumatol [Internet]. 2014;4(5):378–85. Available from: http://www.sciencedirect.com/science/article/pii/S0482500414001144

42. Cummings SR, Nevitt MC, Kidd S. Forgetting falls. The limited accuracy of recall of falls in the elderly. J Am Geriatr Soc. 1988;36(7):613–6.

16

Prevalence and factors associated with diagnosis of early rheumatoid arthritis in the south of Brazil

Rafael Kmiliauskis Santos Gomes[1,2,4*], Ana Carolina de Linhares[3] and Lucas Selistre Lersch[3]

Abstract

Background: Rheumatoid arthritis (RA) is an autoimmune inflammatory disease characterized by peripheral and symmetrical polyarthritis. It can be divided into Very Early Rheumatoid Arthritis (VERA) diagnosed up to 3 months of symptoms and late onset (Late Early Rheumatoid Arthritis – LERA), diagnosed between 3 and 12 months. Currently, it is recommended to evaluate the patient with joint symptoms as early as possible, and the first 12 weeks of manifestations represent the ideal phase for the diagnosis, favoring a better evolution of the treatment. The present study aimed to determine the prevalence of early diagnosis of rheumatoid arthritis, mean time of diagnosis and to determine possible associated factors in the municipality of Blumenau, Santa Catarina, Brazil.

Methods: A cross-sectional study using the 1987 American College of Rheumatology diagnostic criteria to select patients attended at primary or secondary health care units in Blumenau, Santa Catarina, southern Brazil, in 2014. Diagnostic time was verified by self-report of the time elapsed between the onset of symptoms and the diagnosis made by a rheumatologist. To test the associations, the chi-square test, the Wald linear trend test and the Poisson regression analysis were used.

Results: The mean time of diagnosis was 28 months. The prevalence of diagnosis up to 3 and 12 months was 27. 7% and 64.8%, respectively. Obesity was associated with time diagnosis in both periods. The 0–4 years category of the variable education was associated only with the period up to 12 months.

Conclusion: The mean time of diagnosis was similar to the national context. Among socioeconomic factors, lower education was associated with the diagnosis of late onset RA. The anthropometric variable presented a progressive increase in the prevalence due to the longer time to diagnosis.

Keywords: Rheumatoid arthritis, Prevalence, Diagnosis, Epidemiology

Background

Rheumatoid arthritis (RA) is an inflammatory autoimmune disease characterized by peripheral and symmetric polyarthritis [1]. It can be divided into Very Early Rheumatoid Arthritis (VERA) diagnosed up to 3 months of symptoms and late onset (Late Early Rheumatoid Arthritis - LERA), diagnosed between 3 and 12 months [2]. It is estimated that the disease affects between 0.5 and 1% of the adult world population. Its complications can lead to deformity and destruction of joints, due to the erosion of bone and cartilage [3]. These complications can cause severe joint damage with loss of functional capacity, so the importance of early diagnosis and immediate treatment [4].

Currently, it is recommended to evaluate a patient with joint symptoms as early as possible, since the critical period of the first 12 weeks of manifestations represents the ideal phase for the diagnosis, favoring a better evolution of the treatment [5, 6],. Despite this, the world reality differs from that recommended. In Saudi Arabia, an average time of approximately 30 months was verified [7], whereas in England, the ERAN study found a period of approximately 4 months for the diagnosis [8]. In Brazil, a study from São Paulo verified that the average

* Correspondence: gomesmed2002@ibest.com.br
[1]Specialty Center of the City of Blumenau, Blumenau, Santa Catarina State (SC), Brazil
[2]Specialty Center of the City of Brusque, Brusque, SC, Brazil
Full list of author information is available at the end of the article

waiting time between the beginning of the symptoms and rheumatologic evaluation was on average 39 months [9] This situation could be modified with early referral to the specialist and immediate diagnosis of the disease [10].

A Canadian study showed that younger, higher socioeconomic level and female subjects consulted more quickly with specialists, so they were diagnosed earlier [11]. Another study, conducted in Venezuela, showed a significant difference in diagnosis time between private and public health centers. This demonstrates that several factors influence the establishment of the diagnostic interval and initiation of therapy in patients with RA [12].

The prognostic consequences of diagnostic delay may be irreversible, such as deformities and functional limitation by persistent inflammation and progressive joint damage [13]. One can also cite the presence of work incapacity [9] and for daily tasks [14]. Another consequence would be the greater refractoriness of conventional synthetic disease-modifying antirheumatic drugs (csDMARD), leading to an increased risk of immunobiological use, depending on the severity and progression of the disease [15]. This would increase the costs of drug treatment, mainly affecting the Unified Health System (SUS) [16].

The present study aimed to determine the prevalence of early diagnosis of rheumatoid arthritis, the mean time of diagnosis and to determine possible associated factors in the city of Blumenau, Santa Catarina, Brazil.

Methods

This cross-sectional, population-based study was conducted between July 2014 and January 2015 with individuals 20 years of age or older with rheumatoid arthritis according to the American College of Rheumatology criteria of 1987, of both sexes, resident in the municipality of Blumenau, southern region of Brazil.

The formula for calculating the sample size required to estimate the prevalence of an event in a simple random sample was used considering the following parameters: 0.5% RA prevalence (1110 patients), 50% prevalence of exposure and unknown outcome, 5% sample error and 95% confidence level. The participants were recruited from all primary care centers (Unidades Básicas de Saúde – UBS), the specialty outpatient clinic and the specialty pharmacy of the municipality. Sample loss occurred when households were visited twice, once on the weekend and again in the evening, and no resident was at home, the resident had moved or refused to participate in the study on both occasions. The data collection team consisted of a local supervisor docente and 8 medical academics of the Regional University of Blumenau (Universidade Regional de Blumenau – FURB) previously trained to conduct structured interviews at

home and, if necessary, by telephone. Quality control was performed in 20% of respondents, who were interviewed for the second time using a short questionnaire.

The dependent variable was the diagnostic time of rheumatoid arthritis analyzed in two periods: up to 3 months and 12 months. The independent variables were defined as: a) demographic factors: sex, age in completed years, ranging from 20 to 39, 40-49 for adults and $\geq$ 60 years for the erderly b) socioeconomic factors: education in years of completed study, divided into 0–4, 5–8 and $\geq$ 9 years, current monthly personal income in minimum wages before diagnosis of the disease categorized in the first tertile (lowest), second tertile and third tertile (highest); c) anthropometric factors: body mass index (BMI - kg / m^2) subdivided according to the World Health Organization (WHO) in $\leq$24.9 for ideal weight, between 25 and 29.9 for overweight and $\geq$ 30 for obesity; d) disease-related factors: total disease time in months diagnosed by the rheumatologist, categorized between 0 and 24 months and > 24 months of disease, type of medical care in the last 12 months, classified in three groups, the Unified Health System (Sistema Único de Saúde – SUS; free, public healthcare system), Public-Private Healthcare (supplementary healthcare system), and the private healthcare (fee-for-service care) defined according to the Ministry of Health (Ministério da Saúde – MS), number of consultations with rheumatologist in the last 12 months, categorized between 0 and 2 and $\geq$ 3 consultations, current use of cs DMARD, current use of biological disease-modifying antirheumatic drugs (bDMARD) - tumor necrosis factor inhibitors / TNFi (adalimumab, etanercept, infliximab), HAQ (Health Assessment Questionnaire), ranging from 0 to 1 (mild impairment), 1.1 to 2 (moderate) and 2.1 to 3 (severe), the presence of bone erosions in the radiography of hands; and e) labor factor: current professional situation (working, health insurance, disability retirement, retirement for time of service).

The data was entered in a system developed for this study with output in the format of the excel table and later the final file was exported to Stata 10.0 program (Stata Corp., College Station, USA). The variables of interest were analyzed for their distributions using average, standard deviation, median for continuous variables; and frequency and percentage for the categorical ones.

To test the association between symptom time and diagnosis of rheumatoid arthritis in months with independent variables, the chi-square test and, where appropriate, Wald's linear trend test were used. Then, the Poisson regression analysis was performed to verify the association of the factors studied with the dependent variable, estimating the crude and adjusted prevalence ratios (PR), the respective 95% confidence intervals and the value of p.

Table 1 Description of the sample and the prevalence of the diagnostic time of up to 3 and 12 months of symptons according to the independente variables in patients with rheumatoid arthritis of Blumenau, Santa Catarina, Brazil, 2014

Variables	Sample		Diagnostic up to 3 months			Diagnostic up to 12 months		
	N	%	Prevalence(%)	CI 95%	p	Prevalence(%)	CI 95%	p
Total	296	100,0	27,7%	(22,5–32,8)		64,8%	(59,3-70,3)	
Sex (n = 296)					0,098[a]			0,708[a]
Male	48	16,2	37,5	(23,2-51,7)		62,5	(48,2-76,7)	
Female	248	83,8	25,8	(20,3–31,2)		65,3	(59,3-71,2)	
Age in years (n = 287)					0,227[b]			0,893[b]
20–39	16	5,6	12,5	(5, 7–30,7)		62,5	(35,8-89,1)	
40–59	146	50,9	26,7	(19,4–33,9)		65,7	(57,9-73,5)	
≥ 60	125	43,5	29,6	(21,5–37,7)		64,1	(55,4-72,5)	
Education in completed years (n = 284)					0,447[b]			0,093[b]
0–4	106	37,3	27,4	(18,6–36,2)		70,5	(61,5-79,5)	
5–8	76	26,7	21,1	(11,6–30,4)		64,4	(53,4-75,4)	
> 9	102	35,9	32,1	(23,1- 41,1)		59,4	(49,9-68,9)	
Current monthly personal income in minimum wages (n = 248)					0,799[b]			0,493[b]
Third tertile (higher)	82	33,1	28,5	(18,7–38,4)		59,5	(48,8-70,2)	
Second tertile	82	33,1	25,6	(15,9–35,2)		65,8	(55,3-76,3)	
First tertile (lower)	84	33,8	26,8	(17,1–36,6)		64,6	(54,1-75,2)	
Body mass index (Kg/m^2) (n = 285)					0,012[b]			0,001[b]
≤ 24,9	110	38,6	36,3	(27,2-45,4)		75,4	(67,2-83,6)	
25–29,9	113	39,7	24,7	(16,7–32,8)		61,9	(52,8-71,1)	
≥ 30	62	21,7	19,3	(9,2–29,3)		51,6	(38,8-64,4)	
Type of service in the last 12 months (n = 269)					0,166[b]			0,515[b]
Public healthcare system	113	42,1	23,8	(15,9–31,8)		64,6	(55,7-73,4)	
Supplementary healthcare system	84	31,2	27,3	(17,7–37,1)		65,4	(55,2-75,7)	
Fee-for-service care	72	26,7	33,3	(22,3-44,3)		69,9	(58,6-80,2)	
Total number of consultations with a rheumatologist in the last 12 months (n = 281)					0,165[b]			0,069[b]
0–1	42	15,0	33,3	(18,4-48,2)		69,1	(54,4-83,6)	
2–3	126	44,9	23,0	(15,5 –30,4)		58,7	(50,0-67,4)	
≥ 4	113	40,1	30,9	(22,3-39,6)		69,9	(61,3-78,4)	
Disease time in months (n = 235)					0,193[a]			0,102[a]
0–24	37	15,7	37,8	(21,4-54,2)		75,6	(61,1-90,1)	
> 24	198	84,3	27,2	(21,1–33,5)		61,6	(54,7-68,4)	
Use of cs DMARD (n = 296)					0,396[a]			0,994[a]
Yes	202	68,2	29,2	(22,8–35,5)		64,8	(58,2-71,4)	
No	94	31,7	24,4	(15,6–33,3)		64,8	(55,1-74,7)	
Use of TNFi (ADA + ETA+IFX) (n = 288)					0,960[a]			0,592[a]
Yes	75	26,1	28,0	(17,5–38,4)		61,3	(50,1-72,6)	
No	213	73,9	27,6	(21,6–33,7)		64,7	(58,3-71,2)	
HAQ (n = 165)					0,904[b]			0,211[b]
0–1 (mild)	65	39,4	24,6	(13,8–35,3)		55,3	(42,9-67,7)	
1,1–2 (moderate)	59	35,7	32,2	(19,9-44,4)		69,4	(57,3-81,5)	
2,1–3 (severe)	41	24,9	24,3	(10,6–38,1)		65,8	(50,7-81,0)	

Table 1 Description of the sample and the prevalence of the diagnostic time of up to 3 and 12 months of symptons according to the independente variables in patients with rheumatoid arthritis of Blumenau, Santa Catarina, Brazil, 2014 *(Continued)*

Variables	Sample		Diagnostic up to 3 months			Diagnostic up to 12 months		
	N	%	Prevalence(%)	CI 95%	p	Prevalence(%)	CI 95%	p
Presence of radiological changes (erosions) in hands (n = 237)					0,814[a]			0,665[a]
No	89	37,5	26,9	(17,5–36,3)		66,2	(56,2-76,3)	
Yes	148	62,5	28,3	(21,1–35,7)		63,5	(55,6-71,3)	
Current professional situation (237)					0,325[b]			0,132[b]
Working	77	32,5	23,3	(13,7 – 33,1)		59,7	(48,5 – 70,9)	
Health insurance	29	12,2	24,1	(7,5 – 40,7)		55,1	(35,9 – 74,4)	
Disability retirement	65	27,5	27,6	(16,5 – 38,8)		60,1	(47,7 – 77,2)	
Retirement for time of service	66	27,8	30,3	(18,9 – 41,6)		72,2	(61,9 – 83,7)	

csDMARD conventional synthetic disease-modifying antirheumatic drugs, *TNFi* tumor necrosis factor inhibitors *ADA* adalimumab, *ETA* etanercept, *IFX* infliximab, *HAQ* health assessment questionnaire; CI 95%: confidence interval of 95%
[a]Chi-square test [b]Wald's linear trend test

For the input in the final model, all the variables that presented a value of $p < 0.20$ in the crude analysis were taken into account. The regression model adjusted for those variables that maintained the value of $p \leq 0.05$ or adjusted the final model. For the inclusion of the variables in the regression model, the researchers chose sequentially to include the variables: demographic, socioeconomic, anthropometric, related to the disease and professional situation.

This research was submitted to the research ethics committee of the University of São Paulo (USP) and FURB (protocol n°.339 / 13 and 133/12, respectively) and approved; all participants signed the informed consent form.

Results

A total of 336 patients were identified. After excluding deceased patients and those who refused to participate in the study or patients without data for any variable, 296 patients were included in the study.

The majority of the sample consisted of females (83.8%) and adults (50.9%) with mean age and standard deviation (SD) of 58.1 years (SD: 11.5), ranging from 27 to 89 years. Regarding education, the majority of patients had 0 to 4 years of completed study (37.3%), with a mean of 7.7 years (SD: 4.4). Regarding the disease-related characteristics, the mean disease duration was 126 months (SD: 100), ranging from 0 to 420, mean HAQ of 1.3 (SD: 0.8) and that the majority of the population was using cs DMARD (68.2%). The majority of individuals presented overweight BMI, mean of 26.6 kg / m² (SD: 4.9).

Regarding the factors related to the diagnosis time, it was observed that the sex variable, for diagnosis up to 3 months, prevailed among males; for diagnosis up to 12 months in the female sex. In relation to age, for diagnosis up to 3 months, preponderated in the population of 60 years or more; and for 12 months, from 40 to 59 years. Regarding education, individuals with more than 9 years of study predominated, for diagnosis up to 3 months; for diagnosis up to 12 months, the population with 0 to 4 years of study. Patients with a diagnosis established up to 3 months had income in the third tertile (highest), and for 12 months in the second tertile (intermediate). Regarding the variables related to the disease, it was observed that individuals who had a disease time of less than 24 months had a higher prevalence of early diagnosis for both periods. In addition, there was a progressive increase in the prevalence of obese individuals over time. Regarding the total number of consultations with rheumatologists in the last 12 months, the majority of patients diagnosed up to 3 months had 0 to 1 consultation, and those diagnosed up to 12 months, consumed a greater number of consultations, 4 or more (Table 1).

It was verified in the crude regression analysis that the dependent variable up to 3 months showed a tendency of association with sex and age, whereas education only for up to 12 months. Regarding the anthropometric variable, it was observed that in the two time intervals analyzed, the BMI was associated with the category of values ≥ 30, since the longer the diagnosis, the greater the prevalence of obese individuals. The care performed by the SUS showed an associative tendency of lower prevalence with diagnosis in the very early period of the disease in relation to the private care. Patients diagnosed in both periods used fewer consultations than the reference category (2 to 3 visits in 12 months). Regarding the current professional situation, among the patients diagnosed up to 12 months, there was a trend of increasing form 11% to 34% in the health insurance in relation to the patients who remained working. Of the individuals diagnosed for up to 3 months, 16% had a prevalence of disease time greater than 24 months, whereas for the interval of up to 12 months, the prevalence increased to 57%.

Table 2 Crude and adjusted regression analysis of diagnostic time up to 3 months and independent variables in patients with rheumatoid arthritis in Blumenau, Santa Catarina, Brazil, 2014

Variables	Crude analysis			Adjusted analysis		
	(PRc)	CI 95%	p	(PRa)	CI 95%	p
Sex (n = 296)			0,146			0,154**
Male	0,84	(0,6-1,0)		0,85	(0,6-1,0)	
Female	1			1		
Age in years (n = 287)			0,200			0,267**
20–39	1			1		
40–59	0,83	(0,6-1,0)		0,84	(0,6-1,0)	
≥ 60	0,80	(0,6-1,0)		0,81	(0,6-1,0)	
Education in completed years (n = 284)			0,459*			0,314**
0–4	0,93	(0,7-1,1)		0,90	(0,7-1,0)	
5–8	1,08	(0,9-1,2)		1,07	(0,9-1,2)	
> 9	1			1		
Current monthly personal income in minimum wages (n = 248)			0,801*			0,622**
Third tertile (higher)	1			1		
Second tertile	1,01	(0,8-1,2)		1,01	(0,8-1,2)	
First tertile (lower)	0,97	(0,8-1,1)		0,95	(0,7-1,1)	
Body mass index (Kg/m²) (n = 285)			0,010			0,031
≤ 24,9	1			1		
25–29,9	1,18	(0,9-1,4)		1,16	(0,9-1,4)	
≥ 30	1,26	(1,0-1,5)		1,23	(1,0-1,5)	
Type of servicee in the last 12 months (n = 269)			0,177			0,623**
Public healthcare system	0,87	(0,7-1,0)		0,95	(0,7-1,1)	
Supplementary healthcare system	0,95	(0,8-1,1)		0,96	(0,8-1,1)	
Fee-for-service care	1			1		
Total number of consultations with a rheumatologist in the last 12 months (n = 281)			0,165			0,163**
0–1	0,86	(0,6-1,1)		0,85	(0,6-1,0)	
2–3	1			1		
≥ 4	0,89	(0,7-1,0)		0,89	(0,7-1,0)	
Disease time in months (n = 235)			0,247*			0,605**
0–24	1			1		
> 24	1,16	(0,8-1,5)		1,07	(0,8-1,3)	
Use of csDMARD (n = 296)			0,383*			0,283**
Yes	1			1		
No	1,06	(0,9-1,2)		1,12	(0,9-1,3)	
Use of TNFi (ADA + ETA+IFX) (n = 288)			0,960*			0,277**
Yes	0,99	(0,8-1,1)		0,88	(0,7-1,0)	
No	1			1		
HAQ (n = 165)			0,901*			0,587**
0–1 (mild)	1			1		
1,1–2 (moderate)	0,89	(0,7-1,1)		0,86	(0,6-1,1)	
2,1–3 (severe)	1,01	(0,8-1,2)		0,92	(0,6-1,3)	

Table 2 Crude and adjusted regression analysis of diagnostic time up to 3 months and independent variables in patients with rheumatoid arthritis in Blumenau, Santa Catarina, Brazil, 2014 *(Continued)*

Variables	Crude analysis			Adjusted analysis		
	(PRc)	CI 95%	p	(PRa)	CI 95%	p
Presence of radiological changes (erosions) in hands (n = 237)			0,814*			0,306**
No	1			1		
Yes	0,98	(0,8-1,1)		1,13	(0,8-1,4)	
Current professional situation (237)			0,324*			0,637**
Working	1			1		
Health insurance	0,99	(0,7-1,2)		0,99	(0,7 – 1,4)	
Disability retirement	0,94	(0,7-1,1)		0,89	(0,6 – 1,1)	
Retirement for time of service	0,91	(0,7-1,1)		0,95	(0,7 – 1,2)	

csDMARD conventional synthetic disease-modifying antirheumatic drugs, *TNFi* tumor necrosis factor inhibitors, *ADA* adalimumab, *ETA* etanercept, *IFX* infliximab, *HAQ* health assessment questionnaire, *PRc* crude prevalence ratio, *PRa* adjusted prevalence ratio; CI 95%: confidence interval of 95%
* Value of $p > 0,20$ excluded from the adjusted analysis. ** Value of $p > 0,05$ excluded of final model

In the adjusted analysis, the variables sex, age, total number of consultations, time of disease and current professional situation lost power of association with both diagnostic periods, excluded from the final model. The BMI remained in the final model in the two periods represented by the obesity category, respectively, with a prevalence of 23% and 107% higher in relation to the ideal weight patient. The variable education remained in the model for the diagnosis period up to 12 months, with 59% higher prevalence in the category of 0–4 years of study. (Tables 2 and 3).

Discussion

The present study observed that the mean time from onset of symptoms to diagnosis was 28 months. The prevalence of the diagnosis of very early rheumatoid arthritis was 27.7%, whereas in the late initial period it was 64.8%. Although the majority of the patients received the diagnosis up to 12 months, the others presented a great diagnostic delay, which increased the mean time of diagnosis of the disease.

The research identified that the lower educational level of the patient was directly related to the diagnosis later than 12 months. Also, there was a progressive increase in the prevalence of obesity between the diagnostic periods.

Previous studies conducted in other Brazilian cities showed a diagnostic time of approximately 8 [17], 12 [18] and 39 months [9], showing that the present study is within the national intervals, and presented similarity to a study in Brasília, whose time was 27 months [19]. The international literature offers a variety of data, such as a mean time of 6 months in European countries [20], 30 months in Saudi Arabia [7] and up to 33 months in Colombia [21]. These data show that there are contributing factors for the diagnostic time that differ according to locality. The prevalence of patients diagnosed in the

first 3 months of the symptoms is in line with both national (35.3%) [17] and international data, which show values of 1–50% [22] and 32–38% [23]. The prevalence found in the period was found to be better than that found in Sri Lanka (0.7%) [24], but worse than that found in Uruguay (45%) [25] and Norway (50%) [26].

Possible association factors with RA diagnosis time, including social and demographic profile, were analyzed. It was observed that the sex and age of the patients were not related to the dependent variables, as was found in studies carried out in Belgium [27], Norway [26] and England [28] and contrary to a Canadian study that states that women and younger individuals have less diagnostic time [29]. In the present study, patients with less years of study had a later diagnosis, this data contradicts Venezuelan and Canadian literature, where there was no association with this variable [12, 30]. This may occur due to the possible relationship of lower education and income; and consequent greater use of the public health system, which generates more waiting for consultation with a specialist. In Blumenau, this waiting time for consultation is up to 2 months (unpublished data).

It is known that obesity is a frequent condition in patients with RA [31, 32]. According to the present study, when we compared patients with a later diagnosis in relation to the very early, they were more strongly associated with BMI. For the authors' knowledge, this is the first article to demonstrate this association and should be confirmed in the future research. As justification, it is suggested that patients with greater time to diagnosis have more difficulty controlling the disease and therefore use more drugs, such as glucocorticoid, which may influence the weight gain [33]. The result could also occur due to a more advanced disease, which leads to greater disability, favoring the sedentary lifestyle and increased BMI of the patient.

Table 3 Crude and adjusted regression analysis of diagnostic time up to 12 months and independent variables in patients with rheumatoid arthritis in Blumenau, Santa Catarina, Brazil, 2014

Variables	Crude analysis			Adjusted analysis		
	(RPc)	CI 95%	p	(PRa)	CI 95%	p
Sex (n = 296)			0,704*			0,720**
Male	1,08	(0,7-1,6)		1,07	(0,7-1,6)	
Female	1			1		
Age in years (n = 287)			0,894*			0,920**
20–39	1			1		
40–59	0,91	(0,4-1,7)		0,91	(0,6-1,7)	
≥ 60	0,96	(0,4-1,8)		0,95	(0,4-1,8)	
Education in completed years (n = 284)			0,094			0,041
0–4	1,37	(0,9-2,1)		1,59	(1,1 - 2, 5)	
5–8	1,20	(0,7-1,8)		1,29	(0,7-2,1)	
> 9	1			1		
Current monthly personal income in minimum wages (n = 248)			0,496*			0,741**
Third tertile (higher)	1			1		
Second tertile	0,96	(0,6-1,4)		0,91	(0,5-1,4)	
First tertile (lower)	1,11	(0,7-1,6)		1,07	(0,7-1,6)	
Body mass index (Kg/m^2) (n = 285)			0,001			0,001
≤ 24,9	1			1		
25–29,9	1,55	(1,0-2,3)		1,62	(1,0-2,4)	
≥ 30	1,97	(1,2-2,9)		2,07	(1, 3 - 3,1)	
Type of servicee in the last 12 months (n = 269)			0,515*			0,997**
Public healthcare system	0,86	(0,5-1,3)		1,01	(0,6-1,6)	
Supplementary healthcare system	0,97	(0,6-1,4)		0,90	(0,5-1,4)	
Fee-for-service care	1			1		
Total number of consultations with a rheumatologist in the last 12 months (n = 281)			0,074			0,223**
0–1	0,75	(0,4-1,2)		0,79	(0,4-1,3)	
2–3	1			1		
≥ 4	0,72	(0,5-1,0)		0,79	(0,5-1,1)	
Disease time in months (n = 235)			0,134			0,115**
0–24	1			1		
> 24	1,57	(0,8-2,8)		1,76	(0,8-3,5)	
Use of csDMARD (n = 296)			0,994*			0,744**
Yes	1			1		
No	0,99	(0,7-1,3)		1,08	(0,6-1,7)	
Use of TNFi (ADA + ETA+IFX) (n = 288)			0,588*			0,217**
Yes	0,91	(0,6-1,2)		0,75	(0,4-1,1)	
No	1			1		
HAQ (n = 165)			0,227*			0,867**
0–1 (mild)	1			1		
1,1–2 (moderate)	0,68	(0,4-1,1)		0,78	(0,6-1,1)	
2,1–3 (severe)	0,76	(0,4-1,2)		0,82	(0,6-1,3)	

Table 3 Crude and adjusted regression analysis of diagnostic time up to 12 months and independent variables in patients with rheumatoid arthritis in Blumenau, Santa Catarina, Brazil, 2014 *(Continued)*

Variables	Crude analysis			Adjusted analysis		
	(RPc)	CI 95%	p	(PRa)	CI 95%	p
Presence of radiological changes (erosions) in hands (n = 237)			0,668*			0,877**
No	1			1		
Yes	1,08	(0,7-1,5)		1,03	(0,6-1,6)	
Current professional situation (237)			0,125			0,088**
Working	1			1		
Health insurance	1,11	(0,6-1,8)		1,34	(0,8 – 2,1)	
Disability retirement	0,99	(0,6-1,4)		0,85	(0,5 – 1,3)	
Retirement for time of service	0,67	(0,4-1,1)		0,68	(0,4 – 1,1)	

csDMARD conventional synthetic disease-modifying antirheumatic drugs, *TNFi* tumor necrosis factor inhibitors, *ADA* adalimumab, *ETA* etanercept, *IFX* infliximab, *HAQ* health assessment questionnaire, *PRc* crude prevalence ratio; PRa: adjusted prevalence ratio; CI 95%: confidence interval of 95%
* Value of $p > 0,20$ excluded from the adjusted analysis. ** Value of $p > 0,05$ excluded of final model

As for the time of disease, an average of 126 months was found, higher than that found in another Brazilian study that was 92 months [34]. There was no statistical association between diagnosis time and disease time, but patients with a recent disease had an earlier diagnosis, whereas patients with a longer disease period (> 2 years) had a later diagnosis, as observed in international studies [22, 35].

The symptoms of RA can be initially attenuated with symptomatic drugs, however, the specific treatment for the disease is done with cs DMARD and, when they do not achieve adequate control of disease activity, TNFi drugs, which are bDMARD medications [36, 37]. In this study, there was no significant association in the use of cs DMARD and / or TNFi and time to diagnosis. Despite this, it was possible to observe that patients diagnosed up to 3 months would have less need to use cs DMARD when compared to those diagnosed up to 12 months. This finding was also found in the Leiden cohort (Netherlands), stating that there was a higher remission rate without the use of cs DMARD in patients evaluated within 3 months [5]. Regarding the use of TNFi, in earlier diagnosis, there would be less need to use, as found in an Italian study [22].

In the present study, patients had an average of 3.4 consultations in the last year with a rheumatologist, similar to the national data [16, 38]. No statistical association was found regarding the number of consultations with rheumatologists in the last year and the diagnostic interval. However, it was observed that when the diagnosis was made within 3 months, patients consumed fewer visits in the last year compared to those diagnosed within 12 months. This is probably due to better control of the disease when diagnosed earlier, requiring fewer consultations during the year.

It was seen that as the time to diagnosis increased, the prevalence of patients with an intermediate or worse HAQ also increased, although there was no association with the dependent variable. A study conducted between 2007 and 2009 with 1795 patients also showed that individuals diagnosed earlier were able to maintain lower values of HAQ in their follow-up [22]. Non-association could be attributed to a smaller sample of patients when compared to the other variables.

The presence of radiological alterations in hands was observed in the majority of the patients, a result that may have occurred because most of the patients in the sample had more disease time and therefore the availability of resources was more precarious than the ones we have currently, and could favor greater joint damage. In addition, it was initially observed that the later the diagnosis, the greater the prevalence of erosions in the patients hands, as evidenced in a work performed with patients in the state of São Paulo [39].

The results showed a trend that the later the diagnosis, the lower the prevalence of patients being able to retire due to length of service. Brazilian literature confirms this information when it cites that the delay in diagnosis increases the individual's incapacity to work [9]. Regarding the type of care, most of the patients in the sample used the SUS in the last year. In spite of this, there was a tendency of a higher prevalence of the diagnosis of very early RA in the private service when compared to SUS of the order of 13%. As justification, it is assumed that individuals diagnosed earlier would have a higher economic level to obtain faster service.

Some limitations should be considered in this research. The transversal design of the study makes it impossible to determine cause and effect between the exploratory variables and the outcome. Based on the obtained results, the possibility of characteristic reverse causality in cross-sectional studies is highlighted. Other factors to take into account concern the possibility of memory bias in collecting some information attenuated by the common feature of RA being a chronic injury. The agreement between the answers of the first and the second questionnaire including the dependent variable was 82% (unpublished data).

Conclusion

Therefore, this research reinforces the need to know the factors that may delay the earlier diagnosis of RA; and thus decrease the chances of the best results for the patient. It was evidenced that the socioeconomic factor, lower education, was associated with a later initial diagnosis. As a result of the longer diagnosis time there was a progressive increase in the prevalence of obesity among patients. We suggest that more studies be carried out regarding this theme in order to know the local realities, in order to speed up the access of care of the individuals affected by the disease, reinforcing the importance of the early diagnosis.

Abbreviatons

bDMARD: Biological disease-modifying antirheumatic drugs; BMI: body mass index; csDMARD: Conventional synthetic disease-modifying antirheumatic drugs; FURB: Blumenau Regional University Foundation; HAQ: Health Assessment Questionnaire; LERA: Late Early Rheumatoid Arthritis; MS: Ministry of Health; PR: Prevalence ratios; RA: Rheumatoid arthritis (RA); SD: Standard deviation; SUS: Unified Health System; TNFi: Tumor necrosis factor inhibitors; USP: University of São Paulo; VERA: Very Early Rheumatoid Arthritis; WHO: World Health Organization

Authors' contributions

RKSG contributed to elaboration, literature review, statistical analysis and article writing. ACL e LSL contributed to writing and literature review. All approved final version for submission in journal.

Author details

[1]Specialty Center of the City of Blumenau, Blumenau, Santa Catarina State (SC), Brazil. [2]Specialty Center of the City of Brusque, Brusque, SC, Brazil. [3]School of Medicine, Regional University of Blumenau (Universidade Regional de Blumenau – FURB), Blumenau, Brazil. [4]Centro de Referência Policlínica Lindolf Bell, Rua: Dois de Setembro, 1234 - Itoupava Norte, 3° andar, sala 1. CEP, Blumenau, SC 89052-003, Brazil.

References

1. American College of Rheumatology Subcommitte on Rheumatoid Arthritis Guidelines. Guidelines for the management of rheumatoid arthritis. Arthritis Rheumatology. 2002;46:328–46.
2. Da Mota Licia Maria Henrique, Laurindo Ieda Maria Magalhães e Dos Santos Neto Leopoldo Luiz. Artrite reumatoide inicial: conceitos. Rev Assoc Med Bras 2010; 56(2):227–229.
3. Da Henrique MLM, Alfonso CB, Viegas BC, Alves PI, Stange R-FL, Barros BM, et al. Guidelines for the diagnosis of rheumatoid arthritis. Rev Bras Reumatol. 2013;53(2):141–57.
4. Cheung PP, Dougados M, Andre V, Balandraud N, Chales G, Chary-Valckenaere I, et al. Improving agreement in assessment of synovitis in rheumatoid arthritis. Joint Bone Spine. 2013;80(2):155–9.
5. der Linden Michael V, Saskia le C, Karim R, der Woude Diane V, Rachel K, Tom H, der Helm-van Mil Annette V. Long-term impact of delay in assessment of patients with early arthritis. Arthritis Rheumatology. 2010; 62(12):3537–46.
6. Nell VP, Machold KP, Eberl G, Stamm TA, Uffmann M, Smolen JS. Benefit of very early referral and very early therapy with disease-modifying antirheumatic drugs in patients with early rheumatoid arthritis. Oxford J. 2004;43:906–14.
7. Hussain W, Noorwali A, Janoudi N, Baamer M, Kebbi L, Mansafi H, et al. From symptoms to diagnosis: an observational study of the journey of rheumatoid arthritis patients in Saudi Arabia. Oman Med J. 2016;31(1):29–34.
8. Kiely P, Williams R, Walsh D, Young A. Contemporary patterns of care and disease activity outcome in early rheumatoid arthritis: the ERAN cohort. Rheumatology. 2009;48:57–60.
9. Melo V, Aguiar F, Baleroni T, Novaes G. Análise temporal entre início dos sintomas, avaliação reumatológica e tratamento com drogas modificadoras de doença em pacientes com artrite reumatoide. Ver Fac Ciênc Méd Sorocaba. 2008;10(2):12–5.
10. Combe B, Landewe R, Lukas C, Bolosiu HD, Breedveld F, Dougados M, et al. EULAR recommendations for the management of early arthritis: report of a task force of the European Standing Committee for International Clinical Studies Including Therapeutics (ESCISIT). Ann Rheum Dis. 2007;66(1):34–5.
11. Feldman DE, Bernatsky S, Haggerty J, Leffondré K, Tousignant P, Leffondré K, et al. Delay in consultation with specialists for persons with suspected new-onset rheumatoid arthritis: a population based study. Arthritis Rheum. 2007;57:1419–25.
12. Rodríguez-Polanco E, Al Snih S, Kuo YF, Millán A, Rodríguez MA Lag time between onset of symptoms and diagnosis in Venezuelan patients with rheumatoid arthritis. Rheumatol Int 2011; 31(5):657–65.
13. Da Mota LM, Cruz BA, Brenol CV, Pereira IA, Fronza LS, Bertolo MB, et al. Consensus of the Brazilian Society of Rheumatology for diagnosis and early assessment of rheumatoid arthritis. Rev Bras Reumatol. 2011;51(3):199–219.
14. James F, Patricia S, Halsted KGH. Measurement of patient outcome in arthritis. Arthritis Rheum. 1980;23:137–45.
15. Ministério da Saúde. Portaria SCTIE no 66, de 6 de novembro de 2006. Protocolo Clínico e Diretrizes Terapêuticas – artrite reumatoide. Diário Oficial da União 2006.
16. Bagatini BF, Raquel BC, Estima MAC, Nair LS, Rocha FM. Estudo de custo-análise do tratamento da artrite reumatoide grave em um município do Sul do Brasil. Cad Saúde Pública. 2013;29(1):81–91.
17. Da Mota Licia M, Ieda L, Leopoldo N. Características demográficas e clínicas de uma coorte de pacientes de artrite reumatoide inicial. Rev Bras Reumatol. 2010;50(3):235–48.
18. David Juliano M, Mattei Rodrigo A, Mauad Juliana L, Almeida Lauren G, Nogueira Marcio A, Poliana M, et al. Estudo clínico e laboratorial de pacientes com artrite reumatoide diagnosticados em serviço de reumatologia em Cascavel, PR, Brasil. Rev Bras Reumatol. 2013;53(1):57–65.
19. Cunha BM, de Oliveira SB, dos Santos-Neto LL. Coorte Sarar: atividade de doença, capacidade funcional e dano radiológico em pacientes com artrite reumatoide submetidos à artroplastia total de quadril e joelho. Rev Bras Reumatol. 2015;55(5):420–6.
20. Karin R, Rebecca S, Kanta K, Andrew F, Jacqueline D, Hans B, et al. Delays in assessment of patients with rheumatoid arthritis: variations across Europe. Ann Rheum Dis. 2011;70:1822–5.
21. Ruiz O, Salazar JC, Londoño PJ, Saiibi DL, Molina JF, Santos P, et al. Cambio en la capacidad funcional, calidad de vida y actividad de la enfermedad, en un grupo de pacientes colombianos con artritis reumatoide refractaria al tratamiento convencional, que recibieron terapia con infliximab como medicamento de rescate. Revista Med. 2009;17(1):40–9.
22. Elisa G, Fausto S, Laura BS, Alessandro C, Francesca B-P, Roberto C, et al. Very early rheumatoid arthtitis as a predictor of remission: a multicentre real life prospective stydy. Ann Rheum Dis. 2013;72:858–62.
23. Jessica N, Elisabeth B, Floris G, Cornelia A, Tom H, Marcel P, et al. Improved early identification of arthritis: evaluating the efficacy of early Artrhitis recognition clinics. Ann Rheum Dis. 2013;72:1295–301.
24. Atukaorala I, Wljewickrama P, Gunawardena MPH, Atukorala K, Weerathunga D, Dharmasena D. The community prevalence of early rheumatoid arthritis and health seeking behavior of affected individuals. Int J Epidemiol. 2015;44(1): 2016–207.
25. Palleiro D. Diagnostic delay in rheumatoid arthritis. J Clin Rheumatol. 2006;12:41.
26. Palm O, Purinszky E. Women with early rheumatoid arthritis are referred later than men. Ann Rheum Dis. 2005;64:1227–8.
27. De Cock D, Meyfroidt S, Joly J, Van Der Elst K, Westhovens R, Verschueren P. A detailed analysis of treatment delay from the onset of symptons in early rheumatoid arthritis patients. Scand J Rheumatol 2014;43:1–8.
28. Kumar K, Daley DM, Carruthers D, Situnayake C, Gordon K, Grindulis CD, et al. Delay in presentation to primary care physicians is the main reason why patients with rheumatoid arthritis are seen later by rheumatologists. Rheumatology. 2007;46:1438–40.
29. Feldman Debbie E, Sasha B, Jeannie H, Karen L, Pierre T, Yves R, et al. Delay in consultation with specialists for persons with suspected new-onset rheumatoid arthritis: a population-based study. Arthritis Care & Research. 2007;57(8):1419–25.
30. Cheryl B, Juan X, Pope Janet E, Gilles B, Carol H, Boulos H, et al. Factors associated with time to diagnosis in early rheumatoid arthritis. Rheumatol Int. 2014;34:85–92.

31. Junior RSD, Ferraz AL, Oesterreich AS, Schmitz WO, Shinzato MM. Caracterização de pacientes com artrite reumatoide quanto a fatores de risco para doenças vasculares cardíacas no Mato Grosso do Sul. Rev Bras Reumatol. 2015;55(6):493–500.

32. Rachel Z, Marcia D, Thelma S. Perfil nutricional na artrite reumatoide. Rev Bras Reumatol. 2013;54(1):68–72.

33. Michael G, Joshua B. The obesity epidemic and consequences for rheumatoid arthritis. Curr Rheumatol Rep. 2016;18(1):6.

34. Almeida Maria do Socorro TM, Almeida João Vicente M, Bertolo Manuel B. Características demográficas e clínicas de pacientes com artrite reumatoide no Piauí, Brasil – avaliação de 98 pacientes. Rev Bras Reumatol. 2014;54(5):360–5.

35. Jennifer A, George W, Verhoeven Arco C, Felson David T. Factors predicting response to treatment in rheumatoid arthritis: the importance of disease duration. Arthritis & Rheumatism. 2000;43:22–9.

36. Jasvinder S, Kenneth S, Louis B Jr, Elie A, Raveendhara B, Matthew S, et al. 2015 American College of Rheumatology Guideline for the treatment of rheumatoid arthritis. Arthritis Care Res. 2015;67(10):1335–486.

37. Monika S, John W, David S, Angela Z, Pamela R, Robert L, et al. Economic aspects of treatment options in rheumatoid arthritis: a systematic literature review informing the EULAR recommendations for the management of rheumatoid arthritis. Ann Rheum Dis. 2010;69:996––1004.

38. Vaz Andrey E, Faria Wilmar A Jr, Lazarski Cristina FS, Do Carmo Humberto Franco, Da Rocha Hermínio Maurício. Perfil epidemiológico e clínico de pacientes portadores de artrite reumatóide em um hospital escola de medicina em Goiânia, Goiás, Brasil. Medicina (Ribeirão Preto) 2013;46(2):141–153.

39. Louzada-Junior P, Souza BDB, Toledo RA, Ciconelli RM. Análise descritiva das características demográficas e clínicas de pacientes com artrite reumatoide no estado de São Paulo, Brasil. Rev Bras Reumatol. 2007;47(2):84–90.

17

Methotrexate use, not interleukin 33, is associated with lower carotid intima-media thickness in patients with rheumatoid arthritis

Maria Raquel Costa Pinto[1]*⬥, Adriana Maria Kakehasi[1], Adriano José Souza[2], Wilson Campos Tavares Jr[3], Monaliza Angela Rocha[1], Cyntia Gabriele Michel Cardoso Trant[1] and Marcus Vinicius Andrade[1]

Abstract

Background: Rheumatoid arthritis is a risk factor for early mortality due to cardiovascular disease. Interleukin-33 appears to protect against the development of atherosclerosis. The purpose of this study was to investigate the relationship between serum levels of interleukin-33 and its soluble receptor with the presence of subclinical carotid atherosclerosis in rheumatoid arthritis patients.

Methods: Rheumatoid arthritis patients without atherosclerotic disease were subjected to clinical and laboratory assessments, including carotid ultrasound. Interleukin-33 and its soluble receptor serum levels were measured by ELISA.

Results: 102 patients were included. The prevalence of carotid plaques was 23.5% and the median intima-media thickness was 0.7 mm. The median interleukin-33 and its soluble receptor concentration was 69.1 and 469.8 pg/ml. No association was found between serum interleukin-33 or its soluble receptor and intima-media thickness or plaque occurrence. Each 0.1 mm increase of intima-media thickness raised the odds of plaque occurrence by 5.3-fold, and each additional year of rheumatoid arthritis duration increased the odds of plaque occurrence by 6%. Each additional year in patients age and each one-point increase in the Framingham Risk Score were associated with a 0.004 mm and 0.012 mm increase in intima-media thickness. Methotrexate use was associated with a 0.07 mm reduction in intima-media thickness.

Conclusions: Interleukin-33 and its soluble receptor were not associated with subclinical atherosclerosis. Traditional risk factors for atherosclerosis and rheumatoid arthritis duration were associated with intima-media thickness and plaque occurrence; methotrexate use was associated with a lower intima-media thickness.

Keywords: Rheumatoid arthritis, Cardiovascular diseases, Interleukins, Methotrexate

Background

Rheumatoid arthritis (RA) is an autoimmune inflammatory disease that can lead to articular destruction. Fibroblast-like synoviocytes are local producers of inflammatory interleukins, including interleukin 33 (IL-33). IL-33 is a member of the IL-1 family that modulates the immune response by inducing cytokine production by type 2 T helper lymphocytes (Th2). IL-33 is a ligand for receptor ST2, a member of the IL1R/TLR superfamily. Increased levels of soluble ST2 (sST2) were found in inflammatory conditions, and it is involved in the attenuation of the Th2-induced inflammatory response, probably via IL-33 sequestration. IL-33/ST2 signaling behaves as an intracellular system with participation in antigen-antigen response, autoimmunity, fibrosis processes and possibly RA pathogenesis. The active form of IL-33 is released after cell damage and it promotes macrophage activation, neutrophil migration to articular sites and production of metalloproteinases and cytokines by fibroblast-like synoviocytes. IL-33 stimulates naïve CD4 + T cells to differentiate into Th2 and induces the production of IL-5 and IL-3. IL-33 also promotes

---
* Correspondence: dramariaraquel@gmail.com
[1]School of Medicine, Federal University of Minas Gerais (Universidade Federal de Minas Gerais – UFMG), Avenida Alfredo Balena, 190, Bairro Santa Efigênia, Belo Horizonte, Minas Gerais CEP 30130-100, Brazil
Full list of author information is available at the end of the article

autoantibody-mediated mast cell activation and degranulation [1, 2]. Significantly higher IL-33 levels were found in serum and synovial fluid of RA patients when compared with controls. IL-33 levels were correlated to IL-1β, IL-6, C-reactive protein, DAS28, rheumatoid factor and anti-CCP. Treatment with antirheumatic agents reduced serum IL-33 levels [3–5]. Thus, IL-33 may be an acceptable biomarker and potential therapeutic target for RA.

IL-33/ST2 signaling also appears to play a role in atherosclerosis [6]. IL-33 and ST2 are expressed in human venous and coronary artery endothelium [7, 8]. Administration of IL-33 to apolipoprotein E-deficient mice reduced atherosclerotic plaque development. In contrast, mice treated with sST2 developed larger plaques. These results suggest that IL-33/ST2 may have protective effects in relation to atherosclerosis [7]. On the other hand, some studies showed that IL-33 may, on the contrary, be associated with progression of atherosclerotic plaques by increasing vascular permeability, inflammatory cytokine production and expression of the adhesion molecules in coronary artery [8, 9].

RA is an independent risk factor for early mortality and is associated with a high risk of death from cardiovascular disease (CVD), even after adjustment for traditional risk factors for coronary atherosclerotic disease [10–12]. The cause of the early and accelerated atherosclerosis has not been fully elucidated, but the combination of traditional and non-traditional risk factors is likely to be relevant [10, 13, 14]. Circulating inflammatory mediators may affect the arterial wall during the various stages of atherosclerosis development [15]. Several investigators reported that the association between systemic inflammation markers and vascular abnormalities was only found in the presence of traditional risk factors [16, 17].

Assessment of the carotid arteries using high-resolution ultrasound is one of the noninvasive procedures used to evaluate early preclinical atherosclerosis. Increased intima-media thickness (IMT) and presence of plaques are independently associated with cardiovascular risk factors and generalized atherosclerosis [18]. They are strong predictors of future cardiovascular events in overall population and in high-risk patients, such as those with RA [19–22].

Our study investigated the possible association between serum IL-33 and sST2 levels and subclinical carotid atherosclerosis in RA patients.

Methods
Patients
Adults with RA, defined according to the American College of Rheumatology (ACR) or ACR/European League Against Rheumatism classification criteria, with symptoms lasting for more than 6 months were invited to participate in the study. The exclusion criteria consisted of past or present angina, acute myocardial infarction, coronary revascularization procedures, coronary stenosis on angiography, stroke or transient ischemic attack, carotid stenosis and peripheral arterial insufficiency on angiography or ultrasonography; the presence of heart failure, atrial fibrillation, and implanted pacemaker or defibrillator; the presence of other connective tissue disorders (overlap syndromes), except for secondary Sjögren syndrome; and the presence of signs and symptoms of infection or recent history of infection.

Methods
The participants were subjected to a clinical evaluation that included a count of the number of swollen and painful joints. Disease-related information, laboratory test data, current and previous treatment records and the cumulative prednisone dose were obtained through interviews and a review of medical records.

Systemic arterial hypertension was defined as a systolic arterial pressure ≥ 140, diastolic arterial pressure ≥ 90 or the use of antihypertensive medication. Smoking was defined as the use of any amount of tobacco in the past 30 days, and ex-smokers were defined as those who abstained from tobacco use in the past 30 days. A family history of early CVD was defined as the presence of atherosclerotic artery disease among parents, siblings or children before the age of 55 for males and 65 for females [23]. Dyslipidemia was defined as the use of hypolipidemic agents, triglycerides > 150 mg/dl, high-density lipoprotein (HDL) cholesterol < 50 mg/dl for women and < 40 mg/dl for men, or low-density lipoprotein (LDL) cholesterol > 160 mg/dL [23]. The LDL cut-off value was determined using cardiovascular risk stratification and the Framingham Risk Score [24], as recommended by the Brazilian Society of Cardiology [23]. Central obesity was defined as a waist circumference ≥ 94 cm for men and ≥ 80 cm for women. Metabolic syndrome was defined according to the criteria established by the International Diabetes Federation [25].

Hand/wrist and forefoot anteroposterior radiographs were taken within 12 months prior to or after the assessment. A single radiologist blinded to the patients' data analyzed the radiographs by calculating the total Sharp/van der Heijde modified score. The intra-rater agreement was good (intraclass correlation coefficient: 0.958).

The participants were assessed using the Health Assessment Questionnaire Disability Index (HAQ-DI) validated for the Portuguese language and two 0–100 mm visual analog scales for pain and global disease activity. CDAI and DAS28, which are composite disease activity indices consisting of four variables, were calculated using the erythrocyte sedimentation rate (ERS) measured on the day of assessment and the patient-reported visual analog scale for disease activity.

IL-33 and sST2 measurements
Blood samples were collected from a peripheral vein, and the serum was separated from the sample. IL-33

and sST2 were measured using an enzyme-linked immunosorbent assay (ELISA) according to the manufacturer's instructions (Human IL-33 DuoSet Economy Pack and sST2 DuoSet-ELISA sandwich assay, R&D System Inc., Minneapolis, MN, USA).

Carotid ultrasound

The subclinical atherosclerosis of carotid arteries was assessed using B-mode ultrasound to detect atherosclerotic plaques and measure IMT according to previously established guidelines [22, 26]. A high-resolution Philips iE33 ultrasound machine with a 3-to-9 MHz linear probe and artery specific software was used. The left and right common internal and external carotid arteries were transversely and longitudinally scanned for atherosclerotic plaques, which were defined as focal structures protruding into the artery lumen that measured at least 0.5 mm and were greater than 50% of the adjacent IMT or showed an IMT over 1.5 mm. The IMT was measured on the posterior wall of the left and right distal common carotid arteries at a plaque-free site one to two centimeters from the artery bifurcation. Images were obtained with adequate gain and depth adjustments along the longitudinal axis at a site where the artery segment was the most perpendicular to the ultrasound beam. Anterior, posterior or sternocleidomastoid access was utilized. The most rectilinear images with well-defined double-line patterns were selected for measurement. After completion of the test, IMT measurements were made on a 10-mm common carotid artery segment using automatic border (lumen-intima and media-adventitia) detection software. The average of the measurements was calculated for the right and left arteries separately. For each patient, the highest average IMT calculated on the right or left artery was used in the statistical analysis. The parameters used to classify IMT as abnormal comprised the values obtained in the Multi-Ethnic Study of Atherosclerosis [22]. Values above the 75th percentile for sex, age, race, and IMT in the right or left artery were considered as abnormal.

A single professional with extensive technical experience who was blinded to the clinical status of the participants performed all of the tests. The intra-rater agreement was good (intraclass correlation coefficient of 98.7% for IMT measurements and a Kappa coefficient of 100% for plaque detection).

Statistical analysis

A descriptive analysis was performed using frequency distribution tables and central tendency measurements. All of the statistical analyses were performed with SPSS version 15.0 software.

A univariate analysis was used to investigate factors associated with the presence of atherosclerotic plaques. A Pearson's chi-square or Fisher's exact test was used to compare categorical variables, and Student's t-test or the non-parametric Mann-Whitney test was used to compare numerical variables. Distribution normality was assessed using the Kolmogorov-Smirnov test. Binary logistic regression was used in the multivariate analysis. Using the final model, the adjusted odd ratios (OR) with corresponding 95% confidence interval (95%CI) were calculated. The model goodness of fit was assessed using the Hosmer-Lemeshow test.

A univariate analysis was used to investigate factors associated with IMT. The Mann-Whitney or Kruskal-Wallis test was used to compare categorical variables, and the Spearman's correlation coefficient was used to compare numerical variables. Non-parametric tests were selected because the IMT distribution was slightly skewed. A linear regression model was used in the multivariate analysis. The goodness of fit of the final model was assessed using the coefficient of determination (R^2) and diagnostic plots. The data were not transformed to obtain a normal distribution because the distribution of the model residuals for IMT was very close to normality.

An analysis of the residual plots indicated that the model was appropriate for the data.

Predictive variables with a p-value < 0.15 in the univariate analysis were included in the multivariate model using forward stepwise selection. The significance level for the final model was set at 5%.

Results

Patient clinical and laboratory characteristics

Between March 2012 and August 2013, a total of 102 patients were included in the study. The demographic and clinical characteristics of the patients and their medication use are provided in Table 1.

Based on their Framingham Risk Scores [24], 64 (62.7%) participants were at high cardiovascular risk, and only 22 (21.6%) patients met the LDL therapeutic goal established by the Brazilian Society of Cardiology Guideline [23] (Table 1). The median (interquartile range) IMT of the common carotid artery was 0.7 (0.6–0.8) mm. The IMT was elevated in 18.6% of patients. Atherosclerotic plaques were detected in 24 (23.5%) participants (Table 2). A total of 36 participants (35.3%) exhibited atherosclerotic plaques and/or increased IMT.

The serum IL-33 and sST2 levels were above the limit of detection in 68 (66.7%) and 101 (99%) participants, respectively (Table 2). No correlation was found between IL-33 and sST2 levels (r = 0.123; $p = 0.319$).

Factors associated with the occurrence of atherosclerotic plaques

The participants with atherosclerotic plaques had an older average age (59.9 versus 54.2 years old; $p = 0.014$) and longer mean disease duration (21.9 versus 16.3 years;

Table 1 Demographic, clinical and laboratory characteristics of participants

Variable	Value
Age (years - mean ± SD)	55.5 ± 10
Age at onset of symptoms (years - mean ± SD)	37.9 ± 11.9
Disease length (years - mean ± SD)	17.6 ± 9.5
Female gender (n (%))	94 (92.5)
Postmenopausal (n (% female participants))	71 (75.5)
Non-white ethnicity (n (%))	74 (72.5)
Seropositive RA (n (%))[a]	84 (82.4)
Extra-articular involvement[b] (n (%))	23 (22.5)
DAS28 (mean ± SD)	4 ± 1.4
CDAI (mean ± SD)	13.4 ± 11.7
HAQ-DI (median (IQR))	0.8 (0.3–1.4)
Sharp/van der Heijde score [c] (median (IQR))	38 (10–75.5)
SAP/DAP (mmHg - mean ± SD)	123 ± 13 / 77.5 ± 8.6
Waist circumference (cm - mean ± SD)	94.5 ± 10.8
BMI (mean ± SD)	27.5 ± 4.7
Medications in use (n patients (%))	
Oral hypoglycemic agents and/or insulin	14 (13.7)
Hypolipidemic agents	28 (27.5)
Antihypertensives	54 (52.9)
DMARDs	91 (89.2)
Methotrexate	66 (64.7)
Leflunomide	42 (41.2)
Anti-TNFα	15 (14.7)
Nonsteroidal anti-inflammatory drugs	22 (21.6)
Prednisone	62 (60.8)
Prednisone daily dose (mg - median (IQR))	2.5 (0–5)
Prednisone cumulative dose (g - mean ± SD)	21.8 ± 15.7
Laboratory tests	
HDL (mg/dL – mean ± SD)	58.4 ± 16.1
LDL (mg/dL – mean ± SD)	110.6 ± 28
TC/HDL (median (IQR))[d]	3.5 (2.8–4.1)
Triglycerides (mg/dL - median (IQR))	112 (81–165.5)
Fasting glucose (mg/dL - median (IQR))	89 (79–97)
CRP (mg/L - median (IQR))	8.3 (4.9–16.9)
ESR (mm/h - median (IQR))	22 (15–32)
Traditional risk factors for CAD (n (%))	
Current smoker	12 (11.8)
Diabetes mellitus	17 (16.7)
Family history of early CVD	18 (17.6)
Metabolic syndrome	53 (52)
Systemic arterial hypertension	60 (58.8)
Dyslipidemia	65 (63.7)
Central obesity	88.2 (90)

Table 1 Demographic, clinical and laboratory characteristics of participants (Continued)

Variable	Value
Global Risk Score (Framingham) (Ref. 67) (median (IQR))	7.1 (4.1–11.6)
High cardiovascular risk (Ref. 65) (n (%))	64 (62.7)
LDL within therapeutic goal (BSC) (Ref. 65) (n (%))	22 (21.6)

SD standard deviation, *RA* rheumatoid arthritis, *DAS28* Disease Activity Score based on 28 joints, *CDAI* Clinical Disease Activity Index, *HAQ-DI* Health Assessment Questionnaire Disability Index, *IQR* interquartile range, *BMI* body mass index, *DMARDs* disease-modifying antirheumatic drugs, *CAD* coronary artery disease, *CRP* C-reactive protein, *ESR* erythrocyte sedimentation rate, *CVD* cardiovascular disease; and *BSC* Brazilian Society of Cardiology
[a] number of patients with positive rheumatoid factor and/or anti-CCP in any titer at any time during the clinical course of disease
[b] number of patients with extra-articular involvement at any time during the clinical course of disease
[c] total Sharp/Van der Heijde modified score (0–448)
[d] total cholesterol-to-HDL ratio

$p = 0.011$). The prevalence of atherosclerotic plaques was higher in postmenopausal women than in non-postmenopausal women (29.6% versus 8.7%; $p = 0.043$). The median IMT was higher in patients with atherosclerotic plaques (0.8 mm versus 0.6 mm; $p = 0.001$). No patient with LDL values within the therapeutic goal range exhibited plaques, while the prevalence of plaques in the remaining participants was 30% ($p = 0.003$). The Framingham Risk Score values were higher for patients with atherosclerotic plaques (8.7 versus 6.3, $p = 0.048$) (Table 3).

There was no association between IL-33 and sST2 levels and the occurrence of atherosclerotic plaques ($p > 0.05$) (Table 3). None of the other factors we assessed correlated with plaque occurrence.

The multivariate analysis showed that each 0.1-mm increase in IMT caused a 5.3-fold increase in the odds for plaque occurrence (OR: 53.2; 95%CI 2.88–983.37). Each additional year of disease duration increased the odds of plaque occurrence by 6% (OR: 1.06; 95%CI 1.01–1.12).

Table 2 Results of carotid artery ultrasounds and IL-33 and sST2 measurements

Variable	Value
IMT - CCA (mm - median (IQR))	0.7 (0.6–0.8)
Increased IMT (n (%))	19 (18.6)
Atherosclerotic plaque (n (%))	24 (23.5)
IL-33 (pg/mL - median (IQR))[a]	32.1 (0–78.7)
IL-33 (pg/mL - median (IQR))[b]	69.1 (31.6–114.5)
sST2 (pg/mL - median (IQR))[c]	469.8 (336.3–651)
IL-33/sST2 (median (IQR))[d]	0.1 (0–0.3)

IMT intima-media thickness, *CCA* common carotid artery; and *IQR* interquartile range. According to the manufacturer, the minimum detectable concentration of IL-33 and sST2 was 23.4 and 31.2 pg/ml, respectively
[a] levels below the limit of detection were considered as zero
[b] only considering the 68 participants with levels above the limit of detection
[c] only considering the 101 participants with levels above the limit of detection
[d] IL-33-to-sST2 ratio

Table 3 Comparison of patients with and without atherosclerotic plaques

Variable	Plaques absent (n = 78)	Plaques present (n = 24)	p-value
Age (years - mean ± SD)	54.2 ± 9.8	59.9 ± 9.7	0.014[a]
Disease length (years - mean ± SD)	16.3 ± 9.7	21.9 ± 8	0.011[a]
Postmenopausal (n (%)): No	21 (91.3)	2 (8.7)	0.043[b]
Yes	50 (70.4)	21 (29.6)	
LDL within goal (Ref. 65) (n (%)) No	56 (70)	24 (30)	0.003[b]
Yes	22 (100)	0 (0)	
Global CVR score (median (IQR))	6.3 (2.9–11.6)	8.7 (6.2–11.8)	0.048[c]
IMT (mm - median (IQR))	0.6 (0.6–0.8)	0.8 (0.7–0.9)	0.001[c]
IL-33 (n (%))[d]: positive	52 (76.5)	16 (23.5)	1[b]
negative	26 (76.5)	8 (23.5)	
IL-33 (pg/mL - median (IQR))[e]	33.1 (0–78.7)	12.1 (0–85.8)	0.856[c]
IL-33 (pg/mL - median (IQR))[f]	69.1 (33.1–124.3)	70.6 (12.1–90.1)	0.745[c]
sST2 (pg/mL - median (IQR))[g]	461.7 (316.6–651)	485.9 (372.9–649)	0.675[c]
IL-33/sST2 (median (IQR))[h]	0.1 (0–0.3)	0.1 (0–0.3)	0.965[c]

[a]t-test; [b]chi-square; [c]Mann-Whitney test

SD standard deviation, *NPJ* number of painful joints upon physical examination, *IQR* interquartile range, *SAH* systemic arterial hypertension, *CVR* cardiovascular risk, *NSAIDs* nonsteroidal anti-inflammatory drugs; and *IMT* intima-media thickness

[d]IL-33 positive: serum IL-33 ≥ 23.4 pg/mL; and IL-33 negative: serum IL-33 < 23.4 pg/mL

[e]levels below the limit of detection were considered as zero

[f]only considering the 68 participants with levels above the limit of detection

[g]data from the 101 participants with detectable levels

[h]IL-33-to-sST2 ratio

Factors associated with intima-media thickness

Significant direct correlations were found between IMT and patient age (r = 0.613; $p < 0.001$), disease duration (r = 0.224; $p = 0.024$) and age at onset of RA symptoms (r = 0.334; $p = 0.001$). Similarly, IMT correlated with systolic arterial pressure (r = 0.282; $p = 0.004$), fasting glucose (r = 0.264; $p = 0.008$) and Framingham Risk Score (r = 0.591; p < 0.001). IMT inversely correlated with daily prednisone dose (r = − 0.205; $p = 0.039$) (Table 4).

The IMT was higher in patients with a history of extra-articular involvement ($p = 0.014$), systemic arterial hypertension ($p = 0.001$), diabetes mellitus ($p = 0.003$), and metabolic syndrome ($p = 0.037$). Within women, the IMT was higher in those who were postmenopausal (p

Table 4 Correlation of IMT with clinical and laboratory characteristics

Variable	Coefficient[a]	p-value
Age (years)	0.613	< 0.001
Disease length (years)	0.224	0.024
Age at onset of symptoms (years)	0.334	0.001
Time since onset of symptoms to 1st rheumatology visit (years)	0.204	0.040
Fasting glucose (mg/dL)	0.263	0.008
SAP (mmHg)	0.282	0.004
Global Cardiovascular Risk Score	0.591	< 0.001
Current prednisone daily dose	−0.205	0.039
IL-33 (pg/mL)[b]	−0.77	0.439
IL-33 (pg/mL)[c]	−0.035	0.775
sST2 (pg/mL)[d]	0.002	0.981
IL-33/sST2**	− 0.071	0.566

[a]Spearman's correlation coefficient

IMT intima-media thickness, *IQR* interquartile range, *SD* standard deviation, *CRP* C-reactive protein; and *SAP* systemic arterial pressure

[b]levels below the limit of detection were considered as zero

[c]only considering the 68 participants with levels above the limit of detection

[d]data from the 101 participants with detectable levels

[e]IL-33-to-sST2 ratio

= 0.001). The IMT was also higher in patients with a high cardiovascular risk according to the Framingham Risk Score ($p < 0.001$). In contrast, patients using methotrexate (MTX) and those with LDL values within the therapeutic goal range had a lower IMT ($p = 0.005$ and 0.012, respectively) (Table 5).

None of the other factors we assessed, including serum IL-33 and sST2 levels and the IL-33/sST2 ratio, were associated with IMT (Tables 4 and 5).

The variables remaining in the final model, i.e., those associated with IMT, included age ($p = 0.024$; 95%CI 0–0.007), Framingham Risk Score ($p < 0.001$; 95%CI 0.007–0.016) and MTX use ($p = 0.015$; 95%CI -0.117 to −0.013). Each additional year of patient age was associated with a 0.004 mm increase in IMT. Each one-point increase in the Framingham Risk Score was associated with a 0.012 mm increase in IMT. Patients using MTX at the time of assessment exhibited a 0.065 mm reduction in IMT. The model explained 45.2% of the data variability and had a satisfactory goodness of fit as evidenced by the diagnostic plots.

Discussion

We did not find an association between IL-33 or its soluble receptor and the presence of subclinical atherosclerosis in our RA patients. Due to the possible fluctuations in IL-33 and sST2 levels during the course of the disease, a single measurement may not accurately reflect the role of these factors in vascular morphology abnormalities and plaque development over time. IL-33 is released after the occurrence of cell damage and then binds to its receptor and promotes cell activation; thus, IL-33 and sST2 may only have a significant effect during acute cardiovascular events. Therefore, the main limitation of the present study was to make a single serum measure of IL-33 and sST2. A single dosage may not be the most appropriate to study the association of the biomarkers in question with the development of atherosclerosis over time.

IL-33 and sST2 are involved in the pathogenesis of RA [1] and can serve as markers of inflammation and disease activity [3, 5]. Similarly, IL-33 and sST2 participate in atherosclerosis development and cardiac remodeling

Table 5 Correlation of IMT with demographic, clinical and laboratory characteristics

Variable		IMT (mm - median (IQR))	P-value
Postmenopausal	No	0.60 (0.55–0.65)	0.001[a]
	Yes	0.71 (0.6–0.8)	
Extra-articular involvement	No	0.65 (0.58–0.76)	0.014[a]
	Yes	0.72 (0.63–0.88)	
SAH	Absent	0.60 (0.55–0.71)	0.001[a]
	Present	0.72 (0.63–0.81)	
Using antihypertensives	No	0.62 (0.56–0.71)	0.001[a]
	Yes	0.73 (0.63–0.81)	
Diabetes mellitus	Absent	0.65 (0.58–0.76)	0.003[a]
	Present	0.84 (0.63–0.95)	
Using hypoglycemic agents/insulin	No	0.65 (0.58–0.76)	0.001[a]
	Yes	0.84 (0.7–1.02)	
LDL within goal	No	0.7 (0.6–0.8)	0.012[a]
	Yes	0.6 (0.6–0.7)	
Metabolic syndrome	Absent	0.64 (0.58–0.74)	0.037[a]
	Present	0.71 (0.6–0.84)	
Using methotrexate	No	0.75 (0.62–0.87)	0.005[a]
	Yes	0.63 (0.58–0.73)	
CVR classification[c]	High	0.73 (0.61–0.84)	< 0.001[b]
	Intermediate	0.71 (0.64–0.77)	
	Low	0.6 (0.54–0.64)	
IL-33 positive[d]	No	0.69 (0.59–0.85)	0.449[a]
	Yes	0.66 (0.59–0.78)	

[a]Mann-Whitney test; [b]Kruskal-Wallis test
IMT intima-media thickness, *IQR* interquartile range, *SAH* systemic arterial hypertension; and *CVR* cardiovascular risk
[c]according to the Global Risk Score (Framingham)
[d]IL-33 positive: serum IL-33 ≥ 23.4 pg/mL

[6, 27]. The relationship between serum IL-33 and its soluble receptor with atherosclerosis in RA patients requires further study. It is not currently possible to determine if IL-33 participates in both RA and atherosclerosis via antagonistic effects on vessels, acts as a marker of inflammation in RA and/or exerts protective effects against atherosclerosis. Indeed, thorough research on the complex interactions between IL-33/sST2, atherosclerosis and RA is necessary.

The serum IL-33 level was undetectable in approximately one-third of patients. In a study by Matsuyama and colleagues, the IL-33 level was above the limit of detection in only 50.8% of patients, and 94% of the participants used disease-modifying antirheumatic drugs (DMARDs) [3]. Therefore, the low IL-33 levels found in our study may be due to the use of at least one DMARD in 90% of patients.

In the present study, 36 (35.3%) participants had increased IMT and/or atherosclerotic plaques. Due to its independent association with generalized atherosclerosis and future cardiac events, IMT was selected as an indirect marker of early vascular morphology abnormalities in RA patients without a history of manifest atherosclerotic disease [18–22]. Similarly, plaque occurrence was investigated because it can be used to identify individuals at higher risk of coronary events in populations without coronary atherosclerotic disease [28]. Awareness of the presence of asymptomatic vascular morphological abnormalities may motivate patients to change their lifestyle and improve their adherence to treatment [29].

Both RA-related, e.g., disease duration and MTX use, and traditional, e.g., age and Framingham Risk Score, risk factors for coronary atherosclerotic disease were associated with the presence of subclinical atherosclerosis. These findings agree with the hypothesis that the interaction between RA-related and traditional risk factors increases a patient's cardiovascular morbidity and mortality in comparison to the overall population [10, 13, 14, 16].

Patients with atherosclerotic plaques had a longer RA disease duration and higher median IMT. Indeed, longer disease duration has been associated with plaque occurrence in RA [30]. Thus, disease duration may serve as an indirect marker of cumulative inflammation. Cross-sectional studies conducted in the overall population found a positive correlation between common carotid artery IMT and the presence of carotid plaques [29, 31, 32]. This association was also detected in populations of RA patients [30, 33].

MTX use was protective against intima-media thickening. This finding is in agreement with previous studies and with the fact that MTX has been shown to have cardioprotective effects. MTX also improves the lipid profile, mainly by increasing HDL levels. However, this improved lipid profile could be due to the control of inflammation or a direct effect of the drug [34, 35].

Age is an essential determinant of CVD [11]. In addition, age is one of the strongest determinants of IMT, which increases 0.01 to 0.02 mm per year in the overall population [31, 36]. In agreement with previous studies in RA patients, we determined that IMT increased with age [30, 34, 37, 38]. Our multivariate analysis did not reveal any significant correlations between IMT and any other single traditional risk factor. However, an independent correlation was found between IMT and Framingham Risk Score, which combines several risk factors.

RA-related chronic inflammation plays a crucial role in accelerated atherosclerosis [15]. Similar to previous studies, none of the inflammation or disease activity markers that we tested (ESR, C-reactive protein, DAS28 and CDAI) correlated with plaque occurrence or IMT [30, 37, 38]. A possible explanation for this lack of association is that RA-related inflammation fluctuates, and thus, the assessment of biomarkers in cross-sectional studies may not accurately reflect the cumulative effect of chronic inflammation on the vascular wall [34, 39].

Distinct factors were independently associated with IMT and the presence of carotid plaques. This discrepancy suggests that although IMT and plaque occurrence are correlated phenomena, they correspond to different stages and aspects of atherogenesis and thus have different determinants [28, 29, 32, 40]. Diffuse adaptive thickening of the carotid wall, which occurs in response to aging and systemic arterial hypertension, is a more accurate reflection of arteriosclerosis than plaque formation. The latter is a focal process related to atherosclerotic phenomena, such as inflammation, oxidation and endothelial dysfunction [28, 40]. In the present study, systolic arterial pressure and systemic arterial hypertension were associated with IMT in our univariate analysis but were not robust enough to constitute independent factors in the final model.

Conclusions

In view of the current evidence of IL-33/sST2 system participation in the pathogenesis and evolution of both RA and atherosclerotic disease, this study was designed. However, no association between IL-33/sST2 serum levels and subclinical atherosclerosis in patients with established RA was found. Traditional risk factors for atherosclerosis and rheumatoid arthritis duration were associated with intima-media thickness and plaque occurrence; methotrexate use was associated with a lower intima-media thickness. All these factors were previously described as being associated with subclinical atherosclerosis in RA. There have been few clinical studies evaluating the relationship between IL-33 and subclinical atherosclerosis. The importance of determining the role of specific cytokines in RA and their relationship to cardiovascular disease lies in the fact that this understanding may present in the future a clinical application in determining risk and prognostic markers, as well as identifying new therapeutic targets.

Abbreviations

ACR: American College of Rheumatology; CI: Confidence interval; CVD: Cardiovascular disease; DMARDs: Disease-modifying antirheumatic drugs; ELISA: Enzyme-linked immunosorbent assay; ERS: Erythrocyte sedimentation rate; HAQ-DI: Health Assessment Questionnaire Disability Index; HDL: High-density lipoprotein cholesterol; IL: Interleukin; IMT: Intima-media thickness; LDL: Low-density lipoprotein; MTX: Methotrexate; OR: Odd ratios; RA: Rheumatoid arthritis; sST2: Soluble ST2 receptor; Th2: Type 2 T helper lymphocytes

Acknowledgements

Not applicable.

Authors' contributions

MRCP, AMK and MVA designed the study and wrote the paper. MRCP and AMK worked on the background research and on the analysis and interpretation of the results. MRCP, AJS, WCT, MAR, CGMCT and MVA worked on the acquisition of data. All authors read and approved the final manuscript.

Author details

[1]School of Medicine, Federal University of Minas Gerais (Universidade Federal de Minas Gerais – UFMG), Avenida Alfredo Balena, 190, Bairro Santa Efigênia, Belo Horizonte, Minas Gerais CEP 30130-100, Brazil. [2]Conrad Diagnostic Imaging (Conrad Diagnóstico por Imagem), Rua Rio Grande do Norte, 77, Bairro Santa Efigênia, Belo Horizonte, MG CEP: 30130-130, Brazil. [3]Ecoar Diagnostic Medicine (Ecoar Medicina Diagnóstica), Avenida do Contorno, 6760, Bairro Santo Antônio, Belo Horizonte, MG CEP: 30110-044, Brazil.

References

1. Schmitz J, Owyang A, Oldham E, Song Y, Murphy E, McClanahan TK, et al. IL-33, an interleukin-1-like cytokine that signals via the IL-1 receptor-related protein ST2 and induces T helper type 2-associated cytokines. Immunity. 2005;23(5):479–90.
2. Verri WA, Souto FO, Vieira SM, Almeida SC, Fukada SY, Xu D, et al. IL-33 induces neutrophil migration in rheumatoid arthritis and is a target of anti-TNF therapy. Ann Rheum Dis. 2010;69(9):1697–703.
3. Matsuyama Y, Okazaki H, Tamemoto H, Kimura H, Kamata Y, Nagatani K, et al. Increased levels of interleukin 33 in sera and synovial fluid from patients with active rheumatoid arthritis. J Rheumatol. 2010;37(1):18–25.
4. Hong YS, Moon SJ, Joo YB, Jeon CH, Cho ML, Ju JH, et al. Measurement of interleukin-33 (IL-33) and IL-33 receptors (sST2 and ST2L) in patients with rheumatoid arthritis. J Korean Med Sci. 2011;26(9):1132–9.
5. Kageyama Y, Torikai E, Tsujimura K, Kobayashi M. Involvement of IL-33 in the pathogenesis of rheumatoid arthritis: the effect of etanercept on the serum levels of IL-33. Mod Rheumatol. 2012;22(1):89–93.
6. Miller AM, Liew FY. The IL-33/ST2 pathway--a new therapeutic target in cardiovascular disease. Pharmacol Ther. 2011;131(2):179–86.
7. Miller AM, Xu D, Asquith DL, Denby L, Li Y, Sattar N, et al. IL-33 reduces the development of atherosclerosis. J Exp Med. 2008;205(2):339–46.
8. Choi YS, Choi HJ, Min JK, Pyun BJ, Maeng YS, Park H, et al. Interleukin-33 induces angiogenesis and vascular permeability through ST2/TRAF6-mediated endothelial nitric oxide production. Blood. 2009;114(14):3117–26.
9. Demyanets S, Konya V, Kastl SP, Kaun C, Rauscher S, Niessner A, et al. Interleukin-33 induces expression of adhesion molecules and inflammatory activation in human endothelial cells and in human atherosclerotic plaques. Arterioscler Thromb Vasc Biol. 2011;31(9):2080–9.
10. Salmon JE, Roman MJ. Subclinical atherosclerosis in rheumatoid arthritis and systemic lupus erythematosus. Am J Med. 2008;121(10 Suppl 1):S3–8.
11. Kremers HM, Crowson CS, Therneau TM, Roger VL, Gabriel SE. High ten-year risk of cardiovascular disease in newly diagnosed rheumatoid arthritis patients: a population-based cohort study. Arthritis Rheum. 2008;58(8):2268–74.
12. Peters MJ, van Halm VP, Voskuyl AE, Smulders YM, Boers M, Lems WF, et al. Does rheumatoid arthritis equal diabetes mellitus as an independent risk factor for cardiovascular disease? A prospective study. Arthritis Rheum. 2009; 61(11):1571–9.
13. Frostegård J. Atherosclerosis in patients with autoimmune disorders. Arterioscler Thromb Vasc Biol. 2005;25(9):1776–85.
14. Liang KP. Cardiovascular risk in rheumatoid arthritis (RA): does it matter if RA is diagnosed in early or late age? J Rheumatol. 2013;40(12):1945–7.
15. Sattar N, McCarey DW, Capell H, McInnes IB. Explaining how "high-grade" systemic inflammation accelerates vascular risk in rheumatoid arthritis. Circulation. 2003;108(24):2957–63.
16. del Rincón I, Freeman GL, Haas RW, O'Leary DH, Escalante A. Relative contribution of cardiovascular risk factors and rheumatoid arthritis clinical manifestations to atherosclerosis. Arthritis Rheum. 2005;52(11):3413–23.
17. Zampeli E, Protogerou A, Stamatelopoulos K, Fragiadaki K, Katsiari CG, Kyrkou K, et al. Predictors of new atherosclerotic carotid plaque development in patients with rheumatoid arthritis: a longitudinal study. Arthritis Res Ther. 2012;14(2):R44.
18. Hodis HN, Mack WJ, LaBree L, Selzer RH, Liu CR, Liu CH, et al. The role of carotid arterial intima-media thickness in predicting clinical coronary events. Ann Intern Med. 1998;128(4):262–9.
19. O'Leary DH, Polak JF, Kronmal RA, Manolio TA, Burke GL, Wolfson SK. Carotid-artery intima and media thickness as a risk factor for myocardial infarction and stroke in older adults. Cardiovascular health study collaborative research group. N Engl J Med. 1999;340(1):14–22.
20. Sandoo A, van Zanten JJ, Metsios GS, Carroll D, Kitas GD. The endothelium and its role in regulating vascular tone. Open Cardiovasc Med J. 2010;4:302–12.
21. Lorenz MW, von Kegler S, Steinmetz H, Markus HS, Sitzer M. Carotid intima-media thickening indicates a higher vascular risk across a wide age range: prospective data from the carotid atherosclerosis progression study (CAPS). Stroke. 2006;37(1):87–92.
22. Stein JH, Korcarz CE, Hurst RT, Lonn E, Kendall CB, Mohler ER, et al. Use of carotid ultrasound to identify subclinical vascular disease and evaluate cardiovascular disease risk: a consensus statement from the American Society of Echocardiography carotid intima-media thickness task force. Endorsed by the Society for Vascular Medicine. J Am Soc Echocardiogr. 2008;21(2):93–111 quiz 89-90.
23. Xavier HT, Izar MC, Faria Neto JR, Assad MH, Rocha VZ, Sposito AC, et al. V Diretriz Brasileira de Dislipidemias e Prevenção da Aterosclerose. Arq Bras Cardiol. 2013;101(4 Suppl 1):1–20.
24. D'Agostino RB, Vasan RS, Pencina MJ, Wolf PA, Cobain M, Massaro JM, et al. General cardiovascular risk profile for use in primary care: the Framingham heart study. Circulation. 2008;117(6):743–53.
25. Alberti KG, Zimmet P, Shaw J. Metabolic syndrome--a new world-wide definition. A consensus statement from the international diabetes federation. Diabet Med. 2006;23(5):469–80.
26. Touboul PJ, Hennerici MG, Meairs S, Adams H, Amarenco P, Bornstein N, et al. Mannheim carotid intima-media thickness and plaque consensus (2004-2006-2011). An update on behalf of the advisory board of the 3rd, 4th and 5th watching the risk symposia, at the 13th, 15th and 20th European stroke conferences, Mannheim, Germany, 2004, Brussels, Belgium, 2006, and Hamburg, Germany, 2011. Cerebrovasc Dis. 2012;34(4):290–6.
27. Kunes P, Holubcová Z, Koláčková M, Krejsek J. The counter-regulation of atherogenesis: a role for interleukin-33. Acta Med (Hradec Kralove). 2010; 53(3):125–9.
28. Plichart M, Celermajer DS, Zureik M, Helmer C, Jouven X, Ritchie K, et al. Carotid intima-media thickness in plaque-free site, carotid plaques and coronary heart disease risk prediction in older adults. The Three-City study. Atherosclerosis. 2011;219(2):917–24.
29. Ebrahim S, Papacosta O, Whincup P, Wannamethee G, Walker M, Nicolaides AN, et al. Carotid plaque, intima media thickness, cardiovascular risk factors, and prevalent cardiovascular disease in men and women: the British regional heart study. Stroke. 1999;30(4):841–50.
30. Gonzalez-Juanatey C, Llorca J, Testa A, Revuelta J, Garcia-Porrua C, Gonzalez-Gay MA. Increased prevalence of severe subclinical atherosclerotic findings in long-term treated rheumatoid arthritis patients without clinically evident atherosclerotic disease. Medicine (Baltimore). 2003;82(6):407–13.
31. Veller MG, Fisher CM, Nicolaides AN, Renton S, Geroulakos G, Stafford NJ, et al. Measurement of the ultrasonic intima-media complex thickness in normal subjects. J Vasc Surg. 1993;17(4):719–25.
32. Zureik M, Ducimetière P, Touboul PJ, Courbon D, Bonithon-Kopp C, Berr C, et al. Common carotid intima-media thickness predicts occurrence of carotid atherosclerotic plaques: longitudinal results from the aging vascular study (EVA) study. Arterioscler Thromb Vasc Biol. 2000;20(6):1622–9.

33. Pereira I, Laurindo I, Burlingame R, Anjos L, Viana V, Leon E, et al. Auto-antibodies do not influence development of atherosclerotic plaques in rheumatoid arthritis. Joint Bone Spine. 2008;75(4):416–21.

34. Ristić GG, Lepić T, Glisić B, Stanisavljević D, Vojvodić D, Petronijević M, et al. Rheumatoid arthritis is an independent risk factor for increased carotid intima-media thickness: impact of anti-inflammatory treatment. Rheumatology (Oxford). 2010;49(6):1076–81.

35. Westlake SL, Colebatch AN, Baird J, Kiely P, Quinn M, Choy E, et al. The effect of methotrexate on cardiovascular disease in patients with rheumatoid arthritis: a systematic literature review. Rheumatology (Oxford). 2010;49(2):295–307.

36. Howard G, Sharrett AR, Heiss G, Evans GW, Chambless LE, Riley WA, et al. Carotid artery intimal-medial thickness distribution in general populations as evaluated by B-mode ultrasound. ARIC investigators. Stroke. 1993;24(9): 1297–304.

37. Kumeda Y, Inaba M, Goto H, Nagata M, Henmi Y, Furumitsu Y, et al. Increased thickness of the arterial intima-media detected by ultrasonography in patients with rheumatoid arthritis. Arthritis Rheum. 2002; 46(6):1489–97.

38. Alkaabi JK, Ho M, Levison R, Pullar T, Belch JJ. Rheumatoid arthritis and macrovascular disease. Rheumatology (Oxford). 2003;42(2):292–7.

39. Sandoo A, Chanchlani N, Hodson J, Smith JP, Douglas KM, Kitas GD. Classical cardiovascular disease risk factors associate with vascular function and morphology in rheumatoid arthritis: a six-year prospective study. Arthritis Res Ther. 2013;15(6):R203.

40. Kiechl S, Willeit J. The natural course of atherosclerosis. Part I: incidence and progression. Arterioscler Thromb Vasc Biol. 1999;19(6):1484–90.

18

Relationship of rheumatoid arthritis and coronary artery disease in the Korean population

Tae Hyub Lee[1], Gwan Gyu Song[2,3], Sung Jae Choi[2,4], Hongdeok Seok[5] and Jae Hyun Jung[1,4*] (iD)

Abstract

Background: Rheumatoid arthritis (RA) is known to be associated with coronary artery diseases (CAD). Previous studies of the association between RA and CAD were reported mainly in non-Asian groups. We aimed to examine the prevalence of RA and the relationship between RA and CAD in South Korea.

Methods: We conducted a nationwide cross-sectional study by using the Korea National Health and Nutrition Examination Survey, which collected data for four years between 2008 and 2012. A total of 25,828 eligible participants were included. To balance the distribution of baseline characteristics, we used propensity score-matching. A multivariable logistic regression model was employed and we calculated the odds ratios (ORs) and 95% confidence intervals (CI) for the odds of the participants with RA on CAD prevalence.

Results: The prevalence of RA in Korea from 2008 to 2012 was 0.6% and RA was predominant among elderly women. The prevalence of CAD in patients with RA was significantly higher than in general population. After propensity score-matching to balance the confounding factors, RA was significantly associated with CAD (OR 2.97, 95% CI 1.15–7.68, $P = 0.02$).

Conclusions: The prevalence of RA in South Korea was comparable to the worldwide data, and the presence of CAD in RA patients was more than two-fold.

Keywords: Rheumatoid arthritis, Prevalence, Angina pectoris, Myocardial infarction

Background

Rheumatoid arthritis (RA) is a chronic autoimmune inflammatory disease and has been known to increase the risk of cardiovascular diseases (CVD) [1]. RA is associated with increased risks of myocardial infarction (MI), and considered as an independent risk factor for coronary artery diseases (CAD) [2]. Interestingly, clinical manifestations of CAD in patients with RA are somewhat different from those in the general population. CAD in patients with RA presents earlier, silently, and suddenly

[3]. Several mechanisms have been introduced to explain these associations beyond traditional cardiovascular (CV) risk factors such as age, sex, hypertension (HTN), diabetes mellitus (DM), dyslipidemia, obesity, and smoking [4, 5]. The inflammatory pathways have been proposed to be involved in the pathogenesis of both diseases by many in vivo and in vitro studies [6–8]. Additionally, genetic factors are known to enhance the CV risks in RA [9].

Although the relationship between RA and CAD is not fully explained, RA accelerates the process of atherosclerosis and worsens the CV outcomes [10]. Recent meta-analysis showed that CVD mortality in patents with RA is higher than that in the general population [11]. Hence, assessment of CV risks in patients with RA is important, and management of CAD is an essential

---

* Correspondence: mcfriend82@naver.com
[1]College of Medicine, Chung-Ang University, 84 Heukseouk-ro, Donjak-gu, Seoul 06974, South Korea
[4]Division of Rheumatology, Department of Internal Medicine, Korea University Ansan Hospital, 123 Jeokgeum-ro, Danwon-gu, Ansan-si, Gyeonggi-do 15355, South Korea
Full list of author information is available at the end of the article

part of RA treatment. However, CV risks in RA could differ according to race, and the need for population-specific CAD risk stratification in RA was proposed [12]. Epidemiologic studies investigating relationship between RA and CAD have been reported globally and shown different prevalence among the nations [13, 14]. Unfortunately, the association between RA and CAD were reported mainly in non-Asian groups and no data in South Korea have been reported yet [1, 2, 14]. Since some Asians appeared to have a higher risk for CAD, it is necessary to investigate whether CAD is more common in Korean RA patients than in non-RA patients [15]. We, therefore, investigated the prevalence of RA and the association between RA and CAD in South Korea using nationwide data.

Methods

Study design and population

We conducted a nationwide cross-sectional study by using the Korea National Health and Nutrition Examination Survey (KNHANES), which collected data for four years between 2008 and 2012. Voluntary participants, who provided written informed consents, were included in the KNHANES. The Korean Ministry of Health and Welfare conducted the KNHANES, which was a nationwide cross-sectional study. Households were randomly selected for participation, and sampled multi-stage stratification was based on geographical areas. The KNHANES was conducted in accordance with the Helsinki Declaration of 2000. The samples were determined by the household registries of the 2005 National Census Registry.

A total of 36,853 individuals participated in the 2008–2012 KHANES. A total of 11,025 participants who did not complete the health survey section regarding age, smoking, alcohol drinking, RA, HTN, DM, and/or dyslipidemia were excluded. Thus, the total number of eligible individuals was 25,828.

Main variables and covariates

The current diagnosis of RA was based on the self-reported data in response to the questions "Was your RA diagnosed by a physician" and "Are you being treated for RA?" The response was either "Yes" or "No." The participants who responded "Yes" to both questions were considered as RA patients. The presence of CAD was based on a "Yes" response to the questions, "Was your angina pectoris or MI diagnosed by a physician" and "Are you currently being treated for angina pectoris or MI?" Alcohol consumption status was defined as follows: 1) heavy drinkers (consumed an average of ≥ 7 units of alcohol for men and ≥ 5 units for women ≥ 2 days/week), 2) moderate drinkers (consumed more than one glass of alcohol per month over the past year), and 3) nondrinkers

(never drank or had drunk less than one glass of alcohol per month over the past year) [16]. The smoking group comprised current smokers, and the nonsmoking group comprised former smokers and those who had never smoked. For obesity classification, we classified the participants into three groups: 1) low weight group for body mass index (BMI) lower than $18.5 \, \text{kg/m}^2$, 2) normal weight group for BMI between 18.5 and $25 \, \text{kg/m}^2$, and 3) obese group for BMI higher than $25 \, \text{kg/m}^2$, according to the guidelines of Korean practice [17]. HTN was defined as average systolic blood pressure $\geq 140 \, \text{mmHg}$ or diastolic blood pressure $\geq 90 \, \text{mmHg}$ or taking of antihypertensive medications. Systolic and diastolic blood pressure was measured by standard methods using a sphygmomanometer while the patient was seated. Three measurements were recorded for all subjects at 5-min intervals, and the average of the second and third measurements was used in the analysis. We defined dyslipidemia as follows: hypercholesterolemia, total cholesterol $\geq 200 \, \text{mg/dl}$; hypertriglyceridemia, triglyceride $\geq 150 \, \text{mg/} dl$; and hypo-high-density lipoprotein-cholesterolemia (HDL-C), $< 40 \, \text{mg/dL}$ in men, $< 50 \, \text{mg/dL}$ in women, or currently taking any anti-dyslipidemic drug for the purpose of controlling blood lipid concentrations. Low-density lipoprotein cholesterol (LDL-C) concentration was calculated according to the Friedewald equation, after the exclusion of participants whose triglyceride concentrations exceeded $350 \, \text{mg/dl}$. DM was defined as a fasting plasma glucose (FPG) level $\geq 126 \, \text{mg/dL}$, diagnosis of DM by a clinician, or taking of an oral hypoglycemic agent or injected insulin.

Statistical analysis

According to the Korea Ministry of Health and Welfare and Korea Centers for Disease Control & Prevention guidelines, we used the survey-weighted statistical analyses. Chi-square or Fisher's exact tests were used to compare for categorical variables, t-tests for normal distribution, and Kruskal-Wallis tests for non-normal distribution of continuous variables to compare the demographic variables. We calculated the odds ratios (ORs) and 95% confidence intervals (CI) for CAD risk according to RA. We used the multivariable logistic regression model in which we adjusted for the confounding variables of age, sex, alcohol consumption and smoking status, BMI, HTN, dyslipidemia, and DM. The SPSS ver. 23.0 (SPSS Inc., Chicago, IL, USA) was used for all statistical analyses, and the IBM SPSS Statistics Version 23 - Essentials for R Version 23.0.0 (SPSS Inc., Chicago, IL, USA) was used for propensity score-matched analysis. A P value < 0.05 was considered significant.

Propensity score-matching

To balance the distribution of baseline characteristics, we used propensity score-matching. We estimated a propensity score for each study participant using the multivariable logistic regression model. In the model, potential confounders and variables associated with CAD, such as age, sex, alcohol consumption and smoking status, BMI, HTN, dyslipidemia, and DM were included. We then created an exchangeable comparison group of the patients with RA by matching each with one patient without RA. Our propensity score model discriminated well between the RA and non-RA groups. The model was fit to the data during all steps of the regression analyses (Hosmer and Lemeshow goodness-of-fit test $\chi^2 = 4.56$; $P = 0.95$, and relative multivariate imbalance L1 after matching = 0.714). We then used the propensity score to match each patient with RA to another patient without RA, who had a similar propensity score, matching 238 of those patients with RA to another 238 patients without RA. Our assessment of the covariate balance after matching focused on these standardized differences. Before matching, the mean propensity score for the patients with RA was 0.009, and for the patients without RA was 0.022. After matching, the mean propensity score for the patients with RA was 0.022, and for the patients without RA was 0.022.

Results

Prevalence of RA
Of the 25,828 KNHANES participants included in the present study, 10,915 were men (42.3%), 14,913 were women (57.7%), and 238 were patients with RA (0.9%).

Baseline patient characteristics between the RA and non-RA groups were significantly different (Table 1). Old age and female gender were dominant in the RA group. While non-drinkers were more in the RA group, current smoker was more in the non-RA group. Prevalence of HTN, dyslipidemia, DM, and CAD were also higher in RA group than in the non-RA group. The overall adjusted prevalence of RA in Korea from 2008 to 2012 was 0.6% (95% CI 0.5–0.7%). The prevalence of RA increased with age (Table 2).

Association between RA and CAD
After propensity score-matching for all confounding variables such as age, sex, alcohol consumption, smoking status, BMI, HTN, dyslipidemia, and DM, baseline characteristics in the two groups were similar (Table 3). In an analysis with propensity score-matching, the prevalence of CAD was significantly higher in RA patients (OR 2.97, 95% CI 1.15–7.68, $P = 0.02$; Table 4).

Discussion
This nationwide study investigated the prevalence of RA in Korea and the association between RA and CAD. In this study, the prevalence of RA in Korea from 2008 to 2012 was 0.6%. RA was dominant among the aged women, and patients in the RA groups had more frequencies of HTN, dyslipidemia, and DM. Although smoking is known to be a risk factor for RA, in this study, current smokers were more common in the non RA group. This result is probably due to the fact that

Table 1 Baseline characteristics of the study participants

Variables	Frequency			Weighted frequency*		
	RA group $n = 238$	Non-RA group $n = 25,590$	P	RA group $n = 938,122$	Non-RA group $n = 147,771,248$	P
Age, years[†]	64.40 ± 13.17	49.87 ± 16.67	< 0.001	61.39 ± 14.71	44.96 ± 15.96	< 0.001
Female sex, n (%)	201 (84.5)	14,712 (57.5%)	< 0.001	801,097 (85.4)	74,517,785 (50.4%)	< 0.001
Alcohol Intake			< 0.001			< 0.001
Nondrinker, n (%)	219 (92.0)	20,159 (78.8)		851,124 (90.7)	112,482,020 (76.1)	
Moderate drinker, n (%)	13 (5.5)	3560 (13.9)		58,045 (6.2)	24,128,683 (16.3)	
Heavy drinker, n (%)	6 (2.5)	1871 (7.3)		28,953 (3.1)	11,160,544 (7.6)	
Current smoker, n (%)	19 (8.0)	5265 (20.6)	< 0.001	79,400 (8.5)	37,895,669 (25.6)	< 0.001
Degree of obesity			0.43			< 0.001
Low, n (%)	11 (4.6)	1189 (4.6)		50,925 (5.4)	7,230,860 (4.9)	
Normal, n (%)	142 (59.7)	16,262 (63.5)		552,121 (58.9)	93,306,408 (63.1)	
Obese, n (%)	85 (35.7)	8139 (31.8)		335,076 (35.7)	47,233,980 (32.0)	
Hypertension, n (%)	93 (39.1)	5643 (22.1)	< 0.001	335,843 (35.8)	25,000,131 (16.9)	< 0.001
Dyslipidemia, n (%)	33 (13.9)	2466 (9.6)	0.03	120,048 (12.8)	11,675,583 (7.9)	< 0.001
Diabetes mellitus, n (%)	42 (17.6)	2087 (8.2)	< 0.001	171,300 (18.3)	9,271,183 (6.3)	< 0.001
Coronary artery disease, n (%)	17 (7.1)	452 (1.8)	< 0.001	62,174 (6.6)	1871,935 (1.3)	< 0.001

[†]Data are presented as mean ± standard deviation
*Weighted population according to individual weight provided by national surveys
RA: rheumatoid arthritis

Table 2 Prevalence of rheumatoid arthritis in Korea

Age	Prevalence of RA		Weighted prevalence of RA, n (%)	
	Female, n (%)[†]	Overall, n (%)[‡]	Female, n (%)[†]	Overall, n (%)[‡]
Overall age	201 (84.5)	238 (0.9)	801,096 (85.4)	938,122 (0.6)
Age, years				
< 40	12 (80.0)	15 (0.2)	69,025 (81.6)	84,589 (0.1)
40–49	16 (88.9)	18 (0.4)	100,034 (87.2)	114,741 (0.4)
50–59	30 (85.7)	35 (0.8)	144,675 (81.2)	178,109 (0.7)
60–69	61 (89.7)	68 (1.6)	190,633 (90.2)	211,309 (1.3)
≥ 70	82 (80.4)	102 (2.6)	296,729 (84.9)	349,374 (2.6)

[†]Data show the percentage of female
[‡]Data show the proportion with RA in the total population
RA: rheumatoid arthritis

most of the RA patients were middle-aged women and smoking prevalence of middle-aged women is low in Korea. The prevalence of CAD in patients with RA was significantly higher than in general population. After the propensity score-matching, RA was significantly correlated with CAD.

Epidemiologic studies investigating RA showed a prevalence of 0.3–6.0%, which varied according to their countries [18–23]. An averaged prevalence of 0.5–1.1% was reported in the European and general populations of the United States; however, native Americans showed a higher prevalence of 5.3–6.0% [13]. Studies carried out in developing countries reported a lower RA prevalence of 0.1–0.5%. In Asia, most studies reported a prevalence of 0.1–0.3%; in

contrast, one previous study suggested a relatively higher prevalence of 2.0–4.7% [24]. In this study, the prevalence of RA was 0.6%, which was comparable to that of the western population but higher than that of the other Asian populations. Early diagnosis of RA and higher life expectancy in Korea than in other Asian countries is considered to be responsible for the increased prevalence of RA.

The prevalence of RA was generally two to threefold higher in women [13]. In this study, RA was more prevalent in women; the sex ratio was about 4:1, with greater predominance in women than reported in other studies. Majority of the studies also revealed that RA onset peaked in the fifth decade or later [25–28]. In this study, the prevalence of RA increased with age; however, the exact disease onset could not be assessed.

We have shown that the prevalence of CAD in RA patients was higher than in non-RA patients using propensity score-matching. Previous studies reported that RA directly affected the coronary arteries and raised the risk of CVD by 2-fold [29, 30]. A recent study investigating co-morbidities in patients with RA suggested that the prevalence of CAD might be increased in Korean patients with RA [31]. In our study, we assessed and compared the risks of CAD on RA, using propensity-score matching between patients with RA and without RA. Therefore, we consider that this study is novel in assessing the risks of CAD on RA in an Asian population.

Regarding the relationship between RA and CAD, traditional risk factors could not fully explain the elevated risk of CVD in patients with RA. In addition to traditional risk factors, nontraditional risk factors were additively associated with atherosclerosis and CVD in RA patients. The most likely mechanism is high-grade inflammation in RA. Studies investigating the relationship between RA and CAD suggested a direct link between the degree of inflammation and the risk of CV events [32]. Pro-inflammatory cytokines, such as tumor necrosis factor-α and interleukin-6 were well known to contribute to atherosclerosis development and played an

Table 3 Baseline characteristics of the study participants after propensity score-matching

Variables	RA group n = 238	Non-RA group n = 238	P
Age, years[†]	64.40 ± 13.17	64.07 ± 13.32	0.79
Female sex, n (%)	201 (84.5)	201 (84.5)	0.99
Alcohol Intake			0.48
Nondrinker, n (%)	219 (92.0)	225 (94.5)	
Moderate drinker, n (%)	13 (5.5)	10 (4.2)	
Heavy drinker, n (%)	6 (2.5)	3 (1.3)	
Current smoker, n (%)	19 (8.0)	20 (8.4)	0.99
Degree of obesity			0.83
Low, n (%)	11 (4.6)	14 (5.9)	
Normal, n (%)	142 (59.7)	140 (58.8)	
Obese, n (%)	85 (35.7)	84 (35.3)	
Hypertension, n (%)	93 (39.1)	97 (40.8)	0.78
Dyslipidemia, n (%)	33 (13.9)	43 (18.1)	0.26
Diabetes mellitus, n (%)	42 (17.6)	37 (15.5)	0.62
Coronary artery disease, n (%)	17 (7.1)	6 (2.5)	0.03

[†] Data are presented as mean ± standard deviation
RA: rheumatoid arthritis

Table 4 Influence of rheumatoid arthritis on coronary artery disease

Variables	OR before PS-matching			OR after PS-matching		
	OR	95% CI	P for trend	OR	95% CI	P for trend
RA[†]	4.28	2.59–7.07	< 0.001	2.97	1.15–7.68	0.02
Age	1.08	1.07–1.08	< 0.001	1.05	1.01–1.10	0.01
Female sex	0.69	0.57–0.83	< 0.001	1.98	0.46–8.65	0.36
Alcohol Intake						
Nondrinker	1.00			1.00		
Moderate drinker	0.54	0.39–0.76	< 0.001	–	–	–
Heavy drinker	0.99	0.70–1.40	0.95	–	–	–
Current smoker	0.60	0.46–0.78	< 0.001	1.07	0.24–4.75	0.93
Degree of obesity						
Low	1.00			1.00		
Normal	2.04	1.05–3.98	0.04	0.56	0.12–2.61	0.46
Obese	3.49	1.78–6.81	< 0.001	0.57	0.11–2.86	0.50
Hypertension	5.71	4.73–6.89	< 0.001	3.67	1.48–9.09	0.005
Dyslipidemia	4.79	3.90–5.88	< 0.001	4.51	1.90–10.71	< 0.001
Diabetes mellitus	4.78	4.77–4.79	< 0.001	4.28	1.81–10.15	< 0.001

[†]Adjusted for age, sex, alcohol intake and smoking status, body mass index, hypertension, dyslipidemia and diabetes mellitus
RA: rheumatoid arthritis; PS: propensity score; OR: odds ratio; 95% CI: 95% confidence interval

important role in accelerating atherosclerosis in patients with RA [33]. Indeed, high-grade inflammation could increase metabolic risks such as insulin resistance, and directly impair endothelial function. Endothelial dysfunction promoted by such pro-inflammatory cytokines was characterized by decreased nitric oxide bioavailability [34, 35]. Further, oxidative stress and T cells were suggested to play a key role in inflammation and atherosclerosis development in patients with RA [36]. A recent study on anti-inflammatory therapy targeting the interleukin-1β innate immunity pathway with canakinumab suggests that reducing inflammation without affecting lipid levels reduces the risk of cardiovascular disease [37]. Consequently, further investigation of the role of anti-inflammatory therapy in patients with RA and CAD is required.

Some limitations are present in this study. First, the cross-sectional design precludes conclusions about causal relationships; thus, further prospective studies and intervention trials should be undertaken to establish a causal association between RA and CAD. The relationship of RA to CAD is important, since these two diseases possess common inflammatory pathways. Second, the current diagnostic status of RA and CAD was based on self-reports. Consequently, these data may have been influenced by systematic errors in individuals' consideration, which may have led to non-differential misclassification or overestimation. In particular, osteoarthritis (OA) can be confused with RA. However, in case of OA diagnosis in KNHANES, it is possible to prevent misdiagnosis to some extent because OA diagnosis was based on patients' pain and radiologic examinations.

Conclusions

The present study found that the prevalence of RA was 0.6%, which was similar to that reported worldwide, and the presence of RA was associated with an approximately 2-fold increased prevalence of CAD. Therefore, patients with RA would be better to be examined for CAD for early diagnosis and management.

Abbreviations
BMI: body mass index; CAD: coronary artery diseases; CVD: cardiovascular diseases; DM: diabetes mellitus; FPG: fasting plasma glucose; HDL-C: high-density lipoprotein-cholesterol; HTN: hypertension; LDL-C: low-density lipoprotein cholesterol; MI: myocardial infarction; OA: osteoarthritis; RA: rheumatoid arthritis

Acknowledgements
Not applicable.

Authors' contributions
THL: Study design; Manuscript preparation; Elaboration of article; Data analysis and interpretation. GGS: Elaboration of article and critical review; Data analysis and interpretation. SJC: Elaboration of article and critical review; Data analysis and interpretation. HS: Data collection; Data analysis and interpretation. JHJ: Study design; Manuscript preparation; Elaboration of article and critical review; Data interpretation. All authors read and approved the final manuscript to be published.

Author details
[1]College of Medicine, Chung-Ang University, 84 Heukseouk-ro, Donjak-gu, Seoul 06974, South Korea. [2]Korea University College of Medicine, 73 Inchon-ro, Seongbuk-gu, Seoul 02841, South Korea. [3]Department of Rheumatology, Korea University Guro Hospital, 148 Gurodong-ro, Guro-gu, Seoul 08308, South Korea. [4]Division of Rheumatology, Department of Internal Medicine, Korea University Ansan Hospital, 123 Jeokgeum-ro, Danwon-gu, Ansan-si, Gyeonggi-do 15355, South Korea. [5]Department of Occupational and Environmental Medicine, Busan Adventist Hospital, Sahmyook Medical Center, 170 Daeti-ro, Seo-gu, Busan 49230, South Korea.

References

1. Lindhardsen J, Ahlehoff O, Gislason GH, Madsen OR, Olesen JB, Torp-Pedersen C, et al. The risk of myocardial infarction in rheumatoid arthritis and diabetes mellitus: a Danish nationwide cohort study. Ann Rheum Dis. 2011;70:929–34.
2. Solomon DH, Karlson EW, Rimm EB, Cannuscio CC, Mandl LA, Manson JE, et al. Cardiovascular morbidity and mortality in women diagnosed with rheumatoid arthritis. Circulation. 2003;107:1303–7.
3. Gabriel SE. Why do people with rheumatoid arthritis still die prematurely? Ann Rheum Dis. 2008;67:iii30–4.
4. Gkaliagkousi E, Gavriilaki E, Doumas M, Petidis K, Aslanidis S, Stella D. Cardiovascular risk in rheumatoid arthritis: pathogenesis, diagnosis, and management. J Clin Rheumatol. 2012;18:422–30.
5. Willers J, Hahn A. Cardiovascular risk in patients with rheumatoid arthritis: assessment of several traditional risk parameters and a German risk score model. Rheumatol Int. 2012;32:3741–9.
6. Mason JC, Libby P. Cardiovascular disease in patients with chronic inflammation: mechanisms underlying premature cardiovascular events in rheumatologic conditions. Eur Heart J. 2015;36:482–9.
7. Liao KP, Solomon DH. Mechanistic insights into the link between inflammation and cardiovascular disease: rheumatoid arthritis as a human model of inflammation. Circ Cardiovasc Imaging. 2014;7:575–7.
8. Ross R. Atherosclerosis--an inflammatory disease. N Engl J Med. 1999;340: 115–26.
9. Gonzalez-Gay MA, Gonzalez-Juanatey C, Lopez-Diaz MJ, Piñeiro A, Garcia-Porrua C, Miranda-Filloy JA, et al. HLA-DRB1 and persistent chronic inflammation contribute to cardiovascular events and cardiovascular mortality in patients with rheumatoid arthritis. Arthritis Rheum. 2007;57:125–32.
10. Tournadre A, Mathieu S, Soubrier M. Managing cardiovascular risk in patients with inflammatory arthritis: practical considerations. Ther Adv Musculoskelet Dis. 2016;8:180–91.
11. Avina-Zubieta JA, Thomas J, Sadatsafavi M, Lehman AJ, Lacaille D. Risk of incident cardiovascular events in patients with rheumatoid arthritis: a meta-analysis of observational studies. Ann Rheum Dis. 2012;71:1524–9.
12. Kurian AK, Cardarelli KM. Racial and ethnic differences in cardiovascular disease risk factors: a systematic review. Ethn Dis. 2007;17:143–52.
13. Alamanos Y, Drosos AA. Epidemiology of adult rheumatoid arthritis. Autoimmun Rev. 2005;4:130–6.
14. Naranjo A, Sokka T, Descalzo MA, Calvo-Alén J, Hørslev-Petersen K, Luukkainen RK, et al. Cardiovascular disease in patients with rheumatoid arthritis: results from the QUEST-RA study. Arthritis Res Ther. 2008;10:R30.
15. Solomon A, Tsang L, Woodiwiss AJ, Millen AM, Norton GR, Dessein PH, et al. Cardiovascular disease risk amongst African black patients with rheumatoid arthritis: the need for population specific stratification. Biomed Res Int. 2014; 2014:826095.
16. Seok H, Yoon JH, Lee W, Lee JH, Jung PK, Kim I, et al. The association between concealing emotions at work and medical utilization in Korea. Ann Occup Environ Med. 2014;26:31.
17. Kim MK, Lee WY, Kang JH, Kang JH, Kim BT, Sim SM, et al. 2014 clinical practice guidelines for overweight and obesity in Korea. Endocrinol Metab (Seoul). 2014;29:405–9.
18. Riise T, Jacobsen BK, Gran JT. Incidence and prevalence of rheumatoid arthritis in the county of Troms, northern Norway. J Rheumatol. 2000;27:1386–9.
19. Symmons D, Turner G, Webb R, Asten P, Barrett E, Lunt M, et al. The prevalence of rheumatoid arthritis in the United Kingdom: new estimates for a new century. Rheumatology (Oxford). 2002;41:793–800.
20. Stojanović R, Vlajinac H, Palić-Obradović D, Janosević S, Adanja B. Prevalence of rheumatoid arthritis in Belgrade, Yugoslavia. Br J Rheumatol. 1998;37:729–32.
21. Spindler A, Bellomio V, Berman A, Lucero E, Baigorria M, Paz S, et al. Prevalence of rheumatoid arthritis in Tucuman. Argentina J Rheumatol. 2002;29:1166–70.
22. Pountain G. The prevalence of rheumatoid arthritis in the Sultanate of Oman. Br J Rheumatol. 1991;30:24–8.
23. Lau E, Symmons D, Bankhead C, MacGregor A, Donnan S, Silman A. Low prevalence of rheumatoid arthritis in the urbanized Chinese of Hong Kong. J Rheumatol. 1993;20:1133–7.
24. Shichikawa K, Inoue K, Hirota S, Maeda A, Ota H, Kimura M, et al. Changes in the incidence and prevalence of rheumatoid arthritis in Kamitonda, Wakayama, Japan, 1965-1996. Ann Rheum Dis. 1999;58:751–6.
25. Symmons DP, Barrett EM, Bankhead CR, Scott DG, Silman AJ. The incidence of rheumatoid arthritis in the United Kingdom: results from the Norfolk arthritis register. Br J Rheumatol. 1994;33:735–9.
26. Doran MF, Pond GR, Crowson CS, O'Fallon WM, Gabriel SE. Trends in incidence and mortality in rheumatoid arthritis in Rochester, Minnesota, over a forty-year period. Arthritis Rheum. 2002;46:625–31.
27. Söderlin MK, Börjesson O, Kautiainen H, Skogh T, Leirisalo-Repo M. Annual incidence of inflammatory joint diseases in a population based study in southern Sweden. Ann Rheum Dis. 2002;61:911–5.
28. Guillemin F, Briançon S, Klein JM, Sauleau E, Pourel J. Low incidence of rheumatoid arthritis in France. Scand J Rheumatol. 1994;23:264–8.
29. Dregan A, Charlton J, Chowienczyk P, Gulliford MC. Chronic inflammatory disorders and risk of type 2 diabetes mellitus, coronary heart disease, and stroke: a population-based cohort study. Circulation. 2014;130:837–44.
30. Meune C, Touze E, Trinquart L, Allanore Y. High risk of clinical cardiovascular events in rheumatoid arthritis: levels of associations of myocardial infarction and stroke through a systematic review and meta-analysis. Arch Cardiovasc Dis. 2010;103:253–61.
31. Jeong H, Baek SY, Kim SW, Eun YH, Kim IY, Kim H, et al. Comorbidities of rheumatoid arthritis: results from the Korean National Health and nutrition examination survey. PLoS One. 2017;12:e0176260.
32. Gargiulo P, Marsico F, Parente A, Paolillo S, Cecere M, Casaretti L, et al. Ischemic heart disease in systemic inflammatory diseases. An appraisal Int J Cardiol. 2014;170:286–90.
33. Sattar N, McCarey DW, Capell H, McInnes IB. Explaining how "high-grade" systemic inflammation accelerates vascular risk in rheumatoid arthritis. Circulation. 2003;108:2957–63.
34. Roldan CA, Joson J, Sharrar J, Qualls CR, Sibbitt WL Jr. Premature aortic atherosclerosis in systemic lupus erythematosus: a controlled transesophageal echocardiographic study. J Rheumatol. 2010;37:71–8.
35. Sandoo A. Veldhuijzen van Zanten JJ, Metsios GS, Carroll D, Kitas GD. Vascular function and morphology in rheumatoid arthritis: a systematic review. Rheumatology (Oxford). 2011;50:2125–39.
36. Korbecki J, Baranowska-Bosiacka I, Gutowska I, Chlubek D. The effect of reactive oxygen species on the synthesis of prostanoids from arachidonic acid. J Physiol Pharmacol. 2013;64:409–21.
37. Ridker PM, Everett BM, Thuren T, MacFadyen JG, Chang WH, Ballantyne C, et al. Antiinflammatory therapy with canakinumab for atherosclerotic disease. N Engl J Med. 2017;377:119–31.

19

Real - rheumatoid arthritis in real life - study cohort: A sociodemographic profile of rheumatoid arthritis in Brazil

Nathália de Carvalho Sacilotto[1][*][iD], Rina Dalva Neubarth Giorgi[1], Ana Beatriz Vargas-Santos[2], Cleandro Pires de Albuquerque[3], Sebastião Cezar Radominski[4], Ivânio Alves Pereira[5], Maria Fernanda Brandão Resende Guimarães[6], Manoel Barros Bértolo[7], Paulo Louzada Jr[8], Maria de Fátima Lobato da Cunha Sauma[9], Karina Rossi Bonfiglioli[10], Claiton Viegas Brenol[11], Licia Maria Henrique da Mota[3] and Geraldo da Rocha Castelar-Pinheiro[2]

Abstract

Background: In Brazil, socioeconomic differences in the incidence of rheumatoid arthritis (RA) have been demonstrated, which are important in the formulation of hypotheses regarding the association between environmental factors, lifestyle and the risk of disease development. This study examines how the socioeconomic condition of the patient with RA in Brazil, assessed according to social class, educational level, employment situation and use of caregivers, affects the times between the beginning of symptoms and diagnosis and the beginning of the use of disease-modifying antirheumatic drugs, as well as the presence of erosive disease and functional status.

Methods: This work is part of a multicentric study called REAL - Rheumatoid Arthritis in Real Life in Brazil, which is a prospective observational cohort study.

Results: As described in the REAL study, we included a total of 1115 patients. It was noted that patients with an educational classification of up to second grade incomplete presented with erosion percentages above those with a higher grade complete. Patients with caregivers presented a higher percentage of erosion than patients without caregivers. We verified that patients from economic classes above B2 presented fewer occurrences of erosion than those from classes C2, D-E. We also analyzed the average time differences from the beginning of symptoms and diagnosis and the beginning of treatment, according to academic level, erosion and economic classification. Patients with first grade complete showed an HAQ-DI averages higher than those with second grade complete. The patients who had employment showed lower HAQ-DI averages than patients who were not employed. The patients with erosion showed an HAQ-DI value higher than those without erosion. Patients with caregivers showed an HAQ-DI average higher than that of without caregivers.

(Continued on next page)

* Correspondence: nath-cs@uol.com.br
[1]Hospital do ServidorPúblicoEstadual de São Paulo, Rua Pedro de Toledo, 1800, Vila Clementino, São Paulo, SP 04039-000, Brazil
Full list of author information is available at the end of the article

(Continued from previous page)

Conclusion: This study showed that the therapeutic window of RA is not being reached, and therefore we should have a policy to expand and ensure access to public health for all patients, especially those with lower levels of education and income.

Keywords: Rheumatoid arthritis, Demographic profile, Public health

Background

Rheumatoid arthritis (RA) is an autoimmune disease associated with periods of inflammation and progressive joint damage, possibly leading to a reduction in movement and premature death [1].

Socioeconomic differences in the incidence of RA, which are important in the formulation of hypotheses regarding the association between environmental factors, lifestyle and the risk of disease development, have been demonstrated. Studies show that patients with a higher socioeconomic level have half the risk of RA development than patients with a lower level [2, 3], as well as a better outcome inclusively proved by a lower index in the Health Assessment Questionnaire-Disability Index (HAQ-DI) [4]. A better educational level and nonmanual work were associated with a lower risk of RA development [2].

Such socioeconomic differences are also important from the perspective of public health. It is estimated that 20–70% of patients who are employed at the beginning of an RA diagnosis are unable to continue their work activities 7–10 years into the evolution of the disease, which can have negative consequences, including a reduction in social activities, quality of life and socioeconomic conditions [5].

However, the economic impact of RA must also be assessed by the productivity of patients who continue to work that can be adversely affected by absences related to the disease or limits in working capacity, which is also important in the assessment of the functional class [6, 7]. Such limitations have shown themselves to be one of the principal economic consequences of RA and can be reduced by aggressive and early treatment during the initial phase of the disease [1].

This study examines how the socioeconomic condition of the patient with RA in Brazil, assessed according to social class, educational level, employment situation and use of caregivers, affects the time between the beginning of symptoms and diagnosis and the beginning of the use of disease-modifying antirheumatic drugs (DMARD), as well as the presence of erosive disease and functional status, as measured by the HAQ-DI.

Methods

This work is part of a Brazilian multicentric study called REAL-Rheumatoid Arthritis in Real Life in Brazil, which is a prospective observational cohort study of patients with RA from 11 public healthcare centers in different geographic regions of Brazil that are specialized in RA management. For the present article, a cross-sectional cohort was analyzed, corresponding to the initial assessment of the participants, who were accompanied afterwards for a 12-month period [8].

Each center was expected to enroll 100 patients consecutively. The inclusion criteria were as follows: 1) fulfillment of the 1987 American Rheumatism Association (ARA) or the 2010 American College of Rheumatology (ACR)/European League Against Rheumatism (EULAR) classification criteria for rheumatoid arthritis; 2) age of 18 years or older; and 3) documented medical record data of at least 6 months of follow up in their healthcare center prior to study enrollment.

All data were collected on an electronic medical chart and gathered in a centralized dataset.

We described the following characteristics: clinical, laboratory, radiographic, therapeutic and quality of life characteristics and patient adherence to treatment.

Most data were collected during the medical appointments, with previous medical records used as secondary sources. For the assessment of the clinical and demographic profiles in the present study, the following assessments were used:

- School level: divided into below literacy level, first grade not complete, first grade complete, second grade not complete, second grade complete, higher grade not complete, higher grade complete and postgraduate.
- Employment situation: divided into retired, housewife, receiving disability benefit or retired temporarily by INSS (National Social Security Institute), unemployed, unemployed looking for work in the last 3 months, formally employed worker, self-employed worker, unregistered self-employed worker, and informally employed, completed by means of an individual questionnaire after explanations [8]. Only one option could be chosen.
- Time from symptoms to diagnosis, in months.
- Time from symptoms to first DMARD, in months.
- Economic Classification: determined by the Brazilian Economic Classification Criterion (BECC), a score

system updated in 2015 that includes variables such as the number of household electrical appliances, level of education of the householder and access to public services [8]. The score range is stratified from A to D-E, with each stratum corresponding to an estimated household income.

- Functional capacity assessed according to the HAQ-

    DI – Health Assessment Questionnaire - Disability Index.
- The presence of erosion was documented according to the existence or lack of bone erosions in X-rays of the hands and feet. The X-rays interpretation was not standardized but individualized at each center, by certified and qualified rheumatologists.
- Necessity of caregivers.

All the patients agreed to participate in the study and signed an informed consent form.

Statistical methodology

Initially, the information was analyzed descriptively. The categorical variables were presented as absolute and relative frequencies and the numeric variables were presented as average and standard deviation for normally distributed data, and minimum, maximum, 1st quartile. Median and 3rd quartile for skewed/non-normally distributed data.

The associations between categorical variables were assessed by the Chi-squared test. To evaluate differences in distributions, we used adjusted standardized residuals, and local absolute differences were considered significant if larger than 1,96.

For the comparison of two groups, Student's t test was used. For comparisons of more than 2 groups the nonparametric Kruskal-Wallis test was used because of the violation of the distribution normality assumption as assessed by the Kolmogorov-Smirnov test. While we used the Kruskal-Wallis test to check differences in averages, we subsequently used the multiple comparisons test of Dunn-Bonferroni to identify categories with distinct averages maintaining levels of global significance.

For all the statistical tests, we used a significance level of 5%.

The statistical analyses were achieved by use of the statistics software SPSS 20.0.

Results

As described in The REAL Study, we included a total of 1115 patients with RA in Brazil. Approximately 90% were female, with a mean age of 56.7 years and a median disease duration of 12.7 years. The majority of subjects were white, with minorities from Asian and Brazilian-Indian origins making up 1% of the sample. The median BMI was 27 kg/m^2, with 64% of the patients classified as

overweight or obese. Approximately 40% of the patients were either current or former smokers. The seropositivity rate was similar between rheumatoid factor and anti-citrullinated protein antibody, but it is important to highlight that the latter was assessed in less than half of the patients, of whom only 7% were seronegative in both immunological tests. Almost half of the patients were taking glucocorticoids, 96.5% were taking DMARDs (conventional synthetic, targeted synthetic and/or biological) of these 35.7% were taking biologics DMARDs. Of these taking biologics, 15.6% were on monotherapy. Median DAS28-ESR (Disease Activity Score 28 - erythrocyte sedimentation rate) was 3.5, with 58.7% of patients presenting moderate or high disease activity. When assessed by CDAI (Clinical Disease Activity Index), the median score represented low disease activity (CDAI = 9), with 46.7% of subjects classified as presenting moderate to high disease activity [8].

The educational level and employment status distribution of our patients are shown in Fig. 1. Of note, among the patients who were retired, and among the patients receiving disability benefit or temporarily retired by INSS, 56 and 82%, respectively, were as such due to RA. According to the BECC, patients were classified as approximately 1% in class A, 4% in class B1, 19% in class B2, 27% in class C1, 31% in class C2 and 18% in classes D and E. Of note, 45% of patients did not present with erosive disease and 95% did not have caregivers.

According to Table 1, we found an association between erosion and academic level ($p = 0.001$), employment situation ($p < 0.001$), use of caregivers ($p = 0.042$) and economic classification ($p < 0.001$). Accordingly, it was also noted that patients with up to a second grade incomplete education level presented erosion percentages above those with a higher grade complete. Patients with caregivers also presented a higher percentage of erosion (67.2%) than those without a caregiver (54.2%). Additionally, we verified that patients from economic classes B2 and higher presented fewer occurrences of erosion than those from classes C2, D-E.

According to Table 2, significant differences were found in the average time from the beginning of symptoms and diagnosis according to academic level, erosion and economic classification. We observed that the below literacy-level patients presented a higher average than patients with a higher grade complete or a postgraduate education, which were similar to each other. There were no differences in the averages between the other academic levels. In addition to this finding, patients with erosion had a longer average time from the beginning of the symptoms and diagnosis than those without erosion. Of note, the patients from classes D - E presented a longer average than the patients from classes B2 and C1,

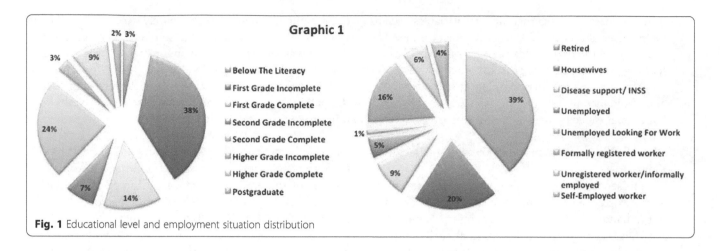

Fig. 1 Educational level and employment situation distribution

which did not differ from each other. We could not find differences in averages for the A, B1 and C2 classes from those for the others. Neither employment status nor the need of caregivers were associated with the time between symptoms and RA diagnosis.

As seen in Table 3, we found differences in average times for the beginning of treatment in terms of level of schooling, erosion and economic classification. As such, we observed that the below literacy-level patients had an average time higher than those patients with first grade complete that, in turn, presented an average higher than the patients with a higher grade complete. We did not find differences in averages in the other levels of education. In addition to this finding, patients with erosion presented a higher mean time to the beginning of the first DMARD treatment than that of patients without erosion. It was also noted that patients from the D - E classes showed a higher average than that from class C2

Table 1 Erosion

| | Erosion | | | | Total | | p |
| | No | | Yes | | | | |
	N	%	N	%	N	%	
School grade level	**494**	45.1%	**601**	54.9%	**1.095**	**100%**	0.001
Below literacy level	13	36.1%	23	63.9%	36	100%	
First grade not complete	172	40.6%	252	59.4%	424	100%	
First grade complete	61	41.2%	87	58.8%	148	100%	
Second grade not complete	26	35.1%	48	64.9%	74	100%	
Second grade complete	134	51.0%	129	49.0%	263	100%	
Higher grade not complete	15	50.0%	15	50.0%	30	100%	
Higher grade complete	60	62.5%	36	37.5%	96	100%	
Postgraduate	13	54.2%	11	45.8%	24	100%	
Employment situation	**493**	45.0%	**602**	55.0%	**1.095**	**100%**	<0.001
Retired	152	36.4%	266	63.6%	418	100%	
Receiving disability benefit or retired temporarily by INSS	44	44.9%	54	55.1%	98	100%	
Unemployed	26	50.0%	26	50.0%	52	100%	
Unemployed looking for work in the last 3 months	3	37.5%	5	62.5%	8	100%	
Housewife	100	44.4%	125	55.6%	225	100%	
Formally employed worker	108	59.7%	73	40.3%	181	100%	
Self-employed worker	27	61.4%	17	38.6%	44	100%	
Unregistered self-employed worker / informally employed	33	47.8%	36	52.2%	69	100%	
Caregiver	**492**	45.1%	**600**	54.9%	**1.092**	**100%**	0.042
No	471	45.8%	557	54.2%	1.028	100%	
Yes	21	32.8%	43	67.2%	64	100%	
Economic Classification	**489**	45.1%	**595**	54.9%	**1.084**	**100%**	<0.001
A	9	56.3%	7	43.8%	16	100%	
B1	22	56.4%	17	43.6%	39	100%	
B2	109	54.2%	92	45.8%	201	100%	
C1	146	49.2%	151	50.8%	297	100%	
C2	134	39.6%	204	60.4%	338	100%	
D-E	69	35.8%	124	64.2%	193	100%	

Table 2 Time from symptoms to diagnosis, in months

	Average	Standard Deviation	Minimum	Maximum	1° quartile	Median	3° quartile	N	p
Total	32.50	51.60	0.00	457	6.00	12.00	36.00	1.079	-
School grade level									<0.001
Below literacy level	65.40	86.70	1.00	372	8.00	24.00	112.00	35	
First grade not complete	33.70	49.90	0.00	360	6.00	12.00	36.00	414	
First grade complete	35.60	50.00	0.00	288	6.00	12.00	48.00	148	
Second grade not complete	28.10	43.60	1.00	256	6.00	12.00	24.00	73	
Second grade complete	29.90	49.70	1.00	348	6.00	12.00	24.00	262	
Higher grade not complete	19.70	32.00	1.00	145	4.80	11.5	19.50	30	
Higher grade complete	29.80	60.70	1.00	457	4.00	12.00	24.00	94	
Postgraduate	14.40	22.60	1.00	84	3.00	6.00	12.00	22	
Employment situation									0.118
Retired	37.20	54.80	0.00	457	6.00	12.00	48.00	415	
Receiving disability benefit or retired temporarily by INSS	31.00	53.50	1.00	372	6.00	12.00	24.00	37	
Unemployed	40.00	73.00	2.00	348	8.00	12.00	27.00	50	
Unemployed looking for work in the last 3 months	26.30	34.70	4.00	108	7.00	12.00	33.00	8	
Housewife	30.30	46.90	1.00	276	6.00	12.00	24.00	221	
Formally employed worker	25.40	43.80	0.00	288	4.80	12.00	24.00	178	
Self-employed worker	32.10	60.60	1.00	360	6.00	12.00	36.00	42	
Unregistered self-employed worker / informally employed	27.50	36.00	1.00	156	5.00	12.00	36.00	67	
Caregiver									0.864
No	32.50	52.30	0.00	457	6.00	12.00	36.00	1012	
Sim	33.60	40.20	1.00	240	9.00	24.00	36.00	63	
Erosão									<0.001
No	21.50	30.40	0.00	240	6.00	12.00	24.00	477	
Yes	41.70	62.90	0.00	457	6.00	12.00	48.00	584	
Economic Classification									0.001
A	27.40	35.90	1.00	120	6.00	12.00	42.00	14	
B1	29.90	33.50	1.00	156	6.00	12.00	48.00	38	
B2	26.40	48.60	1.00	457	5.00	12.00	24.00	196	
C1	26.00	37.70	1.00	269	6.00	12.00	24.00	300	
C2	33.80	53.50	0.00	348	6.00	12.00	30.00	329	
D-E	47.80	69.70	0.00	372	8.30	18.00	48.00	188	

which in turn was higher than those in classes B2 and C1, which did not differ from each other. We did not find any differences in averages in classes A and B1 compared to those in the others. Neither employment status nor the need of caregivers were associated with the average time to the beginning of DMARD treatment.

As shown in Table 4, differences in HAQ averages were found in all demographic characteristics assessed by the study. Accordingly, we observed that patients with first grade completed showed an HAQ-DI average higher than those with second grade completed, but we could not find the difference in averages among the other levels of education. Patients receiving disability benefit from INSS or unemployed showed higher HAQ averages than those retired or unemployed looking for work in the last 3 months. The later two categories, in turn, had higher HAQ averages than the housewives. While the HAQ averages did not differ among the three categories of patients who were still working, they were lower than those from the other employment status categories. HAQ-DI averages were higher in patients with erosions than in those without them, and higher in patients who needed caregivers than in those who didn't. We also noted that patients from class D/E showed an HAQ-DI average higher than that from class C2, which in turn was higher than the average of those from classes C1, B2 and B1, which did not differ from each other. No differences were noted between the class A HAQ-DI average and the averages of the other economical classes.

Discussion

We describe a cohort of 1115 patients selected from different geographic regions of Brazil. The REAL study showed that the demographic, clinical, serological and radiographic characteristics of the patients being followed had several similar but some divergent characteristics from those of previously published North American, European and Latin American cohorts. Particularly notable was the long delay for diagnosis and the high frequency of corticosteroid use and of erosive disease as well as the elevated percentage of patients with moderate or high disease activity. The high frequency of biologic DMARD use, considering the economic limitations in Brazil, is also notable [8].

Table 3 Time from symptoms to first DMARD, in months

	Average	Standard Deviation	Minimum	Maximum	1° quartile	Median	3° quartile	N	p
Total	38.6	62.68	0.00	624.0	6.00	12.00	42.00	995.00	-
School grade level									<0.001
Below literacy level	68.27	85.56	1.00	360	11.5	27.00	116	33.00	
First grade not complete	38.97	59.75	0.00	540	6.00	14.00	48.00	380.00	
First grade complete	43.83	56.87	1.00	288	9.00	24.00	60.00	132.00	
Second grade not complete	26.07	39.60	1.00	256	5.25	12.00	24.0	68.00	
Second grade complete	39.14	72.51	0.00	624	6.00	12.00	36.00	246.00	
Higher grade not complete	19.18	33.2	0.00	144	3.25	6.00	17.50	28.00	
Higher grade complete	33.31	58.57	0.00	327	4.00	12.00	26.00	87.00	
Postgraduate	35.45	79.12	1.00	360	6.00	10.50	33.00	20.00	
Employment situation									0.077
Retired	48.31	77.32	0.00	624	6.00	16.00	60.00	374.00	
Receiving disability benefit or retired temporarily by INSS	31.57	46.92	0.00	256	6.00	12.00	36.00	86.00	
Unemployed	43,0	73.00	2.00	348	6.00	12.00	39.00	50.00	
Unemployed looking for work in the last 3 months	38.13	37.11	4.00	108	8.25	27.00	66.00	8.00	
Housewife	33.33	51.04	1.00	360	6.05	12.00	36.00	209.00	
Formally employed worker	30.79	50.90	0.00	327	5.00	12.00	30.00	165.00	
Self-employed worker	31.62	48.02	1.00	269	7.00	12.00	36.00	39.00	
Unregistered self-employed worker / informally employed	29.92	39.92	1.00	180	6.00	12.00	36.00	63.00	
Caregiver									0.816
No	38.53	63.45	0.00	624	6.00	12.00	39.00	940.00	
Sim	40.63	49.07	0.00	240	8.00	24.00	54.00	51.00	
Erosão									<0.001
No	24.84	38.25	0.00	360	6.00	12.00	24.00	448.00	
Yes	50.8	76.16	0.00	624	6.00	24.00	60.00	531.00	
Economic Classification									<0.001
A	27.57	35.75	1.00	120	6.00	12.00	42.00	14.00	
B1	33.94	39.75	1.00	156	6.00	12.00	48.00	35.00	
B2	29.65	59.93	0.00	624	5.00	12.00	36.00	179.00	
C1	30.75	46.54	0.00	360	6.00	12.00	36.00	279.00	
C2	43.03	70.55	0.00	540	8.00	15.00	45.00	297.00	
D-E	55.07	76.04	1.00	444	12.00	24.00	63.75	178.00	

Table 4 HAQ.

	Average	Standard Deviation	Minimum	Maximum	1° quartile	Median	3° quartile	N	p
Total	0.94	0.77	0.00	3,00	0.25	0.88	1.50	1.116	-
School grade level									<0.001
Below literacy level	1.19	0.87	0.00	2.75	0.28	1.19	1.88	36.00	
First grade not complete	1.02	0.80	0.00	3.00	0.25	0.88	1.63	429.00	
First grade complete	1.03	0.73	0.00	3.00	0.50	0.88	1.50	156.00	
Second grade not complete	0.97	0.79	0.00	3.00	0.25	0.94	1.44	74.00	
Second grade complete	0.80	0.72	0.00	2.75	0.25	0.63	1.25	266.00	
Higher grade not complete	0.85	0.85	0.00	2.88	0.00	0.88	1.38	31.00	
Higher grade complete	0.81	0.69	0.00	2.50	0.13	0.63	1.38	99.00	
Postgraduate	0.62	0.67	0.00	2.75	0.03	0.50	0.84	24.00	
Employment situation									<0.001
Retired	1.05	0.77	0.00	3.00	0.38	1.00	1.63	430.00	
Receiving disability benefit or retired temporarily by INSS	1.32	0.75	0.00	3.00	0.75	1.25	1.88	100.00	
Unemployed	1.24	0.82	0.00	3.00	0.69	1.13	1.88	53.00	
Unemployed looking for work in the last 3 months	1.05	0.8	0.00	2.63	0.50	0.94	1.47	8.00	
Housewife	0.88	0.74	0.00	2.88	0.25	0.75	1.38	227.00	
Formally employed worker	0.66	0.7	0.00	2.75	0.00	0.50	1.00	183.00	
Self-employed worker	0.57	0.66	0.00	2.50	0.00	0.25	0.81	45.00	
Unregistered self-employed worker / informally employed	0.64	0.64	0.00	2.38	0.13	0.50	1.00	69.00	
Caregiver									<0.001
No	0.91	0.75	0.00	3.00	0.25	0.75	1.38	1046.00	
Sim	1.43	0.84	0.00	3.00	0.75	1.38	2.00	66.00	
Erosão									<0.001
No	0.78	0.72	0.00	2.88	0.13	0.63	1.25	494.00	
Yes	1.08	0.79	0.00	3.00	0.38	1.00	1.63	602.00	
Economic Classification									<0.001
A	0.96	0.81	0.00	2.5	0.22	0.81	1.47	16.00	
B1	0.83	0.77	0.00	3.00	0.25	0.63	1.13	39.00	
B2	0.82	0.74	0.00	2.88	0.13	0.63	1.38	203.00	
C1	0.78	0.69	0.00	3.00	0.13	0.63	1.25	302.00	
C2	1.05	0.77	0.00	3.00	0.38	1.00	1.63	345.00	
D-E	1.12	0.83	0.00	3.00	0.38	1.00	1.88	197.00	

Our group study showed that erosion presence, which should be considered a risk factor for higher disease severity leading to a worse overall prognosis [9], is more frequently seen in patients with a lower education level or classified in social classes C2 and D-E. It is also related to a longer time for the diagnosis and thus a delay in the beginning of treatment, which reaches an average of 41.7 and 50.8 months, respectively. Currently, there is a generalization of the concept of initial or early RA and of the existence of a window for a therapeutic opportunity, confirming the notion that early diagnosis and treatment can modify the course of the disease. Not to diagnose, or not to adequately treat a patient with very early symptoms of RA increases the risk of persistent inflammation and progressive joint damage [10], which in turn generates an important socioeconomic impact for the community.

Between January 2005 and October 2006, the QUEST-RA (Quantitative Patient Questionnaires in Standard Monitoring of Patients with RA) project, which included 4363 patients from 15 countries [11], showed that at the moment of the first symptoms, the rates of employment of patients younger than 65 years varied from 57 to 100% (average 86%) in men and from 19 to 87% (average 86%) in women, with the highest rates being seen in countries such as Sweden, Finland, Estonia and Lithuania and the lowest rates in countries such as Turkey, Kosovo, Morocco, Greece and Egypt. In general, more than one-third of the patients cited work disability due to RA because the probability of continuing working for 2 years was 80% and for 5 years was 68%, with similar patterns in countries with a high or low gross domestic product (GDP). The most significant determinant in work incapacity in all countries was the HAQ-DI [12].

An interesting result found in the QUEST-RA study suggests that, when comparing information between countries, patients from countries with a low GDP stay in work with higher levels of incapacity and disease activity than patients from countries with a high GDP [12]. Chung et al. also noted that the withdrawal of patients with RA from the workforce was greater in Finland, regardless of their clinical status, than in the United States, in order to avoid losing their health insurance and having to wait at least one year to be awarded disability payments [13].

These findings indicate that when looking at cases of RA, cultural and economic differences in societies affect work incapacity rates. The availability of biological agents led to expectations of a reduction in such rates; however, accounts of clinical group studies indicate that RA-related work disability continues to be a large problem [12, 14–16].

As such, early diagnosis and adequate therapeutic intervention with DMARDs becomes the principal objective to manage RA to significantly improve the clinical outcome and reduce joint damage [17]. The longest symptom duration allowed and the diagnosis of RA can be defined without the risk of irreversible damage varies greatly in the literature. In the context of the window of opportunity, at the beginning of the 1990s, initial RA was considered having a duration of symptoms of less than 24 months, with great emphasis on the first 12 months of clinical manifestations. At the moment, we aim to evaluate a patient with joint symptoms at the earliest opportunity possible, and the definition of the initial phase of RA includes the first weeks or months of symptoms (generally less than 12 months), highlighting the first 12 weeks of clinical manifestations as early or initial RA as being critical [10]. In Brazil, the group study shows an average of 32.5 months between the time from the onset of symptoms and the diagnosis and 38.6 months for the beginning of treatment. However, for the below literacy-level patients, this average time span extends to 65.4 months, compared with 14.4 months for those patients of postgraduate education, as well as an average of 47.8 months in patients classified as class D/E, compared with 26.4 in those classified in class B2. Such a difference, consequently, is also found in the time to the start of treatment. This information exposes the difficulty patients, principally those from a low educational level and economic classification, have in accessing a specialist at the beginning of the disease.

All the socioeconomic variables evaluated in this study were associated with differences in HAQ-DI. It is important to observe that the lowest HAQ-DI averages were found in patients who were economically active. In the QUEST-RA project, there were some biases found in the interpretation of the HAQ-DI. It is interesting to note that Socio-demographic factors cause relevant response bias in individual items of the health assessment questionnaire, but item bias has minor effect on composite HAQs indicating its overall accuracy across socio-demographic groups [18].

We observed that patients who need a caregiver had the highest HAQ-DI average (1.43) found in the study as a whole. Measurement of physical function at one point in time cannot distinguish impairment caused by the active disease process from chronic irreversible impairment. In this way, differences in the sources of functional limitations should be considered in the interpretation of functional measures, and in their use for prediction and in cost analyses [19].

The World Health Organization (WHO) specifies a series of individual factors in the system that can influence and determine the outcomes in pathologies. These factors include access and use of health services being recognized as independent determinants and are particularly relevant for patients who have chronic diseases.

The large differences in health as a result of the lack of access to care are often avoidable and unfair and so can be referred to as inequalities. However, the concept of equal access to care is complex and difficult to define clearly. Three principal dimensions of access can be identified, as follows: 1 - availability of care, implying a physical presence of doctors and medicine, appointment availability, geographic distribution, capacity of the system, etc.; 2 - accessibility that includes the financing of health caregivers and insurance to cover the costs; and 3- acceptability of the interposition between the provider and the patients' attitudes in relation to the engagement of health caregivers and mutual expectations [12].

The strengths of this study are to evaluate at a national level the characteristics of patients with rheumatoid arthritis, as well as to evaluate possible associations in order to alert the correct management of patients and thus reduce morbidity and mortality, for example through public health measures to aim for the therapeutic window. The limitations of this study are the lack of standardization in X-Ray erosion readings, besides the cross-sectional design, since without a proper follow-up along time, no firm causality conclusions can be drawn. It is important to say that all the sites enrolled in the study are "reference centers", and thus are unlikely to represent the broader management of RA across the country. It is probable that these patients present more severe disease, with a less favorable prognosis. REAL study was designed to be representative of the entire Brazilian population, but one center in the Northeast (representing 27.9% of population) could not participate because of delays in the Ethics Committee approval [8].

Conclusion

This study showed that the therapeutic window of RA is not being reached, and therefore we should have a policy to expand and ensure access to public health for all patients, especially those with lower levels of education and income for early diagnosis and treatment. For better disease control and consequently improve current outcomes such as reduced erosion prevalence and better quality of life for RA patients.

Authors' contributions

All authors made substantial contributions to the acquisition of data, have been involved in drafting the manuscript or revising it critically for important intellectual content, gave final approval of the version to be published and have participated sufficiently in the work to take public responsibility for appropriate portions of the content; and agreed to be accountable for all aspects of the work in ensuring that questions related to the accuracy or integrity of any part of the work are appropriately investigated and resolved.

Author details

[1]Hospital do ServidorPúblicoEstadual de São Paulo, Rua Pedro de Toledo, 1800, Vila Clementino, São Paulo, SP 04039-000, Brazil. [2]Universidade do Estado do Rio de Janeiro, Rio de Janeiro, Brazil. [3]Universidade de Brasília, Federal District, Brazil. [4]Universidade Federal do Paraná, Curitiba, Brazil. [5]Universidade Federal de Santa Catarina, Florianópolis, Brazil. [6]Universidade Federal de Minas Gerais, Belo Horizonte, Brazil. [7]UniversidadeEstadual de Campinas, Campinas, Brazil. [8]Universidade de São Paulo, Ribeirão Preto, Brazil. [9]Universidade Federal do Pará, Belém, Brazil. [10]Universidade de São Paulo, São Paulo, Brazil. [11]Universidade Federal do Rio Grande do Sul, Porto Alegre, Brazil.

References

1. Filipovic I, Walker D, Forster F, Curry AS. Quantifying the economic burden of productivity loss in rheumatoid arthritis. Rheumatology. 2011;50(6):1083–90.
2. Bengtsson C, Nordmark B, Klareskog L, et al. Socioeconomic status and the risk of developing RA: results from the Swedish EIRA study. Ann Rheum Dis. 2005;64(11):1588–94.
3. Liaoa KP, Alfredsson L, Karlsona EW. Environmental influences on risk for rheumatoid arthritis. Curr Opin Rheumatol. 2010;21(3):279–83.
4. Harrison MJ, Farragher TM, Clarke AM, et al. Association of functional outcome with both personal and area-level socioeconomic inequalities in patients with inflammatory polyarthritis. Arthritis Care Res. 2009;61(10):1297–304.
5. Hoving JL, Zwieten MCB, Meer M, et al. Work participation and arthritis: a systematic overview of challenges, adaptations and opportunities for interventions. Rheumatology. 2013;52(7):1254–64.
6. Walker N, Michaud K, Wolfe F. Work limitations among working persons with rheumatoid arthritis: results, reliability, and validity of the work limitations questionnaire in 836 patients. J Rheumatol. 2005;32:1006.
7. Hazes JM, Geuskens GA, Burdorf A. Work limitations in the outcome assessment of rheumatoid arthritis. J Rheumatol. 2005;32:980.
8. Castelar-Pinheiro GR, Vargas-Santos AB, Albuquerque CP, et al. The "REAL" Study: A Nationwide Prospective Study of Rheumatoid Arthritis in Brazil. Adv Rheumatol. 2018;58(9). https://doi.org/10.1186/s42358-018-0017-9.
9. Mota LMH, Cruz BA, Brenol CV, etal. Consenso da Sociedade Brasileira de Reumatologia 2011 para o diagnóstico e avaliação inicial da artrite reumatoide. Rev Bras Reumatol 2011; 51(3): 199–219.
10. Mota LMH, Laurindo IMM, Santos Neto LL. Artrite reumatoide inicial: conceitos. Rev Assoc Méd Bras. 2010;56(2):227–9.
11. Sokka T, Kautiainen H, Toloza S, et al. QUEST-RA: quantitative clinical assessment of patients with rheumatoid arthritis seen in standard rheumatology carein 15 countries. Ann Rheum Dis. 2007;66(11):1491–6.
12. Putrick P, Sokka T, Ramiro S, et al. Impact of socioeconomic gradients within and between countries on health of patients with rheumatoid arthritis (RA): lessons from QUEST-RA. Best Pract Res Clin Rheumatol. 2012;26:705–20.
13. Chung CP, Sokka T, Arbogast PG, Pincus T. Work disability in early rheumatoid arthritis: higher rates but better clinical status in Finland compared with the US. Ann Rheum Dis. 2006;65(12):1653–7.
14. Verstappen SM, Jacobs JW, Hyrich KL. Effect of anti-tumor necrosis factor on work disability. J Rheumatol 2007; 34(11): 2126–2128.
15. Wee MM, Lems WF, Usan H, et al. The effect of biological agents on work participation in rheumatoid arthritis patients: a systematic review. Ann Rheum Dis. 2012;71(2):161–71.
16. Sokka T, Envalds M, Pincus T. Treatment of rheumatoid arthritis: a global perspective on the use of antirheumatic drugs. Mod Rheumatol. 2008;18(3):228–39.
17. Biliavska I, Stamm TA, Martinez-Avila J, et al. Application of the 2010 ACR/EULAR classification criteria in patients with very early inflammatory arthritis: analysis of sensitivity, specificity and predictive values in the SAVE studycohort. Ann Rheum Dis. 2013;72:1335–41.
18. Hifinger M, Norton S, Ramiro S, et al. Equivalence in the health assessment questionnaire (HAQ) acrosssocio-demographic determinants: analyses within QUEST-RA. Semin Arthritis Rheum. 2018;47(4):492–500.
19. Aletaha D, Smolen J, Ward MM. Measuring function in rheumatoid arthritis: identifying reversible and irreversible components. Arthritis Rheum. 2006;54:2784.

20

Levels of CXCL13 and sICAM-1 correlate with disease activity score in patients with rheumatoid arthritis treated with tocilizumab

Katie Tuckwell[1*], Cem Gabay[2], Thierry Sornasse[1], Ruediger Paul Laubender[3], Jianmei Wang[4] and Michael J. Townsend[1]

Abstract

Background: Tocilizumab (TCZ), a humanized monoclonal antibody against the interleukin-6 receptor, has been proven to be a safe and effective treatment for rheumatoid arthritis (RA). Because RA is a heterogenous disease and patient response to treatments can vary, identifying characteristics that predict which patients are more likely to respond to TCZ is important for optimal patient care. Serum levels of C-X-C motif chemokine ligand 13 (CXCL13) and soluble intercellular adhesion molecule-1 (sICAM-1) have been associated with response to TCZ in patients with RA.

Objectives: To evaluate the association of CXCL13 and sICAM-1 with disease activity and response to TCZ in patients with early RA and those with inadequate response to disease-modifying antirheumatic drugs (DMARD-IR).

Methods: Baseline and week 24 serum CXCL13 and sICAM-1 levels were measured using available patient samples from the FUNCTION (early RA) and LITHE (DMARD-IR) trials. Correlations between CXCL13 and sICAM-1 levels and Disease Activity Score in 28 joints calculated with erythrocyte sedimentation rate (DAS28-ESR) at baseline and between change in CXCL13 and sICAM-1 and change in DAS28-ESR at week 24 were estimated. CXCL13 and sICAM-1 changes from baseline to week 24 were compared between treatment arms. The effects of TCZ treatment and baseline DAS28-ESR, CXCL13 and sICAM-1 levels on DAS28-ESR remission and 50% improvement per the American College of Rheumatology (ACR50) response at week 24 were determined.

Results: Overall, 458 patients from FUNCTION and 287 patients from LITHE were included. Correlation of baseline serum CXCL13 and sICAM-1 levels with DAS28-ESR was weak to moderate. CXCL13 and sICAM-1 levels decreased significantly at week 24 in TCZ-treated patients in both the early-RA and DMARD-IR populations. CXCL13 and sICAM-1 changes correlated moderately to weakly with DAS28-ESR changes at week 24 in both populations. The treatment regimen, but not baseline CXCL13 and sICAM-1 levels, had a significant effect on the likelihood of DAS28-ESR remission and ACR50 response.

Conclusions: Although CXCL13 and sICAM-1 are modestly associated with RA disease activity, they do not predict response to TCZ in all RA populations.

Keywords: Biomarkers, CXCL13, Rheumatoid arthritis, Tocilizumab, sICAM-1

* Correspondence: Tuckwell.katie@gene.com
[1]Genentech, Inc., 1 DNA Way, South San Francisco, CA 94080, USA
Full list of author information is available at the end of the article

Introduction

Rheumatoid arthritis (RA) is a pathologically heterogeneous disease, with variability between patients in the number of affected joints, antibody titers, serum cytokine levels, and severity of joint damage. Histological and molecular heterogeneity in synovial tissue of patients with RA has also been demonstrated [1–3]. Genome-wide expression analysis of synovial tissues from a large RA cohort demonstrated distinct molecular and cellular phenotypes, which reflect the heterogeneity present in the RA synovium [4]. Some of the clinical and treatment response heterogeneity may be explained by myeloid-, lymphoid-, and fibroid-dominant synovial subtypes of RA [5]. Although a wide range of treatment options have shown clinical benefit in patients with RA, it is unknown which patients will respond to specific treatments. Synovial tissue is often unavailable before the initiation of treatment; therefore, the use of serum biomarkers to predict which patients will respond to a specific treatment is an area of interest for rheumatologists.

The biomarker C-X-C motif chemokine ligand 13 (CXCL13) is a B-cell chemoattractant that is expressed by follicular dendritic cells in secondary lymphoid tissue and ectopic germinal centers [6]. Studies have shown a correlation between synovial tissue expression of CXCL13 and CXCL13 serum levels [7] and suggested that CXCL13 has a role in RA pathogenesis related to accumulation of B cells in inflamed synovium [8]. CXCL13 has been shown to be associated with the lymphoid phenotype of patients with RA [4]. Soluble intercellular adhesion molecule-1 (sICAM-1) is an adhesion molecule that is upregulated in a variety of cell types in response to TNFα signaling and has been shown to be associated with the myeloid synovial phenotype in patients with RA [4]. CXCL13 (lymphoid) and sICAM-1 (myeloid) were shown to differentially predict response in patients who received the anti–IL-6 receptor antibody tocilizumab (TCZ) as monotherapy and had prior inadequate response to methotrexate (MTX) [4]. In clinical practice, patients vary in terms of duration of RA and previous therapy. Studies are needed to analyze the association of biomarkers with disease activity and treatment response in varied populations of patients who receive TCZ either as monotherapy or in combination with MTX for the treatment of RA. This study aimed to determine whether there is an association of CXCL13 and sICAM-1 with disease activity and response to TCZ in patients with early RA and those with inadequate response to disease-modifying antirheumatic drugs (DMARD-IR).

Materials and methods

Patient inclusion and exclusion criteria and methods for the FUNCTION and LITHE trials were described previously [9, 10]. Patients in FUNCTION had moderate to severe RA of ≤ 2 years' duration (early RA) and had not previously received MTX or biologic agents [9]. Patients in LITHE had moderate to severe RA for ≥ 6 months with an inadequate response to MTX (DMARD-IR) [10]. The FUNCTION and LITHE study protocols were approved by an ethics committee or institutional review board at each participating center before the start of the study. All patients provided written informed consent in accordance with the Declaration of Helsinki.

For the present study, patients from FUNCTION and LITHE placebo (PBO) + MTX arms, TCZ 8 mg/kg monotherapy arm (FUNCTION only), and TCZ 8 mg/kg + MTX arms were selected based on baseline and week 24 serum sample availability. Patients from the TCZ 4 mg/kg arms were not selected. Serum CXCL13 and sICAM-1 levels were measured using a commercial ELLA (automated enzyme-linked immunosorbent assay) and performed in accordance with the relevant national and international regulations and guidance by Microcoat Biotechnologie GmbH (Bernried am Starnberger See, Germany). The CXCL13 assay (ProteinSimple, San Jose, CA, USA) was conducted using 25 μL of serum samples, which were diluted two-fold. The lower limit of quantification as calculated for undiluted serum ranged from 1.14 to 1.58 pg/mL depending on the kit lot of the assay and the upper limit of quantification was 12,220 pg/mL for all kit lots of the assay. The precision, as determined from the analysis of quality control samples, was satisfactory throughout the analytical study and ranged from 0.124 to 10.211% for low quality control (LQC) and from 0.384 to 10.153% for high quality control (HQC). The mean concentration of LQC was 20.387 pg/mL with a coefficient of variation (CV) of 7.4%. The mean concentration of HQC was 974.169 pg/mL with a CV of 5.5%.

The sICAM-1 assay (ProteinSimple, San Jose, CA, USA) was conducted using 5 μL of serum samples, which were diluted 100-fold. The lower limit of quantification as calculated for undiluted serum was 410 pg/mL and the upper limit of quantification as calculated for undiluted serum was 1,563,000 pg/mL. The precision, as determined from the analysis of quality control samples, was satisfactory throughout the analytical study and ranged from 0.064 to 17.640% for LQC and from 0.160 to 11.660% for HQC. The mean concentration of LQC was 114.531 pg/mL with a CV of 9.7%. The mean concentration of HQC was 5240.573 pg/mL with a CV of 6.8%.

Statistical analysis

Baseline clinical characteristics were compared between the FUNCTION biomarker population and the LITHE biomarker population using the Welch t test on transformed data; P values <0.05 were considered statistically significant. Correlations between CXCL13 or sICAM-1 levels and DAS28-ESR scores were evaluated according to the Pearson correlation coefficient. Changes in CXCL13 and sICAM-1 from baseline to week 24 were compared between treatment arms using the Welch t test. The effect of treatment and baseline DAS28-ESR, CXCL13, and sICAM-1 on the likelihood of DAS28-ESR remission and 50% improvement per the American College of Rheumatology (ACR50) response at week 24 was estimated via logistic regression. Log transformation was used for the biomarker values to ensure a more normal distribution of the data. Results were not adjusted for multiple testing.

Results

Overall, 458 of 869 patients from FUNCTION (TCZ 8 mg/kg monotherapy, n = 157; TCZ 8 mg/kg + MTX, n = 160; PBO + MTX, n = 141) and 287 of 791 patients from LITHE (TCZ 8 mg/kg + MTX, n = 137; PBO + MTX, n = 150) were included. Mean disease duration in FUNCTION (early RA) was significantly shorter than in LITHE (DMARD-IR; 0.45 vs 8.65 years; $P < 0.0001$); mean ESR at baseline was significantly higher in patients in FUNCTION than in those in LITHE (Table 1). At baseline, CXCL13 levels correlated moderately with DAS28-ESR in the early-RA population ($r = 0.36$; $P < 0.0001$) and weakly in the DMARD-IR population ($r = 0.21$; $P = 0.0003$) (Fig. 1). Correlation between sICAM-1 levels and DAS28-ESR was low in both the early-RA ($r = 0.14$; $P = 0.0029$) and DMARD-IR populations ($r = 0.17$; $P = 0.0040$).

In the early-RA population, baseline CXCL13 correlated weakly with all 4 components of DAS28-ESR (tender joint count, $r = 0.2$; swollen joint count [SJC], $r = 0.24$; ESR, $r = 0.34$; Patient Global Assessment [PGA], $r = 0.24$; $P < 0.000031$ for all), whereas sICAM-1 only correlated weakly with SJC ($r = 0.15$; $P < 0.0031$) and ESR ($r = 0.17$; $P < 0.00031$). In the DMARD-IR population, baseline CXCL13 correlated weakly with ESR ($r = 0.20$; $P < 0.0031$) and PGA

($r = 0.22$; $P < 0.00031$), and sICAM-1 did not significantly correlate with any of the DAS28-ESR components.

The proportion of patients who achieved ACR50 response and DAS28-ESR remission by study population and treatment arm are shown in Fig. 2. Response to treatment was similar between patients in the present biomarker analysis and the intent-to-treat (ITT) populations in the FUNCTION and LITHE trials (data not shown). CXCL13 decreased significantly at week 24 in all treatment arms in both the early-RA and DMARD-IR populations, with the greatest reductions observed in the TCZ + MTX and TCZ monotherapy arms (Fig. 3a). In the early-RA population, the effect of TCZ monotherapy on CXCL13 was similar to that of TCZ + MTX. sICAM-1 decreased significantly at week 24 in the TCZ monotherapy arm in patients with early RA and the TCZ + MTX arms in both the early-RA and DMARD-IR populations but not in the PBO + MTX arms (Fig. 3b).

Change in CXCL13 correlated moderately with change in DAS28-ESR at week 24 in both the early-RA and DMARD-IR populations ($r = 0.33$; $P < 0.0001$ for both) (Fig. 4). Change in sICAM-1 correlated moderately with change in DAS28-ESR at week 24 in the DMARD-IR population ($r = 0.26$; $P = 0.0002$) but weakly in the early-RA population ($r = 0.16$; $P = 0.0005$). Although the treatment arm had a significant effect on the likelihood of DAS28-ESR remission and achievement of ACR50, the effects of baseline levels of CXCL13 and sICAM-1 were not significant (Additional file 1: Table S1). Furthermore, biomarker categories based on high vs low baseline CXCL13 and sICAM-1 levels did not predict response to TCZ or MTX in the early-RA or DMARD-IR populations (data not shown).

We assessed differences between extreme responders and nonresponders in the FUNCTION and LITHE trials by defining highest DAS28 response as those patients

Table 1 Baseline Clinical Characteristics

Baseline Clinical Characteristics, Mean (SD)	FUNCTION Biomarker Population (n = 458)	LITHE Biomarker Population (n = 287)	P Value*	FUNCTION ITT Population			LITHE ITT Population	
				TCZ 8 mg/kg Monotherapy (n = 292)	TCZ 8 mg/kg + MTX (n = 290)	PBO + MTX (n = 287)	TCZ 8 mg/kg + MTX (n = 398)	PBO + MTX (n = 393)
Disease duration, years	0.45 (0.50)	8.65 (7.80)	< 0.0001	0.5 (0.48)	0.5 (0.53)	0.4 (0.48)	9.3 (8.2)	9.0 (8.1)
TJC68	28.8 (16.9)	29.0 (15.5)	0.5594	28.7 (16.3)	28.7 (16.7)	27.4 (16.5)	29.3 (15.2)	27.9 (14.8)
SJC66	17.3 (11.5)	16.4 (9.5)	0.4889	16.5 (10.1)	17.6 (12.4)	16.2 (10.4)	17.3 (9.5)	16.6 (9.2)
DAS28-ESR	6.7 (1.0)	6.5 (0.9)	0.0013	6.7 (1.0)	6.7 (1.1)	6.6 (1.0)	6.6 (1.0)	6.5 (1.0)
ESR, mm/h	53.0 (28.8)	43.1 (21.4)	< 0.0001	51.3 (28.4)	52.8 (30.2)	50.4 (26.8)	46.3 (24.8)	46.4 (24.7)
CRP, mg/dL	2.5 (2.8)	2.1 (2.5)	0.2702	2.5 (3.2)	2.6 (3.0)	2.3 (2.7)	2.3 (2.6)	2.2 (2.5)
PGA, 100-mm VAS	63.0 (18.8)	62.6 (16.9)	0.7807	63.9 (18.1)	63.6 (18.1)	62.7 (17.3)	62.7 (16.9)	63.1 (17.3)

CRP C-reactive protein, DAS28-ESR Disease Activity Score in 28 joints calculated with erythrocyte sedimentation rate; DMARD-IR inadequate response to disease-modifying antirheumatic drugs; ESR erythrocyte sedimentation rate; ITT intent to treat; PGA Patient Global Assessment; RA rheumatoid arthritis; SJC66 swollen joint count in 66 joints; TJC68 tender joint count in 68 joints; VAS visual analog scale
* P value is for the comparison between the FUNCTION biomarker population and the LITHE biomarker population

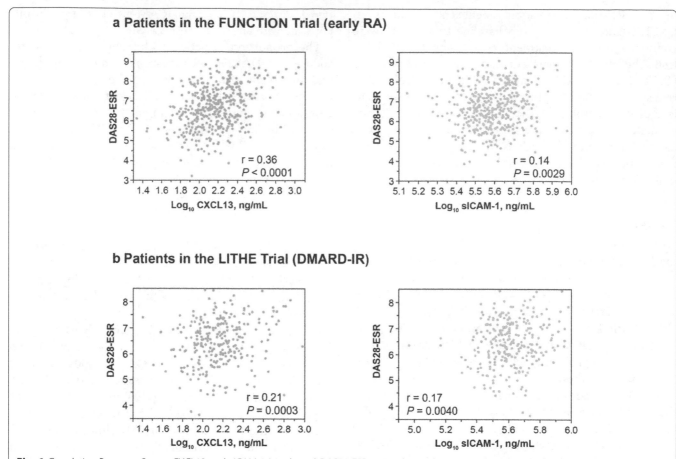

a Patients in the FUNCTION Trial (early RA)

b Patients in the LITHE Trial (DMARD-IR)

Fig. 1 Correlation Between Serum CXCL13 and sICAM-1 Levels and DAS28-ESR at Baseline. **a** Patients in the FUNCTION trial (early RA). **b** Patients in the LITHE trial (DMARD-IR). CXCL13, C-X-C motif chemokine ligand 13; DAS28-ESR, Disease Activity Score in 28 joints calculated with erythrocyte sedimentation rate; DMARD-IR, inadequate response to disease-modifying antirheumatic drugs; RA, rheumatoid arthritis; sICAM-1, soluble intercellular adhesion molecule-1

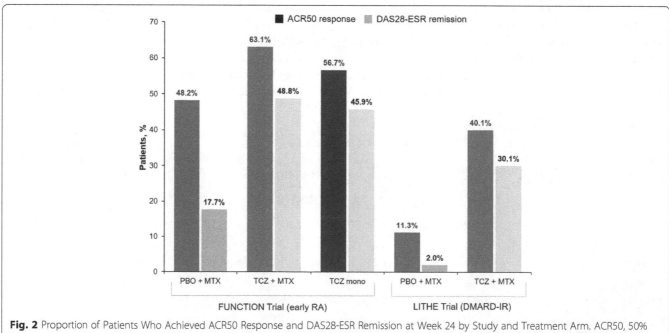

Fig. 2 Proportion of Patients Who Achieved ACR50 Response and DAS28-ESR Remission at Week 24 by Study and Treatment Arm. ACR50, 50% improvement per the American College of Rheumatology; DAS28-ESR, Disease Activity Score in 28 joints calculated with erythrocyte sedimentation rate; DMARD-IR, inadequate response to disease-modifying antirheumatic drugs; mono, monotherapy; MTX, methotrexate; PBO, placebo; RA, rheumatoid arthritis; TCZ, tocilizumab

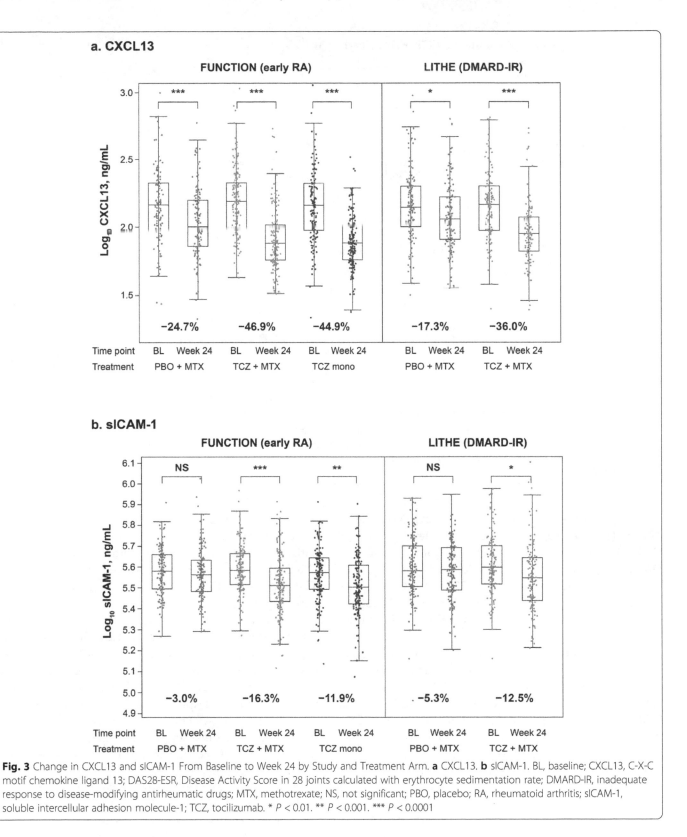

Fig. 3 Change in CXCL13 and sICAM-1 From Baseline to Week 24 by Study and Treatment Arm. **a** CXCL13. **b** sICAM-1. BL, baseline; CXCL13, C-X-C motif chemokine ligand 13; DAS28-ESR, Disease Activity Score in 28 joints calculated with erythrocyte sedimentation rate; DMARD-IR, inadequate response to disease-modifying antirheumatic drugs; MTX, methotrexate; NS, not significant; PBO, placebo; RA, rheumatoid arthritis; sICAM-1, soluble intercellular adhesion molecule-1; TCZ, tocilizumab. * $P < 0.01$. ** $P < 0.001$. *** $P < 0.0001$

who achieve DAS28 remission status at 24 weeks and defining lowest DAS28 response as those patients who failed to achieve a decrease in DAS28 of at least 0.6. In the FUNCTION trial, patients receiving TCZ who achieved remission had a mean (SD) sICAM1 level of 398.89 (99.62) ng/ml and CXCL13 level of 162.64 (109.69) pg/ml, whereas patients who failed to achieve a DAS28 response had a sICAM1 level of 397.34 (117.33) ng/ml and CXCL13 level of 102.63 (33.75) pg/ml. Similarly in the LITHE trial, patients receiving TCZ who

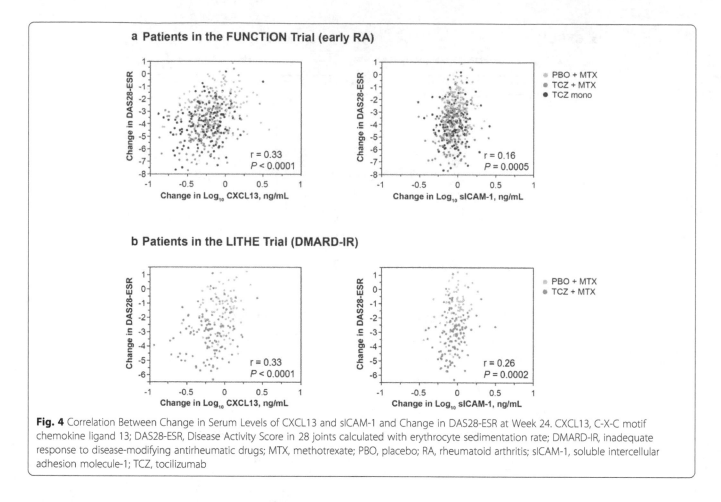

Fig. 4 Correlation Between Change in Serum Levels of CXCL13 and sICAM-1 and Change in DAS28-ESR at Week 24. CXCL13, C-X-C motif chemokine ligand 13; DAS28-ESR, Disease Activity Score in 28 joints calculated with erythrocyte sedimentation rate; DMARD-IR, inadequate response to disease-modifying antirheumatic drugs; MTX, methotrexate; PBO, placebo; RA, rheumatoid arthritis; sICAM-1, soluble intercellular adhesion molecule-1; TCZ, tocilizumab

achieved remission had a mean (SD) sICAM1 level of 421.28 (139.49) ng/ml and CXCL13 level of 165.09 (104.84) pg/ml, whereas patients who failed to achieve a DAS28 response had a sICAM1 level of 426.94 (150.03) ng/ml and CXCL13 level of 176.13 (153.22) pg/ml. Therefore, even in patients with extremes of DAS28 response, baseline levels of CXCL13 and sICAM1 did not differ significantly.

A higher proportion of patients in the ITT population of the LITHE trial were receiving glucocorticoids at baseline (PBO + MTX, 70%; TCZ + MTX, 62%) [10] than patients in the ITT population in the FUNCTION trial (PBO + MTX, 38%; TCZ + MTX, 33%; TCZ mono, 40%) [9]. Inclusion criteria related to glucocorticoids were similar between studies [9, 10].

Discussion

In the present study, the association of CXCL13 with disease activity in RA was stronger in early-RA patients than in DMARD-IR patients. Prior exposure to DMARDs may have affected baseline CXCL13 levels, despite patients having active RA. Furthermore, a study of DMARD-naïve patients with early RA (< 3 months) proposed that high levels of CXCL13 possibly indicated recent inflammation [11]. Changes in CXCL13 and, to a lesser extent, sICAM-1 correlated significantly with changes in DAS28-ESR at week 24. Notably, in early-RA patients, the effect of TCZ monotherapy on changes in CXCL13 was similar to that observed with TCZ + MTX. The decrease in CXCL13 with disease activity was consistent with a previous study analyzing CXCL13 in patients treated with rituximab [7].

In the DMARD-IR patients, CXCL13 levels decreased significantly in patients in the PBO + MTX group. We suspect that this decrease in CXCL13 level is due to the anti-inflammatory effect of methotrexate treatment in these patients, despite their previously reported DMARD-IR status. This effect on the levels of an inflammatory biomarker could reflect better MTX treatment adherence due to the closer medical monitoring while enrolled in a clinical trial.

The results of the present study differed from those of a study of patients with RA (MTX-IR) from the ADACTA trial, which demonstrated that patients with high baseline CXCL13 levels were more likely to respond to TCZ monotherapy than patients with high sICAM-1 levels [4]. The effect of MTX on CXCL13 and sICAM-1 may have contributed to the discordant study results. More patients in the present study received TCZ + MTX ($n = 297$) than TCZ monotherapy ($n = 157$). However, a study of patients with inadequate response to tumor necrosis factor inhibitors who received sarilumab + DMARDs was also unable to fully replicate the biomarker results from ADACTA [12].

Although this study is among the first to evaluate the serum biomarkers CXCL13 and sICAM-1 in early-RA and DMARD-IR patients who received TCZ, it does have limitations. This study used available samples only, which may have resulted in a biased population. However, DAS28 and ACR50 results were similar between patients in the present biomarker study and the ITT populations in the FUNCTION and LITHE trials. In addition, Clinical Disease Activity Index values were not calculated, although they may have been informative because changes in ESR may explain some of the association between decreased CXCL13 and sICAM-1 and decreased disease activity.

Conclusions

In summary, baseline CXCL13 and sICAM-1 levels did not predict response to TCZ at week 24, suggesting that although CXCL13 and sICAM-1 were modestly associated with RA disease activity, they do not predict response to TCZ in all RA populations.

Supplementary information

Additional file 1: Table S1. Online Resource 1 Multivariate Logistic Regression Model for DAS28-ESR Remission and ACR50 Response at Week 24.

Abbreviations

ACR50: 50% improvement per the American College of Rheumatology; CV: Coefficient of variation; CXCL13: C-X-C motif chemokine ligand 13; DAS28-ESR: Disease Activity Score in 28 joints calculated with erythrocyte sedimentation rate; DMARD-IR: Inadequate response to disease-modifying antirheumatic drugs; ESR: Erythrocyte sedimentation rate; HQC: Higher quality control; ITT: Intent to treat; LQC: Lower quality control; MTX: Methotrexate; PGA: Patient global assessment; RA: Rheumatoid arthritis; sICAM-1: Soluble intercellular adhesion molecule-1; SJC: Swollen joint count; TCZ: Tocilizumab

Acknowledgements

Support for third-party writing assistance for this manuscript, furnished by Nicola Gillespie, DVM, of Health Interactions, Inc., was provided by Genentech, Inc.

Authors' contributions

KT analyzed and interpreted study data and contributed to the preparation and writing of the manuscript. CG interpreted the findings and contributed to writing of the manuscript. TS analyzed and interpreted study data and contributed to the preparation and review of the manuscript. RPL and JW contributed to the preparation and review of the manuscript. MJT analyzed and interpreted study data and contributed to the preparation and writing of the manuscript. All authors read and approved the final manuscript.

Author details

[1]Genentech, Inc., 1 DNA Way, South San Francisco, CA 94080, USA. [2]University Hospital of Geneva, Geneva, Switzerland. [3]Roche Diagnostics, Penzberg, Germany. [4]Roche Products, Welwyn Garden City, UK.

References

1. Lindstrom TM, Robinson WH. Biomarkers for rheumatoid arthritis: making it personal. Scand J Clin Lab Invest Suppl. 2010;242:79–84.
2. van Baarsen LG, Bos CL, van der Pouw Kraan TC, Verweij CL. Transcription profiling of rheumatic diseases. Arthritis Res Ther. 2009;11(1):207.
3. van der Pouw Kraan TC, van Gaalen FA, Huizinga TW, Pieterman E, Breedveld FC, Verweij CL. Discovery of distinctive gene expression profiles in rheumatoid synovium using cDNA microarray technology: evidence for the existence of multiple pathways of tissue destruction and repair. Genes Immun. 2003;4(3):187–96.
4. Dennis G Jr, Holweg CT, Kummerfeld SK, Choy DF, Setiadi AF, Hackney JA, et al. Synovial phenotypes in rheumatoid arthritis correlate with response to biologic therapeutics. Arthritis Res Ther. 2014;16(2):R90.
5. Humby F, Kelly S, Hands R, Rocher V, DiCicco M, Ng N, et al. Use of ultrasound-guided small joint biopsy to evaluate the histopathologic response to rheumatoid arthritis therapy: recommendations for application to clinical trials. Arthritis Rheumatol (Hoboken, NJ). 2015;67(10):2601–10.
6. Corsiero E, Bombardieri M, Manzo A, Bugatti S, Uguccioni M, Pitzalis C. Role of lymphoid chemokines in the development of functional ectopic lymphoid structures in rheumatic autoimmune diseases. Immunol Lett. 2012;145(1–2):62–7.
7. Rosengren S, Wei N, Kalunian KC, Kavanaugh A, Boyle DL. CXCL13: a novel biomarker of B-cell return following rituximab treatment and synovitis in patients with rheumatoid arthritis. Rheumatology (Oxford, England). 2011; 50(3):603–10.
8. Armas-Gonzalez E, Dominguez-Luis MJ, Diaz-Martin A, Arce-Franco M, Castro-Hernandez J, Danelon G, et al. Role of CXCL13 and CCL20 in the recruitment of B cells to inflammatory foci in chronic arthritis. Arthritis Res Ther. 2018;20(1):114 -018-1611-2.
9. Burmester GR, Rigby WF, van Vollenhoven RF, Kay J, Rubbert-Roth A, Kelman A, et al. Tocilizumab in early progressive rheumatoid arthritis: FUNCTION, a randomised controlled trial. Ann Rheum Dis. 2016;75(6): 1081–91.
10. Kremer JM, Blanco R, Brzosko M, Burgos-Vargas R, Halland AM, Vernon E, et al. Tocilizumab inhibits structural joint damage in rheumatoid arthritis patients with inadequate responses to methotrexate: results from the double-blind treatment phase of a randomized placebo-controlled trial of tocilizumab safety and prevention of structural joint damage at one year. Arthritis Rheum. 2011;63(3):609–21.
11. Greisen SR, Schelde KK, Rasmussen TK, Kragstrup TW, Stengaard-Pedersen K, Hetland ML, et al. CXCL13 predicts disease activity in early rheumatoid arthritis and could be an indicator of the therapeutic 'window of opportunity'. Arthritis Res Ther. 2014;16(5):434–014 -0434-z.
12. Gabay C, Msihid J, Zilberstein M, Paccard C, Lin Y, Graham NMH, et al. Identification of sarilumab pharmacodynamic and predictive markers in patients with inadequate response to TNF inhibition: a biomarker substudy of the phase 3 TARGET study. RMD Open. 2018;4(1):e000607–2017 eCollection 2018.

21

Burden of rheumatoid arthritis on patients' work productivity and quality of life

Ricardo Machado Xavier[1]*(iD), Cristiano Augusto Freitas Zerbini[2](iD), Daniel Feldman Pollak[3],
Jorge Luis Alberto Morales-Torres[4](iD), Philippe Chalem[5], José Fernando Molina Restrepo[6], Javier Arnaldo Duhau[7],
Jacqueline Rodríguez Amado[8], Maurício Abello[9], Maria Celina de la Vega[10](iD), Adriana Pérez Dávila[11],
Priscila Martin Biegun[12], Maysa Silva Arruda[12] and Cesar Ramos-Remus[13](iD)

Abstract

Background: To determine the burden of Rheumatoid Arthritis (RA) on patients' work productivity and health related quality of life (HRQoL), and examine the influence of several exposure variables; to analyze the progression of RA over 1 year and its impact on work productivity and HRQoL.

Methods: International multicenter prospective survey including patients in 18 centers in Argentina, Brazil, Colombia and Mexico with diagnosis of RA and aged between 21-55 years. The following standard questionnaires were completed at baseline and throughout a 1-year follow-up: WPAI:RA, WALS, WLQ-25, EQ-5D-3 L and SF-36. Clinical and demographic variables were also collected through interview.

Results: The study enrolled 290 patients on baseline visit. Overall mean scores at baseline visit were: WPAI:RA (presenteeism) = 29.5% (SD = 28.8%); WPAI:RA (absenteeism) = 9.0% (SD = 23.2%); WPAI:RA (absenteeism and presenteeism) = 8.6% (SD = 22.6%); WALS = 9.0 (SD = 6.1); WLQ-25 = 7.0% (SD = 5.1%); SF-36 Physical Scale = 39.1 (SD = 10.3) and Mental Scale = 45.4 (SD = 11.3); EQ-5D-3 L VAS = 69.8 (SD = 20.4) and EQ-5D-3 L index = 0.67 (SD = 0.23). Higher educational levels were associated with better results in WLQ-25, while previous orthopedic surgeries reduced absenteeism results of WPAI:RA and work limitations in WLQ-25. Higher disease duration was associated with decreased HRQoL. Intensification of disease activity was associated with decreased work productivity and HRQoL, except in WLQ-25. In the longitudinal analysis, worsening in disease activity was associated with a decrease in both work productivity and HRQoL.

Conclusions: RA patients are dealing with workplace disabilities and limitations and loss in HRQoL, and multiple factors seems to be associated with this. Worsening of disease activity further decreased work productivity and HRQoL, stressing the importance of disease tight control.

Keywords: Rheumatoid arthritis, Quality of life, Work performance, Surveys, Latin America

Introduction

Rheumatoid Arthritis (RA) is an autoimmune disease that causes chronic inflammation and proliferation in the synovial tissue of joints, leading to cartilage damage and joint destruction [1–3]. Irreversible damage occurs early and continue throughout the patient's life [4–6]. RA affects approximately 1% of the United States (US)

population, and this prevalence varies from 0.4 to 1.6% in Latin America population [7–9].

Since RA is not curable, the goals of RA therapy are to reach disease remission or to achieve low disease activity [10, 11]. Aggressive treatment in early RA has shown to reduce functional disability over time, and positively influence employment [12, 13]. Lack of optimal control leads to joint damage and loss of physical function, work impairment, and finally permanent work disability. Unceasing joint injury and irreversible loss of physical functioning will negatively impact patients' work performance and/or employability. A recent study

* Correspondence: rxavier10@gmail.com
[1]Universidade Federal do Rio Grande do Sul, Hospital de Clínicas de Porto Alegre, Porto Alegre, Brazil
Full list of author information is available at the end of the article

showed that work disability rates increases in accordance to disease duration: 35, 39, and 44% after 5, 10, and 15 years of RA diagnosis, respectively [14].

There is still a need of detailed information on how RA patients are successful on preserving employability and how is the current burden of RA on work productivity in Latin America.

Therefore, this study primarily aimed to determine the burden of RA on patients' work productivity and health related quality of life (HRQoL) and to explore the impact of related variables. Additionally, the progression of RA and its impact on work productivity and HRQoL were also investigated.

Methods
Study design and eligibility criteria
PROSE RA study (Patient Reported Outcomes Survey of Employment among patients with RA) is an international multicenter prospective survey. Patients were included from May/2012 to September/2015 in 18 rheumatology public and private clinics from four Latin American countries: Argentina, Brazil, Colombia and Mexico. All sites in Argentina, Colombia and Mexico were private, while 2 out of 3 Brazilian sites were publicly funded. Patients diagnosed with RA identified in outpatient routine visits were invited to participate and were included if they met the eligibility criteria: Age between 21 and 55 years (representing a working age group); documented diagnosis of RA as defined by the revised 1987 classification criteria of the American College of Rheumatology (ACR) [15]; and willing to provide informed consent to participate in the study. Patients not able to give informed consent and/or to complete the study procedures were excluded. Two different analyses were performed: cross-sectional to determine the burden of RA on patients' work productivity and HRQoL (primary) considering the baseline answers to selected patient-reported outcomes (PROs), and longitudinal over 1 year to evaluate the progression of RA and its impact on work productivity and HRQoL (secondary).

Data collection
Five study visits were performed every three months over 1-year follow-up. During each visit, participants answered an interview that assessed data about sociodemographic and clinical characteristics, lifestyle behavior, disease activity, use of Disease-Modifying Antirheumatic Drugs (DMARDs), direct medical resource utilization and medication coverage/insurance. Impact on work productivity and HRQoL was evaluated using standardized instruments: Workplace Activity Limitation Scale (WALS), Work Productivity and Activity Impairment Questionnaire - Rheumatoid Arthritis (WPAI:RA), 25-

Item Work Limitations Questionnaire (WLQ-25), 36-Item Short Form Health Survey (SF-36) and EuroQol 5 Dimensions Questionnaire 3 level version (EQ-5D-3 L). All standardized questionnaires were adequately translated into Brazilian Portuguese and Spanish. Some of the instruments had already been validated with final versions reported in previous publications or by their copyright holders. [16–20] The remaining questionnaires and versions were validated within the scope of the study, using usual methods in the field.

Work productivity
WALS is a 12-item questionnaire that assesses patient's limitation at work without a recall period. Answers options consist of a 4-point Likert scale that ranges from 0 (no difficulties) to 3 (not able to do). Dimensions includes difficulty getting to and from work, lifting, working with hands, crouching/bending/kneeling/reaching, work pace, concentration, standing/sitting for long periods, and meeting work demands. Overall score ranges from 0 to 36 points and higher measures indicate greater limitation [21].

WPAI:RA contains six questions to measure disabilities in paid and unpaid work in the last seven days. Results include four scores that summarize the percentage of: work time missed due to health; impairment while working due to health; activity impairment due to health; and Overall work impairment score due to health problems. The scores ranges from 0 to 100 points and higher measures indicate greater limitation in each domain [22].

WLQ-25 is composed by 25-items and focuses on presenteeism and the proportion of work-time with limitation as opposed to the degree of difficulty or severity of limitations. It assesses four dimensions of presenteeism while at work: physical demands, time management, mental-interpersonal demands and output demands. Questions regarding work productivity and performance over the past 2–4 weeks were answered using a 5-point Likert scale, ranging from 0 (none of the time) to 4 (all of the time). Each scale was scored separately and scores were converted from 0 to 100, where higher scores represent increased limitations [23, 24].

Health-related quality of life
SF-36 is a composed by 36 questions grouped into 8 domains (physical functioning, role-physical, bodily pain, general health, vitality, social functioning, role-emotional, and mental-health). Two summary measures are also provided: Physical Component Summary (PCS) and Mental Component Summary (MCS). The raw score of each dimension was converted into a value from 0 (worst possible health state) to 100 (best possible health state). All scales were standardized to the 1998 general

US population using the norm base scale algorithm. Scale score < 45 can be interpreted as being below the average range for the general population [25].

EQ-5D-3 L assesses health status through 5 domains (mobility, self-care, usual activities, pain/discomfort and anxiety/depression) considering 3 levels: no problems, some problems, extreme problems. Additionally, a Visual Analogue Scale (EQ-VAS) records respondents' self-rated health from "Best imaginable health state"=0 to "Worst imaginable health state"=100. Utility score represents a scale between death = 0 and perfect health = 1 and is derived from the answers to each dimension, calculated using the United Kingdom algorithm [26, 27].

Disease progression

Multi-Dimensional Health Assessment Questionnaire (MDHAQ) was used in the first and last visits to evaluate disease activity, which is a 4-domains measure: physical function (FN), pain (PN), Rheumatoid Arthritis Disease Activity Index (RADAI) and patient global estimate (PTGL). Final disease activity measure was obtained using Rheumatology Assessment Patient Index Data 3 measures (RAPID3), calculated from the answers of three MDHAQ domains (FN, PN and PTGL). RAPID3 score ranges from 0 to 30 points and classify patients into four groups: remission (≤3 points), low severity (3.1 to 6 points), moderate severity (6.1 to 12 points) and high severity (> 12 points) [28]. Disease progression was defined as disease activity modification during the study period, considering the interval between the first and last visits, classified in the following categories: Improvement or maintenance; and Worsen.

Sample size calculation

PROSE RA study was primarily designed to assess how RA impacts on work productivity and HRQoL at baseline and also to analyze association with exposure variables. Thus, sample size was calculated based on assumptions of potential differences between these groups from published data [20, 29–32]. Simulations for a descriptive approach were performed to assure an adequate precision of estimated parameter using two different margins of error: a score difference observed by each subgroup and a fixed value of 5.0% of the maximum in each scale. Considering $a = 0.05$ and a power of 0.80 and adopting a conservative approach, the higher estimated sample size was select ($N = 280$) assuring that the study would have power to detect the smallest difference.

Statistical analysis

Descriptive analysis was performed through means and standard deviation to quantitative variables, and frequency to qualitative variables. Data were tested for normal distribution using the Shapiro-Wilk and Kolmogorov-Smirnov tests. To compare means, variables with normal distribution were analyzed by the Student's t-test and those with non-normal distribution by Mann-Whitney or Wilcoxon nonparametric tests. Linear regression was used to build a multivariate model to assess the association between outcomes and exposure variables, controlled for possible confounders and interactions. Due to the small sample size for each country, bivariate and multivariate analyses were performed considering the entire sample only. Analysis of the impact of disease progression (longitudinal) on work productivity and HRQoL was assessed through the difference on mean scores between study visits 1 and 5. Thus, these differences are shown and tested among disease progression groups: "Improvement or maintenance" and "Worsening".

Only valid answers were used for all PROs. Guidelines [21, 23, 25, 26, 28] from each standardized instruments report different strategies to deal with missing data as follows: MDHAQ (if at least one question left unanswered in any domain, patient excluded from this specific analysis); WALS (patient excluded from specific analysis, if more than two questions left unanswered; values estimated through the mean of answered data, if until two questions left unanswered or the answer of any question "refused"); WPAI:RA (questionnaires with missing answers did not have the corresponding score calculated); WLQ (patient excluded from specific analysis if > 2 questions were left unanswered); SF-36 (missing values estimated through the mean of answered data in the same scale for patients with responses for at least half of the domain questions); and EQ-5D-3 L (patient excluded of specific analysis, if any question left unanswered).

Stata (version MP12) and R Project (version 3.2) were adopted to perform the analysis with a 95% confidence interval and p-value≤0.05.

Ethical approval

Research was reviewed and approved by Independent Ethics Committee according to study site and responsible committees are listed in Additional file 1: Table S1. All procedures were in accordance with the ethical standards from each country and with the Helsinki declaration and its later amendments or comparable ethical standards. Written informed consent and authorization to use and/or disclose his/her anonymised health data was obtained from all participants.

Results

Sociodemographic and clinical characteristics

The study enrolled 290 patients at baseline: 75 (25.9%) from Argentina, 75 (25.9%) from Mexico, 72 (24.8%)

from Colombia and 68 (23.4%) from Brazil. Sociodemographic and clinical characteristics are shown in Tables 1 and 2.

NA = Not applicable.

RA = Rheumatoid Arthritis.

SD = Standard Deviation.

DMARDs = Disease-Modifying Antirheumatic Drugs.

RA = Rheumatoid Arthritis.

RAPID3 = Rheumatology Assessment Patient Index Data 3 measures.

SD = Standard Deviation.

Work productivity at baseline

Table 3 shows descriptive analysis of WALS, WPAI:RA and WLQ-25. Results stratified in accordance with exposure variables for total sample and final models for each questionnaires' measures are shown in Additional file 1: Tables S2 and S3, respectively.

RA = Rheumatoid Arthritis.

SD = Standard Deviation.

WALS=Workplace Activity Limitation Scale.

WLQ-25 = 25-item Work Limitations Questionnaire.

WPAI:RA = Work Productivity and Activity Impairment Questionnaire - Rheumatoid Arthritis.

Overall mean WALS score in total sample was 9.0 (SD = 6.1), ranging from 8.2 (SD = 6.3) in Mexico to 10.6 (SD = 6.8) in Brazil. At least 40.3% of RA patients reported some disability in each of the WALS questions. Main limitations informed in the workplace were difficulty to crouch, bend, kneel or work in awkward positions (84.0%) and to lift, carry or move objects (80.1%). A similar pattern was observed among participating countries. Multivariate analysis showed that higher work limitation according to WALS was observed when patients had medication coverage/insurance (β = 2.35; 95%CI = 0.21 to 4.50; p = 0.031) and increased disease activity level (β = 3.67; 95%CI = 3.01 to 4.34; p < 0.001).

Employment was reported by 60.3% of the total respondents of WPAI:RA - 72.6% in Argentina, 62.5% in Colombia, 57.3% in Mexico and 44.2% in Brazil (data not shown). Considering total sample, the ability to perform usual activities due to RA was the mostly affected category (42.5%; SD = 30.9), and presenteeism was the most impaired productivity dimension (29.5%; SD = 28.8). All participating countries had a comparable pattern. In WPAI:RA final multivariate model, having previous orthopedic surgery (β = − 1.80; 95%CI = -3.28 to − 0.31; p = 0.020), medication coverage/insurance (β = − 2.69; 95%CI = -4.99 to − 0.39; p = 0.024) and consultations in the last 3 months (β = − 1.22; 95%CI = -2.39 to − 0.05; p = 0.042) decreased absenteeism; while reporting having performed ancillary tests increased (β = 1.27; 95%CI = 0.19 to 2.53; p = 0.023). Each disease activity level significantly increased presenteeism (β = 15.91;

95%CI = 12.10 to 19.72; p < 0.001). The "absenteeism and presenteeism" category was decreased by: medication coverage/insurance (β = − 2.70; 95%CI = -4.95 to − 0.45; p = 0.021) and consultations in the last 3 months (β = − 1.26; 95%CI = -2.40 to − 0.11; p = 0.033). Having performed ancillary tests in the last 3 months (β = 1.27; 95%CI = 0.19 to 2.53; p = 0.023) and previous orthopedic surgery (β = 1.80; 95%CI = 0.32 to 3.22; p = 0.019) increased "absenteeism and presenteeism". Impairment in regular daily activities was decreased by overweight/obesity (β = − 7.14; 95%CI = -14.03 to − 0.25; p = 0.042); and increased by disease activity (β = 19.47; 95%CI = 16.67 to 22.28; p < 0.001) and female group (β = 12.14; 95%CI = 1.08 to 23.21; p = 0.032).

For the total sample, WLQ-25 physical demands scale (40.3%) was the most affected due to RA, ranging from 44.0% in Mexico to 35.5% in Colombia. Productivity loss represented by WLQ-25 index was 7.0% (SD = 5.1), ranging from 7.8% (SD = 5.6) in Colombia to 5.9% (SD = 4.5) in Brazil. In multivariate final model, higher educational levels - technical or trade school to complete postgraduate education - (β = − 0.36; 95%CI = -0.70 to − 0.02; p = 0.039) and having undergone a previous orthopedic surgery (β = − 0.50; 95%CI = -1.00 to − 0.01; p = 0.045) decreased productivity losses.

Health-related quality of life

Table 4 shows descriptive analysis of HRQoL measures. These measures were stratified in accordance with exposure variables for total sample and final model for each of the questionnaires' measures are shown in Additional file 1: Tables S4 and S5.

EQ-5D-3 L = EuroQol 5 Dimensions Questionnaire 3 level version.

MCS = Mental Component Score.

PCS=Physical Component Score.

RA = Rheumatoid Arthritis.

SD = Standard Deviation.

SF-36 = 36-Item Short Form Health Survey.

Considering data for general population, seven of eight scales from SF-36 questionnaire in total sample have shown scores slightly below the reference value (lower limit: 45). Value observed in the scale "Vitality" for total sample was the only within the range of 45 and 55. The same pattern was observed in each of the countries, with the exception of Mexico, that has shown scores within the range for the scales "Vitality" (49.8; SD = 10.3) and "Mental Health" (46.7; SD = 11.6). All PCS measures were below the reference value for total sample and also for each country. Mean estimated for MCS was above reference value for total sample, and also in Brazil and Mexico. In the multivariate analysis, patients who had performed ancillary tests in the last 3 months had a decrease in

Table 1 Description of studied sociodemographic characteristics among RA patients at baseline

Characteristic	Argentina (N = 75)		Brazil (N = 68)		Colombia (N = 72)		Mexico (N = 75)		Total (N = 290)	
	N	%	N	%	N	%	N	%	N	%
Age [Mean/SD]	43.4	7.8	45.9	6.8	49.3	8.9	41.6	9.5	43.7	8.4
Gender										
Female	68	90.7	59	86.8	64	88.9	70	93.3	261	90.0
Race										
Mestizo	NA	NA	15	22.1	45	62.5	72	96	132	45.6
Caucasian/White	37	49.3	36	52.9	3	4.2	NA	NA	76	26.2
Hispanic/Latin	37	49.3	NA	NA	21	29.2	NA	NA	58	20.0
African American	NA	NA	14	20.6	1	1.4	–	–	15	5.2
Brazilian Indian	NA	NA	1	1.5	NA	NA	NA	NA	1	0.3
Native American	NA	NA	NA	NA	1	1.4	NA	NA	1	0.3
Other	NA	NA	2	2.9	NA	NA	NA	NA	2	0.7
Marital Status										
Married	41	54.7	35	51.5	30	41.7	41	54.7	147	50.7
Single/Not ever married	20	26.7	19	27.9	24	33.3	18	24.0	81	27.9
Partner/Common law	8	10.7	4	5.9	11	15.3	5	6.7	28	9.7
Divorced	2	2.6	5	7.4	1	1.3	7	9.3	15	5.2
Separated	4	5.3	–	–	3	4.2	1	1.3	8	2.8
Widowed	–	–	3	4.3	3	4.2	2	2.7	8	2.7
Educational level										
Incomplete High School	18	24.0	32	47.1	15	20.8	6	8.0	71	24.5
Complete High School	17	22.7	18	26.5	12	16.7	17	22.7	64	22.1
Technical or trade school	NA	NA	5	7.4	16	22.2	20	26.7	41	14.1
Complete or incomplete graduate degree	35	46.7	4	5.8	20	27.8	18	24.0	77	26.6
Complete postgraduate	2	2.6	4	5.8	9	12.5	4	5.3	19	6.6
Primary occupation										
Professional or technical	16	21.3	4	5.9	18	25.0	13	17.3	51	17.6
Office worker	13	17.3	3	4.4	13	18.1	4	5.3	33	11.4
Service worker	9	12.0	10	14.7	11	15.3	7	9.3	37	12.8
Sales	7	9.3	2	2.9	6	8.3	6	8.0	21	7.2
Manager, official or proprietor	4	5.3	1	1.5	6	8.3	5	6.7	16	5.5
Craftsman or foreman	2	2.7	2	2.9	2	2.8	1	1.3	7	2.4
Operative	1	1.3	3	4.4	3	4.2	1	1.3	8	2.8
Other	12	16.0	6	8.8	11	15.3	34	45.3	69	21.7
NI	11	14.7	37	54.4	2	2.8	4	5.3	54	18.6
Smoking habit										
Nonsmokers	40	53.3	39	57.4	47	65.3	51	68.0	177	61.0
Former smokers	22	29.3	17	25.0	20	27.8	12	16.0	71	24.5
Current smokers	13	17.4	12	17.6	5	6.9	11	14.7	41	14.2

the PCS score ($\beta = -2.33$; 95%CI = -4.17 to -0.49; $p = 0.013$); and each category of disease activity, from remission to high severity, decreased the score of PCS, in at least 7.06 points ($\beta = -7.06$; 95%CI = -7.87 to -6.21; $p < 0.001$) and MCS, in at least 3.34 points ($\beta = -3.34$; 95%CI = -4.72 to -1.96; $p < 0.001$).

EQ-VAS mean score ranged from 64.4 (SD = 21.5) in Brazil to 75.4 (SD = 21.6) in Mexico and for the whole

Table 2 Description of studied clinical characteristics among RA patients at baseline

Characteristic	Argentina (N = 75)		Brazil (N = 68)		Colombia (N = 72)		Mexico (N = 75)		Total (N = 290)	
	N	%	N	%	N	%	N	%	N	%
Clinical characteristics										
Body Mass Index [Mean/SD]	26.8	4.9	29.2	6.1	24.8	3.7	27.6	5.2	27.0	5.3
Comorbidities	53	70.7	59	86.8	40	55.6	40	53.3	192	66.2
Patients who underwent at least one previous orthopedic surgery	18	24.0	12	17.6	11	15.3	7	9.3	48	16.6
Disease characteristics										
Disease duration (years) [Mean/SD]	8.9	9.0	10.8	6.7	8.6	7.3	7.7	7.2	9.0	7.7
Time since symptoms onset (years) [Mean/SD]	9.7	9.0	12	7.8	9.5	7.3	9.4	7.4	10.1	8.0
Patients with medication coverage/insurance	68	90.7	47	69.1	69	95.8	55	73.3	239	82.4
Use of DMARDs	66	88.0	60	88.2	62	86.1	69	92.0	260	89.7
Disease activity (RAPID3 score)										
Remission	9	12.0	3	4.4	6	8.3	15	20.0	33	11.4
Low severity	17	22.7	1	1.5	9	12.5	11	14.7	38	13.1
Moderate severity	14	18.7	23	33.8	21	29.2	21	28.0	79	27.2
High severity	22	29.3	38	55.9	31	43.1	22	29.3	113	39.0
Direct medical resource utilization in the last three months										
Patients with at least one outpatient visit	58	77.3	52	76.5	58	80.5	56	74.7	224	77.2
Patients with at least one visit to perform tests	47	62.7	48	70.6	45	62.5	49	65.3	196	67.9
Patients who underwent at least one surgery (any type)	4	5.3	1	1.5	4	5.6	1	1.3	10	3.4

sample was 69.8 (SD = 20.4). Mean utility score was 0.67 (SD = 0.23) for total sample and ranged from 0.62 (SD = 0.19) to 0.71 (SD = 0.23) among countries. Final multivariate model for EQ-VAS has shown that patients with a longer disease duration ($\geq$9 years) ($\beta = -5.19$; 95%CI = -9.52 to -0.85; $p = 0.019$) and presenting worsening of disease activity level ($\beta = -10.74$; 95%CI = -12.81 to -8.68; p < 0.001) have a decrease in the score. Beside this, use of DMARDs increased EQ-VAS score ($\beta = 8.39$; 95%CI = 1.52 to 15.25; $p = 0.020$).

Regarding utility scores from EQ-5D-3 L instrument, ancillary test multivariate analysis indicates that overweight/obese patients ($\beta = -0.06$; 95%CI = -0.11 to -0.003; $p = 0.039$) and those with a longer disease duration ($\geq$9 years) ($\beta = -0.05$; 95%CI = -0.10 to -0.01; $p = 0.012$) have a decrease in the utility score. Utility score is also reduced with the increase of the disease activity level ($\beta = -0.12$; 95%CI = -0.14 to -0.10; $p < 0.001$). On the other hand, mestizos patients showed an increasing in utility scores ($\beta = 0.06$; 95%CI = 0.01 to 0.11; $p = 0.010$).

Disease progression and impact on work productivity and HRQoL

It was observed a slightly higher mean of RAPID3 score in Visit 1 (10.7; SD = 6.6) than in Visit 5 (9.7; SD = 6.7), but no statistical significant difference was observed between these measures ($p = 0.270$). However, the majority of patients (79.4%) has improved or maintained the disease activity level during the 1-year follow-up period.

Considering differences between the first and last study visits, worsening in the disease activity showed an association with an increase on impact on work productivity and HRQoL. Patients who had improvement/maintenance had also an improvement in the assessed measures and those who worsened also had a worsening in the scores, except for WLQ-25. However, a statistically significant difference was observed only for WALS ($p = 0.001$); WPAI:RA domains "presenteeism" ($p = 0.020$) and "impairment of regular daily activities" ($p = 0.017$); components of SF-36: physical ($p < 0.001$) and mental (p < 0.001); and EQ-5D-3 L utility score ($p = 0.007$) - Table 5.

EQ-5D-3 L = EuroQol 5 Dimensions Questionnaire 3 level version.

HRQoL = Health-Related Quality of Life.

WALS=Workplace Activity Limitation Scale.

WLQ-25 = 25-item Work Limitations Questionnaire.

WPAI:RA = Work Productivity and Activity Impairment Questionnaire - Rheumatoid Arthritis.

SD = Standard Deviation.

SF-36 = 36-Item Short Form Health Survey.

VAS=Visual Analogue Scale.

Table 3 Work productivity assessed through WALS, WPAI:RA and WLQ-25 questionnaires among RA patients at baseline

Work Productivity	Argentina		Brazil		Colombia		Mexico		Total	
	Mean	SD	Mean	SD	Mean	SD	Mean	SD	Mean	SD
WALS	N = 52		N = 22		N = 64		N = 68		N = 206	
1.Get to and from work and maintain punctuality [N/%]	18	34.6	11	50.0	30	46.9	24	35.3	83	40.3
2. Getting to the workplace [N/%]	26	50.0	11	50.0	43	67.2	36	52.9	116	56.3
3. Sitting for long periods of time at your job [N/%]	17	32.7	10	45.5	38	59.4	34	50.0	99	48.1
4. Standing for long periods of time at your job [N/%]	34	65.4	15	68.2	49	76.6	46	67.6	144	69.9
5. Lift, carry or move objects [N/%]	39	75.0	18	81.8	52	81.3	56	82.4	165	80.1
6. Working with your hands [N/%]	35	67.3	17	77.3	45	70.3	30	44.1	127	61.7
7. Crouching, bend, kneel or work in awkward positions [N/%]	43	82.7	20	90.9	52	81.3	58	85.3	173	84.0
8. Stretch out [N/%]	33	63.5	19	86.4	40	62.5	37	54.4	129	62.6
9. With the schedule of hours of work that your job requires [N/%]	18	34.6	12	54.5	30	46.9	30	44.1	90	43.7
10. With the pace of work that your job requires [N/%]	27	51.9	12	54.5	37	57.8	42	61.8	106	51.5
11. Meet your current job demands [N/%]	25	48.1	14	63.6	36	56.3	37	54.4	110	53.4
12. To concentrate and keep your mind on your work [N/%]	19	36.5	12	54.5	7	10.9	25	36.8	92	44.7
Overall score of WALS (0–36)	**8.4**	**5.6**	**10.6**	**6.8**	**9.7**	**6.0**	**8.2**	**6.3**	**9.0**	**6.1**
WPAI:RA	N = 73		N = 52		N = 72		N = 75		N = 272	
Normal Daily Activities										
% Daily activity impairment due to RA	34.0	28.2	56.1	27.4	46.7	29.0	36.5	33.8	42.5	30.9
Professional Activities										
% Impairment while working due to RA (presenteeism)*	23.9	23.9	32.6	26.8	40.5	32.2	23.1	28.5	29.5	28.8
% Work time missed due to RA (absenteeism)*	12.0	27.5	5.8	23.5	7.5	21.6	8.4	18.8	9.0	23.2
% Overall work impairment due to RA (absenteeism and presenteeism)*	10.3	25.0	5.9	23.9	7.6	21.9	8.9	20.3	8.6	22.6
WLQ-25	N = 59		N = 36		N = 43		N = 53		N = 191	
% work impairment due to physical demands	41.1	24.7	37.7	24.1	35.5	24.0	44.0	28.7	40.3	21.4
% work impairment due to time demands	33.5	24.7	29.3	30.6	32.4	26.8	27.9	29.0	30.9	28.0
% work impairment due to output demands	27.6	24.4	18.1	19.3	29.9	25.8	22.7	23.3	24.9	23.8
% work impairment due to mental-interpersonal demands	20.1	21.9	15.2	18.0	20.9	24.8	16.1	20.1	18.2	23.8
WLQ-25 index (%)	**7.5**	**5.1**	**5.9**	**4.5**	**7.8**	**5.6**	**6.5**	**4.9**	**7.0**	**5.1**

Discussion

Our sample was comprised of patients from 4 Latin American countries, mostly middle-aged, female, from multiethnic origin, married with a technical or professional occupation. The educational level was well-distributed in the total sample, but Brazilian patients had a higher frequency of incomplete or complete high school only. This observation may be at least partially explained by the type of funding for study sites in the sample, once only Brazil had publicly-funded healthcare services enrolling patients and those facilities usually attend people with lower income and lower educational level in the country.

The burden of RA on Latin-American patients' work productivity and HRQoL was comprehensively assessed using standard PROs. Thus, it was possible to descriptively compare these data with findings from other contexts and countries. In summary, RA was related with presenteeism, indicating that patients are working with reduced performance and which seems to lead to unemployment [33–36]. For example, WPAI presenteeism measure (percentage of impairment while working due to RA) in our sample was 28.8%, while healthy controls in a previous study in Sweden reported a mean impairment of 20.9%. [37] Regarding HRQoL, physical aspect of the disease seems to be the major impairing condition [38–41]. Although these available data, there are several standard PROs that assess these outcomes from different perspectives, and this study analyzed a unique RA population using these different instruments.

Our results about burden of RA on work productivity assessed at baseline demonstrated an important impact of the disease on patients' life, related to several dimensions according to the instrument, and corroborate international data that patients are working with reduced performance. The overall work impairment due to RA at

Table 4 Health-related quality of life assessed through SF-36 and EQ-5D-3 L questionnaires among RA patients at baseline

Health-related Quality of Life	Argentina		Brazil		Colombia		Mexico		Total	
	Mean	SD	Mean	SD	Mean	SD	Mean	SD	Mean	SD
SF-36	N = 75		N = 68		N = 72		N = 75		N = 290	
Vitality	46.9	10.9	47.0	9.5	47.9	10.2	49.8	10.3	47.9	10.3
Mental health	42.5	11.4	44.3	12.3	43.7	10.4	46.7	11.6	44.3	11.5
Social functioning	41.9	11.6	40.1	11.3	40.6	11.5	44.2	10.9	41.8	11.4
Bodily pain	43.2	10.7	36.6	8.3	39.3	10.1	43.5	10.7	40.8	10.4
Role physical	42.4	11.5	37.0	11.5	39.1	10.7	43.0	9.7	40.5	11.1
General health	41.9	9.7	38.5	11.9	39.5	8.9	41.6	12.2	40.4	10.8
Role emotional	39.9	13.9	41.2	13.5	37.5	11.6	42.1	11.3	40.2	12.7
Physical functioning	38.5	11.0	32.0	8.6	37.6	10.6	40.2	12.2	37.2	11.1
Mental Component Score (MCS)	43.4	11.9	47.3	11.9	43.9	9.9	47.2	11.3	45.4	11.3
Physical Component Score (PCS)	41.8	9.8	33.6	9.6	38.7	9.1	41.5	10.7	39.1	10.3
EQ-5D-3 L	N = 73		N = 68		N = 70		N = 75		N = 286	
Overall Value (0–100)	71.5	16.6	64.4	21.5	67.4	20.2	75.4	21.6	69.8	20.4
Utility Score (0–1)	0.67	0.25	0.62	0.19	0.66	0.25	0.71	0.23	0.67	0.23

baseline in our sample was similar or lower than the observed in previous studies, depending on the characteristics of studied sample [33–35]. The work limitations related to presenteeism were also investigated using WALS measures and our patients are classified as having high severity of work place disability [36]. In the present study, all WLQ-25 subscales at baseline were higher than results observed in US populations of RA patients. A remarkable difference is noted in physical demands scale, indicating that Latin American patients are more limited in work environment mainly in this scale [38, 42].

When HRQoL was assessed at baseline, a major impact on physical aspects was observed, with lower physical SF-36 score (when compared with mental score), as described in the literature. EQ-VAS value estimated in our study was 69.8 (SD = 20.4), which is similar to those reported for Brazilian RA patients (mean score: 63 to 74) [43], and different from Mexican patients (mean score: 49.5) with osteoarthritis, RA or chronic low-back pain [44]. Utility measure calculated was 0.67 and no studies describing utility among Latin American RA patients were found to date. This measure is usually used to define public health policies, resource allocation and

Table 5 Comparison between differences in work productivity and HRQoL scores and disease progression from the first to the last study visit

Outcomes		Disease Progression				
		Improvement or maintenance		Worsening		p-value
		Mean Difference	SD	Mean Difference	SD	
Work Productivity						
WALS		−0.9	4.1	1.9	4.2	**0.001**
WPAI:RA	Absenteeism	−0.7	25.3	5.0	14.7	0.118
	Presenteeism	−3.7	24.9	11.0	21.2	**0.020**
	Absenteeism and Presenteeism	−0.9	26.7	5.0	14.8	0.101
	Impairment of regular daily activities	−5.5	28.4	7.0	27.0	**0.017**
WLQ-25		0.4	7.3	−0.2	8.1	0.723
HRQoL						
SF-36	PCS	2.9	7.1	−1.7	7.1	**< 0.001**
	MCS	1.1	10.3	−4.0	6.6	**< 0.001**
EQ-5D-3 L	Overall VAS Value	5.2	22.8	−1.4	17.7	0.142
	Utility score	0.03	0.25	−0.06	0.18	**0.007**

evaluation of services and programs, as it works as a proxy of how people value changes in health status [45], highlighting the need for these studies in Latin America.

It is known that multiple factors act to generate work impairment and poor HRQoL [46]. Obesity, living without partner, being mestizo, the presence of comorbidities, having medication insurance/coverage, longer disease duration, having performed ancillary test and consultations and a previous orthopedic surgery were associated with a worsening in work productivity and/or HRQoL. An improvement in the assessed PROs scores was associated with a higher educational level, having medication insurance/coverage, being mestizo, having recently performed ancillary test and consultations, a history of previous orthopedic surgery and use of DMARDs. Some variables behaved as protective or risk factors, depending on the instrument assessed, suggesting that these relationships still needs to be further addressed. Also, unexpectedly, obesity and overweight were associated with reduced impairment in regular daily activities in the WPAI analysis, as compared to underweight/normal BMI values. This finding seems in conflict with our observation that obese/overweight individuals have worse quality of life (EQ-5D-3 L utility score) and could not be explained by our data. A similar pattern was observed for the association between greater work limitations according to WALS and medication coverage/insurance. Potential confounders not collected in our study may play in this association.

With exception of WLQ-25, all PROs were associated with disease activity. The hypothesis that the disease activity may have a great impact in these aspects of patients' life arises from the presence of joint damage and loss of physical function in RA, which seems to be a prognostic factor in the ability to keep or get a new job [14, 47]. This relationship was also observed in the longitudinal analysis, and confirms the finding from cross-sectional analysis showing that disease worsening is associated with an increase of the impact on work productivity and a decrease of HRQoL scores. Although no studies in the literature have assessed this relationship over time, this finding corroborates the main goals proposed by EULAR (The European League Against Rheumatism) and ACR (American College of Rheumatology) – o since the disease is not entirely curable, RA therapy must aim to reach disease remission, and if it is not possible, to achieve low disease activity reflecting on patients' professional and personal lives [10, 11]. About this aspect, it is important to notice that in the studied population, most patients had moderate or high disease activity at baseline and maintained it during the 1-year follow-up. Considering the recommendations for strategies of close monitoring and prompt therapy adjustments to achieve low disease activity or remission, this observation suggests that this is a particularly refractory population or that the management could be suboptimal. Further analyses of the data, including medication use, will be done to address this issue.

The aforementioned associations of HRQoL and work productivity among different stratum of study population were not yet well established and, thus, more studies are needed in order to infer a causal relationship [14, 40, 46, 48–53]. However, it is important that healthcare professionals stay alert to those characteristics during RA patients' management and also patients, families and the society, with the aim to minimize its effects on patients' professional and personal lives. It is worth mentioning that health systems should be investing in strategies and technologies targeting disease activity control among RA patients, once this seems to be a variable strongly related to higher burden not only to patients, but also the society. The data presented here will certainly be useful to better estimate the cost-effectiveness of these treatment strategies, invaluable information for optimizing the use limited health resources in relatively low-income countries, particularly nowadays with the growing number of costly anti-rheumatic drugs available.

This was the first study conducted in countries from Latin America with the aim to assess RA patients work productivity and HRQoL. This study adds knowledge in an area scarcely studied and improves global disease comprehension about burden of RA in Latin America.

Conclusion

This study highlights the importance of regular and timely disease management for RA patients, specially focusing on the need to decrease disease activity to promote better results in PROs. An increase in disease activity was responsible for a significant decrease in HRQoL, and a significant increase in workplace disabilities, leading to a more difficult time in maintaining or seeking job opportunities. Also, multiple factors were identified that seem to be associated with work impairment and HRQoL, but as for the protective factors, further research is still needed. This study's results highlight the need for a more comprehensive and holistic approach to RA management and that all relevant stakeholders (from families to HR managers) should be aware of RA's burden in patients' everyday life. Also, it sheds some light in a subject that is often overlooked, adding to the evidence that the burden of RA in QoL is significant. Finally, the knowledge of the burden of disease in Latin America is often limited, and this study contributes to the ever-increasing need to raise awareness so that resource allocation is focused on tackling this issue.

Supplementary information

Additional file 1: Table S1. Independent Ethics Committee/Institutional Review Board approvals. **Table S2.** Work productivity assessed through WALS, WPAI:RA and WLQ-25 questionnaires among several exposure groups of RA patients at baseline. **Table S3.** Final model for the association between work productivity (WALS, WPAI:RA and WLQ-25 scores) and exposure groups at baseline. **Table S4.** Health-related quality of life assessed through SF-36 and EQ-5D-3L questionnaires among several exposure groups of RA patients at baseline. **Table S5.** Final model for the association between health-related quality of life (SF-36 and EQ-5D-3L scores) and exposure groups at baseline.

Abbreviations

ACR: American College of Rheumatology; DMARDs: Disease-Modifying Antirheumatic Drugs; EQ-5D-3 L: EuroQol 5 Dimensions Questionnaire 3 level version; EQ-VAS: EQ Visual Analogue Scale; FN: Physical function; HRQoL: Health related quality of life; MCS: Mental Component Summary; MDHAQ: Multi-Dimensional Health Assessment Questionnaire; PCS: Physical Component Summary; PN: Pain; PROs: Patient-reported outcomes; PROSE RA study: Patient Reported Outcomes Survey of Employment among patients with RA; PTGL: Patient's global assessment; RA : Rheumatoid Arthritis; RADAI: Rheumatoid Arthritis Disease Activity Index; RAPID3: Rheumatology Assessment Patient Index Data 3 measures; SD: Standard Deviation; SF-36: 36-Item Short Form Health Survey; WALS: Workplace Activity Limitation Scale; WLQ-25: 25-Item Work Limitations Questionnaire; WPAI:RA: Work Productivity and Activity Impairment Questionnaire – Rheumatoid Arthritis

Acknowledgments

ANOVA Health Consulting Group provided assistance on study development and manuscript preparation, funded by AbbVie. Maíra Takemoto and Ana Carolina Padula Ribeiro Pereira from ANOVA provided medical writing assistance and editorial support with this manuscript. Diogo Morais from Eurotrials – Scientific Consultants Ltda. provided medical writing assistance and editorial support with this manuscript, funded by AbbVie. AbbVie participated in the study design and conduct, interpretation of data, review, and approval of the content. All the authors had access to all relevant data and participated in writing, review, and approval of this manuscript.

Authors' contributions

All authors meet the ICMJE authorship criteria, giving substantial contribution to the conception or design of the work, data acquisition and analysis, drafting or reviewing the work for intellectual content and giving final approval of the version to be published. The authors agree to be accountable for all aspects of the work in ensuring that questions related to the accuracy or integrity of any part of the work are appropriately investigated and resolved.
All authors have approved the manuscript for submission.

Author details

[1]Universidade Federal do Rio Grande do Sul, Hospital de Clínicas de Porto Alegre, Porto Alegre, Brazil. [2]Centro Paulista de Investigações Clínicas (CEPIC), São Paulo, Brazil. [3]Universidade Federal de São Paulo, São Paulo, Brazil. [4]Morales Vargas Centro de Investigación, Guanajuato, Mexico. [5]Fundación Instituto de Reumatología Fernando Chalem, Bogotá, Colombia. [6]Centro Integral de Reumatología – Reumalab, Medellín, Colombia. [7]Centro de Investigaciones en Enfermedades Reumáticas (CIER), Buenos Aires, Argentina. [8]Desarrollos Biomédicos y Biotecnológicos, Monterrey, Mexico. [9]Circaribe, Barranquilla, Colombia. [10]CEIM Investigaciones Medicas, Buenos Aires, Argentina. [11]Instituto Médico Especializado (IME), Buenos Aires, Argentina. [12]AbbVie Farmacêutica Ltda, São Paulo, Brazil. [13]Unidad de Investigación en Enf. Crónico-Degenerativas, Guadalajara, Mexico.

References

1. Smolen JS, Steiner G. Therapeutic strategies for rheumatoid arthritis. Nat Rev Drug Discov. 2003;2:473–88.
2. Choy EH, Panayi GS. Cytokine pathways and joint inflammation in rheumatoid arthritis. N Engl J Med. 2001;344:907–16.
3. Drosos AA. Newer immunosuppressive drugs: their potential role in rheumatoid arthritis therapy. Drugs. 2002;62:891–907.
4. Goldring SR. Pathogenesis of bone and cartilage destruction in rheumatoid arthritis. Rheumatology (Oxford) 2003;42 Suppl 2:ii11–6.
5. Lee SJ-A, Kavanaugh A. Pharmacological treatment of established rheumatoid arthritis. Best Pract Res Clin Rheumatol. 2003;17:811–29.
6. Lindqvist E. Course of radiographic damage over 10 years in a cohort with early rheumatoid arthritis. Ann Rheum Dis. 2003;62:611–6.
7. Burgos-Vargas R, Catoggio LJJ, Galarza-Maldonado C, Ostojich K, Cardiel MHH. Current therapies in rheumatoid arthritis: a Latin American perspective. Reumatol Clin. 2013;9:106–12.
8. Alarcón GS. Epidemiology of rheumatoid arthritis. Rheum Dis Clin N Am. 1995;21:589–604.
9. Firestein GS. Etiology and pathogenesis of rheumatoid arthritis. In: Kelley's Textbook of Rheumatology. Philadelphia; 1999. p. 851–97.
10. Smolen JS, Landewé R, Breedveld FC, Buch M, Burmester G, Dougados M, et al. EULAR recommendations for the management of rheumatoid arthritis with synthetic and biological disease-modifying antirheumatic drugs: 2013 update. Ann Rheum Dis 2013;0:1–18.
11. Singh JA, Saag KG, Bridges SL, Akl EA, Bannuru RR, Sullivan MC, et al. 2015 American College of Rheumatology Guideline for the treatment of rheumatoid arthritis. Arthritis Rheumatol. 2016;68:1–26.
12. Krishnan E, Fries JF. Reduction in long-term functional disability in rheumatoid arthritis from 1977 to 1998:a longitudinal study of 3035 patients. Am J Med. 2003;115:371–6.
13. Puolakka K, Kautiainen H, Möttönen T, Hannonen P, Korpela M, Julkunen H, et al. Impact of initial aggressive drug treatment with a combination of disease-modifying antirheumatic drugs on the development of work disability in early rheumatoid arthritis: a five-year randomized followup trial. Arthritis Rheum. 2004;50:55–62.
14. Eberhardt K, Larsson B-M, Nived K, Lindqvist E. Work disability in rheumatoid arthritis--development over 15 years and evaluation of predictive factors over time. J Rheumatol. 2007;34:481–7.
15. Arnett FC, Edworthy SM, Bloch DA, McShane DJ, Fries JF, Cooper NS, et al. The American rheumatism association 1987 revised criteria for the classification of rheumatoid arthritis. Arthritis Rheum. 1988;31:315–24.
16. Reilly Associates. WPAI - translations. 2011. Available at: http://www.reillyassociates.net/WPAI_Translations.html.
17. Mapi Trust. Catalogue of questionnaires - HAQ-DI. 2011. Available at: http://www.mapi-trust.org/services/questionnairelicensing/cataloguequestionnaires/54-haq.
18. EuroQol Group. Available EQ-5D versions – EQ-5D. 2019. Available at: https://euroqol.org/eq-5d-instruments/available-eq-5d-versions/.
19. Qualimetrics. SF-36 and SF-36v2 Health Survey. Available at: https://www.optum.com/solutions/life-sciences/answer-research/patient-insights/sf-health-surveys/sf-36v2-health-survey.html. Accessed May 7, 2019.
20. Campolina AG, Bortoluzzo AB, Ferraz MB, Ciconelli RM. Mensuração de preferências em saúde: uma comparação do SF-6D Brasil com derivações do SF-36 em pacientes com artrite reumatóide. Acta Reum Port. 2010;35:200–6.
21. Tang K, Beaton DE, Boonen A, Gignac MAM, Bombardier C. Measures of work disability and productivity. Arthritis Care Res (Hoboken). 2011;63:S337–49.
22. Beck A, Crain AL, Solberg LI, Unutzer J, Glasgow RE, Maciosek MV, et al. Severity of depression and magnitude of productivity loss. Ann Fam Med. 2011;9:305–11.
23. Lerner D, Amick BC, Rogers WH, Malspeis S, Bungay K, Cynn D. The work limitations questionnaire. Med Care. 2001;39:72–85.
24. Lerner DJ, Amick BC, Malspeis S, Rogers WH. A national survey of health-related work limitations among employed persons in the United States. Disabil Rehabil. 2000;22:225–32.
25. Ware JE, Kosinsk M, Turner-Boweker, D.M. Gandek B. User's Manual for the SF-12v2® Health Survey With a Supplement Documenting SF-12® Health Survey.; 2002.
26. The EuroQol Group. EQ-D User Guide.; 2015.
27. Dolan P. Modeling valuations for EuroQol health states valuations modeling. Med Care. 1997;35:1095–108.
28. Pincus T. Scoring Instructions for R808 Multi-Dimensional Health Assessment Questionnaire (MDHAQ) and Rheumatology Assessment Patient Index Data (RAPID3). 2009;40:2009–2010.
29. Beaton DE, Tang K, Gignac M a M, Lacaille D, Badley EM, Anis AH, et al. Reliability, validity, and responsiveness of five at-work productivity measures

in patients with rheumatoid arthritis or osteoarthritis. Arthritis Care Res (Hoboken). 2010;62:28–37.

30. Zhang W, Gignac MAM, Beaton D, Tang K, Anis AH. Productivity loss due to presenteeism among patients with arthritis: estimates from 4 instruments. J Rheumatol. 2010;37:1805–14.

31. Kievit W, Fransen J, Adang EMM, den Broeder AA, Bernelot Moens HJ, Visser H, et al. Long-term effectiveness and safety of TNF-blocking agents in daily clinical practice: results from the Dutch rheumatoid arthritis monitoring register. Rheumatology. 2011;50:196–203.

32. Zhang W, Bansback N, Boonen A, Young A, Singh A, Anis AH. Validity of the work productivity and activity impairment questionnaire--general health version in patients with rheumatoid arthritis. Arthritis Res Ther. 2010;12:R177.

33. Chaparro Del Moral R, Rillo OL, Casalla L, Morón CB, Citera G. Cocco J a M, et al. Work productivity in rheumatoid arthritis: relationship with clinical and radiological features *Arthritis*. 2012;2012:137635.

34. Radner H, Smolen JS, Aletaha D. Remission in rheumatoid arthritis: benefit over low disease activity in patient-reported outcomes and costs. Arthritis Res Ther. 2014;16:R56.

35. Hone D, Cheng A, Watson C, Huang B, Bitman B, Huang X-Y, et al. Impact of etanercept on work and activity impairment in employed moderate to severe rheumatoid arthritis patients in the United States. Arthritis Care Res (Hoboken). 2013;65:1564–72.

36. Gignac M a M, Cao X, Tang K, Beaton DE. Examination of arthritis-related work place activity limitations and intermittent disability over four-and-a-half years and its relationship to job modifications and outcomes. Arthritis Care Res (Hoboken) 2011;63:953–962.

37. Hasselrot K, Lindeberg M, Konings P, Kopp KH. Investigating the loss of work productivity due to symptomatic leiomyoma. PLoS One. 2018;13: e0197958.

38. Walker N, Michaud K, Wolfe F. Work limitations among working persons with rheumatoid arthritis: results, reliability, and validity of the work limitations questionnaire in 836 patients. J Rheumatol. 2005;32:1006–12.

39. Wolfe F, Michaud K, Choi HK, Williams R. Household income and earnings losses among 6,396 persons with rheumatoid arthritis. J Rheumatol. 2005;32: 1875–83.

40. Peláez-Ballestas I, Boonen A, Vázquez-Mellado J, Reyes-Lagunes I, Hernández-Garduño A, Goycochea MV, et al. Coping strategies for health and daily-life stressors in patients with rheumatoid arthritis, Ankylosing spondylitis, and gout: STROBE-compliant article. Medicine (Baltimore). 2015; 94:e600.

41. Contreras-Yáñez I, Cabiedes J, Villa AR, Rull-Gabayet M, Pascual-Ramos V. Persistence on therapy is a major determinant of patient-, physician- and laboratory- reported outcomes in recent-onset rheumatoid arthritis patients. Clin Exp Rheumatol. 2010;28:748–51.

42. Allaire S, Wolfe F, Niu J, Lavalley M, Michaud K. Work disability and its economic effect on 55-64-year-old adults with rheumatoid arthritis. Arthritis Rheum. 2005;53:603–8.

43. Pinheiro G da RC, Khandker RK, Sato R, Rose A, Piercy J. Impact of rheumatoid arthritis on quality of life, work productivity and resource utilisation: an observational, cross-sectional study in Brazil. Clin Exp Rheumatol 2013;31:334–340.

44. Ramos-Remus CR, Hunsche E, Mavros P, Querol J, Suarez R, ProExp Study Group. Evaluation of quality of life following treatment with etoricoxib in patients with arthritis or low-back pain: an open label, uncontrolled pilot study in Mexico. Curr Med Res Opin. 2004;20:691–8.

45. Campolina AG, Ciconelli RM. Qualidade de vida e medidas de utilidade : parâmetros clínicos para as tomadas de decisão em saúde. Rev Panam Salud Pública. 2006;19:128–36.

46. Backman CL. Employment and work disability in rheumatoid arthritis. Curr Opin Rheumatol. 2004;16:148–52.

47. Vollenhoven RF. van, Cifaldi, M.A.; Ray S., Chen N., Weisman MH. Effect of inhibiting joint damage on work performance in patients with early rheumatoid arthritis: results from a companion study to premier. Ann Rheum Dis 2008;67:580.

48. Sokka T, Kautiainen H, Pincus T, Verstappen SMM, Aggarwal A, Alten R, et al. Work disability remains a major problem in rheumatoid arthritis in the 2000s: data from 32 countries in the QUEST-RA study. Arthritis Res Ther. 2010;12:R42.

49. Sokka T. Work disability in early rheumatoid arthritis. Clin Exp Rheumatol. 2003;21:S71–4.

50. Jakobsson U, Hallberg IR. Pain and quality of life among older people with rheumatoid arthritis and/or osteoarthritis: a literature review. J Clin Nurs. 2002;11:430–43.

51. Sherman BW, Lynch WD. The relationship between smoking and health care, workers' compensation, and productivity costs for a large employer. J Occup Environ Med. 2013;55:879–84.

52. Chiu Y-M, Lai M-S, Lin H-Y, Lang H-C, Lee LJ-H, Wang J-D. Disease activity affects all domains of quality of life in patients with rheumatoid arthritis and is modified by disease duration. Clin Exp Rheumatol. 2014;32:898–903.

53. Gerhold K, Richter A, Schneider M, Bergerhausen HJ, Demary W, Liebhaber A, et al. Health-related quality of life in patients with long-standing rheumatoid arthritis in the era of biologics: Data from the German biologics register RABBIT. Rheumatol (United Kingdom) 2015;54:1858–1866.

Permissions

All chapters in this book were first published by BioMed Central; hereby published with permission under the Creative Commons Attribution License or equivalent. Every chapter published in this book has been scrutinized by our experts. Their significance has been extensively debated. The topics covered herein carry significant findings which will fuel the growth of the discipline. They may even be implemented as practical applications or may be referred to as a beginning point for another development.

The contributors of this book come from diverse backgrounds, making this book a truly international effort. This book will bring forth new frontiers with its revolutionizing research information and detailed analysis of the nascent developments around the world.

We would like to thank all the contributing authors for lending their expertise to make the book truly unique. They have played a crucial role in the development of this book. Without their invaluable contributions this book wouldn't have been possible. They have made vital efforts to compile up to date information on the varied aspects of this subject to make this book a valuable addition to the collection of many professionals and students.

This book was conceptualized with the vision of imparting up-to-date information and advanced data in this field. To ensure the same, a matchless editorial board was set up. Every individual on the board went through rigorous rounds of assessment to prove their worth. After which they invested a large part of their time researching and compiling the most relevant data for our readers.

The editorial board has been involved in producing this book since its inception. They have spent rigorous hours researching and exploring the diverse topics which have resulted in the successful publishing of this book. They have passed on their knowledge of decades through this book. To expedite this challenging task, the publisher supported the team at every step. A small team of assistant editors was also appointed to further simplify the editing procedure and attain best results for the readers.

Apart from the editorial board, the designing team has also invested a significant amount of their time in understanding the subject and creating the most relevant covers. They scrutinized every image to scout for the most suitable representation of the subject and create an appropriate cover for the book.

The publishing team has been an ardent support to the editorial, designing and production team. Their endless efforts to recruit the best for this project, has resulted in the accomplishment of this book. They are a veteran in the field of academics and their pool of knowledge is as vast as their experience in printing. Their expertise and guidance has proved useful at every step. Their uncompromising quality standards have made this book an exceptional effort. Their encouragement from time to time has been an inspiration for everyone.

The publisher and the editorial board hope that this book will prove to be a valuable piece of knowledge for researchers, students, practitioners and scholars across the globe.

List of Contributors

Aline Defaveri do Prado
Rheumatology Department, Sao Lucas Hospital, Faculty of Medicine of Pontifical Catholic University of Rio Grande do Sul (PUCRS), Av. Ipiranga, 6690/220, Porto Alegre 90610-000, Brazil
Rheumatology Service, Hospital Nossa Senhora da Conceição – Grupo Hospitalar Conceição (GHC), Av. Francisco Trein, 596 – 2nd floor, Porto Alegre, RS CEP 91350-200, Brazil

Henrique Luiz Staub, Melissa Cláudia Bisi and Inês Guimarães da Silveira
Rheumatology Department, Sao Lucas Hospital, Faculty of Medicine of Pontifical Catholic University of Rio Grande do Sul (PUCRS), Av. Ipiranga, 6690/220, Porto Alegre 90610-000, Brazil

Joaquim Polido-Pereira and João Eurico Fonseca
Rheumatology Research Unit, Instituto de Medicina Molecular, Faculdade de Medicina, Universidade de Lisboa, Lisbon, Portugal
Rheumatology Department, Hospital de Santa Maria, Lisbon Academic Medical Centre, Lisbon, Portugal

Deise Marcela Piovesan
Rheumatology Service, Pontifícia Universidade Católica do Rio Grande do Sul (PUCRS), Ipiranga Avenue, 6690 room 220, Porto Alegre, RS CEP 90610-000, Brazil

Markus Bredemeier
Rheumatology Service, Hospital Nossa Senhora da Conceição – Grupo Hospitalar Conceição (GHC), Av. Francisco Trein, 596 – 2nd floor, Porto Alegre, RS CEP 91350-200, Brazil

Talita Siara Baptista, Laura Petersen and Moises Evandro Bauer
Laboratory of Immunosenescence, Institute of Biomedical Research, Pontificia Universidade Católica do Rio Grande do Sul (PUCRS), Av. Ipiranga, 6690, 2nd floor, Porto Alegre, RS CEP 90610-000, Brazil

José Alexandre Mendonça
Rheumatology Department, Pontifícia Universidade Católica de Campinas (PUCCAMP), Av. John Boyd Dunlop, S/N, Campinas, SP CEP 13034-685, Brazil

Punchong Hanvivadhanakul
Division of Rheumatology, Department of Medicine, Faculty of Medicine, Thammasat University, 99/209 Moo 18, Paholyothin Road, Klong Luang, Pathumthanee 12120, Thailand

Adisai Buakhamsri
Division of Cardiology, Department of Medicine, Faculty of Medicine, Thammasat University, 99/209 Moo 18, Paholyothin Road, Klong Luang, Pathumthanee 12120, Thailand

Denise Blum
Serviço de Reumatologia, Hospital de Clínicas de Porto Alegre, Universidade Federal do Rio Grande do Sul, Porto Alegre, Brazil

Rodrigo Rodrigues
Laboratório de Pesquisa do Exercício, Universidade Federal do Rio Grande do Sul, Porto Alegre, Brazil
Centro Universitário da Serra Gaúcha, Caxias do Sul, Brazil

Jeam Marcel Geremia and Marco Aurélio Vaz
Laboratório de Pesquisa do Exercício, Universidade Federal do Rio Grande do Sul, Porto Alegre, Brazil

Andrese Aline Gasparin and Fernanda Igansi
Universidade Federal do Rio Grande do Sul (UFRGS), Programa de Pós Graduação em Ciências Médicas (PPGCM), Rua Ramiro Barcelos 2400, segundo andar, Porto Alegre 90035-903, Brazil

Nicole Pamplona Bueno de Andrade
Universidade Federal do Rio Grande do Sul (UFRGS), Programa de Pós Graduação em Ciências Médicas (PPGCM), Rua Ramiro Barcelos 2400, segundo andar, Porto Alegre 90035-903, Brazil
Faculdade de Medicina, Universidade Federal do Rio Grande do Sul (UFRGS), Porto Alegre, Alegre, Brazil

Penélope Esther Palominos and Rafael Mendonça da Silva Chakr
Universidade Federal do Rio Grande do Sul (UFRGS), Programa de Pós Graduação em Ciências Médicas (PPGCM), Rua Ramiro Barcelos 2400, segundo andar, Porto Alegre 90035-903, Brazil
Department of Rheumatology, Hospital de Clinicas de Porto Alegre, Rua Ramiro Barcelos 2350, sexto andar, Porto Alegre 90035-903, Brazil

Laure Gossec
Sorbonne Universités, UPMC Univ Paris 06, Institut Pierre Louis d'Epidémiologie et de Santé Publique, GRC-UPMC 08 (EEMOIS); Department of Rheumatology, Pitié Salpêtrière Hospital, AP-HP, 47-83 Boulevard de l'Hôpital, 75013 Paris, France

Geraldo da Rocha Castelar-Pinheiro
Departamento de Medicina Interna, Disciplina de Reumatologia, Universidade do Estado do Rio de Janeiro, Avenida Nossa Senhora de Copacabana, 978, sala 508, Copacabana, Rio de Janeiro, RJ 22060-002, Brazil
Universidade do Estado do Rio de Janeiro, Rio de Janeiro, Brazil
Disciplina de Reumatologia, Departamento de Medicina Interna, Universidade do Estado do Rio de Janeiro, Rio de Janeiro, Brazil

Ana Beatriz Vargas-Santos
Serviço de Reumatologia, Hospital Universitário Pedro Ernesto -Universidade do Estado do Rio de Janeiro, Rio de Janeiro, Brazil
Universidade do Estado do Rio de Janeiro, Rio de Janeiro, Brazil

Cleandro Pires de Albuquerque
Serviço de Reumatologia, Hospital Universitário de Brasília - Universidade de Brasília, Brasília, Brazil
Universidade de Brasília- UnB, Brasília, DF, Brazil

Manoel Barros Bértolo
Disciplina de Reumatologia, Faculdade de Ciências Médicas, Universidade Estadual de Campinas, Campinas, Brazil

Paulo Louzada Júnior
Disciplina de Reumatologia, Faculdade de Medicina da Universidade de Ribeirao Preto, Universidade de Sao Paulo, Ribeirão Preto, Brazil

Sebastião Cezar Radominski
Disciplina de Reumatologia, Faculdade de Medicina da Universidade Federal do Paraná, Universidade Federal do Paraná, Curitiba, Brazil

Maria Fernanda B. Resende Guimarães
Serviço de Reumatologia, Hospital das Clínicas, Universidade Federal de Minas Gerais, Belo Horizonte, Brazil

Karina Rossi Bonfiglioli
Disciplina de Reumatologia, Faculdade de Medicina, Universidade de São Paulo, São Paulo, Brazil

Maria de Fátima Lobato da Cunha Sauma
Disciplina de Reumatologia, Faculdade de Medicina, Universidade Federal do Pará, Belém, Brazil

Ivânio Alves Pereira
Serviço de Reumatologia, Hospital Universitário, Universidade Federal de Santa Catarina, Florianópolis, Brazil

Evandro Silva Freire Coutinho
Departamento de Epidemiologia e Métodos Quantitativos em Saúde, Fundação Osvaldo Cruz, Rio de Janeiro, Brazil

Licia Maria Henrique da Mota
Programa de Pós-graduação em Ciências Médicas, Faculdade de Medicina- Universidade de Brasília; Serviço de Reumatologia, Hospital Universitário de Brasília, Universidade de Brasília, Brasília, Brazil
Rheos, Centro Médico Lúcio Costa, SGAS 610, bloco 1, salas T50- T51, L2 Sul, Asa Sul, Brasília, DF 70200700, Brazil
Universidade de Brasília- UnB, Brasília, DF, Brazil
Serviço de Reumatologia, Hospital Universitário de Brasília - Universidade de Brasília, Brasília, Brazil

Adriana Maria Kakehasi
Disciplina de Reumatologia, Faculdade de Medicina, Universidade Federal de Minas Gerais, Belo Horizonte, Brazil
School of Medicine, Federal University of Minas Gerais (Universidade Federal de Minas Gerais – UFMG), Avenida Alfredo Balena, 190, Bairro Santa Efigênia, Belo Horizonte, Minas Gerais CEP 30130-100, Brazil
Faculdade de Medicina, Universidade Federal de Minas Gerais (UFMG), Belo Horizonte, Brazil
Post Graduate Program in Sciences Applied to Adult Health Care, Federal University of Minas Gerais, Belo Horizonte, Minas Gerais State, Brazil

Ana Paula Monteiro Gomides
Programa de Pós-graduação em Ciências Médicas, Faculdade de Medicina- Universidade de Brasília; Serviço de Reumatologia, Hospital Universitário de Brasília, Universidade de Brasília, Brasília, Brazil
Centro Universitário de Brasília- UniCEUB, Brasília, Brazil

Angela Luzia Branco Pinto Duarte
Universidade Federal de Pernambuco, Recife, Brazil

Bóris Afonso Cruz
Hospital Vera Cruz, Belo Horizonte, Brazil

Claiton Viegas Brenol
Serviço de Reumatologia, Departamento de Medicina Interna, Serviço de Reumatologia, Hospital de Clínicas de Porto Alegre, Universidade Federal do Rio Grande do Sul, Porto Alegre, Brazil
Faculdade de Medicina, Universidade Federal do Rio Grande do Sul (UFRGS), Porto Alegre, Alegre, Brazil

Ieda Maria Magalhães Laurindo
Universidade Nove de Julho, São Paulo, Brazil

Ivanio Alves Pereira
Universidade do Sul de Santa Catarina, Florianópolis, Brazil

Manoel Barros Bertolo
Disciplina de Reumatologia, Faculdade de Ciências Médicas, Universidade Estadual de Campinas, Campinas, Brazil

Mariana Peixoto Guimarães Ubirajara Silva de Souza
Santa Casa de Belo Horizonte, Belo Horizonte, Brazil

Max Vitor Carioca de Freitas
Universidade de Fortaleza, Fortaleza, Brazil

Paulo Louzada-Júnior
Disciplina de Reumatologia, Faculdade de Medicina de Universidade de Ribeirão Preto, Universidade de São Paulo, Ribeirão Preto, Brazil

Elis Carolina de Souza Fatel
Postgraduate Program, Health Sciences Center, State University of Londrina, Londrina, Paraná, Brazil
Department of Nutrition, University of Fronteira Sul, Rodovia PR 182 Km 466, CEP 85770-000, Realeza, Paraná Postal Code 253, Brazil

Flávia Troncon Rosa
Postgraduate Program, Experimental Pathology, State University of Londrina, Londrina, Paraná, Brazil

Andréa Name Colado Simão
Department of Pathology, Clinical Analysis and Toxicology, University Londrina, Londrina, Paraná, Brazil

Isaias Dichi
Department of Internal Medicine, University of Londrina, Londrina, Paraná, Brazil

Graziela Sferra da Silva and Mariana de Almeida Lourenço
Faculty of Medicine of Marilia (Famema), Marília, SP, Brazil

Rafael Kmiliauskis Santos Gomes
Specialty Center of the City of Blumenau, Blumenau, Santa Catarina State (SC), Brazil
Specialty Center of the City of Brusque, Brusque, SC, Brazil
Centro de Referência Policlínica Lindolf Bell, Rua: Dois de Setembro, 1234 – Itoupava Norte, 3° andar, sala 1, Blumenau, SC CEP: 89052-003, Brazil

Luana Cristina Schreiner, Mateus Oliveira Vieira and Patrícia Helena Machado
School of Medicine, Regional University of Blumenau (Universidade Regional de Blumenau – FURB), Blumenau, Brazil

Moacyr Roberto Cuce Nobre
Clinical Epidemiology Unit, Heart Institute, University Hospital, School of Medicine, University of São Paulo (Universidade de São Paulo – USP), São Paulo, SP, Brazil

Sara de Brito Rocha, Danielle Cristiane Baldo and Luis Eduardo Coelho Andrade
Rheumatology Division, Escola Paulista de Medicina, Universidade Federal de São Paulo, Disciplina de Reumatologia, Rua Botucatu 740, 3o andar, São Paulo, SP, Brazil

Maria Fernanda Brandão de Resende Guimarães
Serviço de Reumatologia, Hospital das Clínicas, Universidade Federal de Minas Gerais (UFMG), Rua Adolfo Pereira, 262, apto 901, Belo Horizonte, MG 30310-350, Brazil

Carlos Ewerton Maia Rodrigues
Programa de Pós-graduacão em Ci ncias Médicas, Universidade de Fortaleza (UNIFOR), Fortaleza, Brazil

Kirla Wagner Poti Gomes
Universidade de Fortalea e Hospital Geral de Fortaleza-HGF, Fortaleza, Brazil

Carla Jorge Machado
Faculdade de Medicina, Universidade Federal de Minas Gerais (UFMG), Belo Horizonte, Brazil

Susana Ferreira Krampe
Faculdade de Medicina, Universidade Federal do Rio Grande do Sul (UFRGS), Porto Alegre, Alegre, Brazil

Ana Paula Monteiro Gomides
Universidade de Brasília- UnB, Brasília, DF, Brazil

Ana Beatriz Vargas Santos and Geraldo da Rocha Castelar Pinheiro
Universidade do Estado do Rio de Janeiro, Rio de Janeiro, RJ, Brazil

Jéssica Martins Amaral
Post Graduate Program in Sciences Applied to Adult Health Care, Federal University of Minas Gerais, Avenida Alfredo Balena, 190 room 193 Santa Efigênia, Belo Horizonte, Minas Gerais, Brazil

Maria José Menezes Brito
Applied Nursing Department, Nursing School Federal University of Minas Gerais, Belo Horizonte, Minas Gerais, Brazil

Mariana de Almeida Lourenço and Flávia Vilas Boas Ortiz Carli
Marília School of Medicine, R. Pedro Martins, 209. Marília/SP – Brazil, Marília, São Paulo CEP 17519-430, Brazil

Marcos Renato de Assis
Marília School of Medicine, R. Pedro Martins, 209. Marília/SP – Brazil, Marília, São Paulo CEP 17519-430, Brazil
Faculty of Medicine of Marilia (Famema), Marília, SP, Brazil

Ana Carolina de Linhares and Lucas Selistre Lersch
School of Medicine, Regional University of Blumenau (Universidade Regional de Blumenau – FURB), Blumenau, Brazil

Maria Raquel Costa Pinto, Monaliza Angela Rocha, Cyntia Gabriele Michel Cardoso Trant and Marcus Vinicius Andrade
School of Medicine, Federal University of Minas Gerais (Universidade Federal de Minas Gerais – UFMG), Avenida Alfredo Balena, 190, Bairro Santa Efigênia, Belo Horizonte, Minas Gerais CEP 30130-100, Brazil

Adriano José Souza
Conrad Diagnostic Imaging (Conrad Diagnóstico por Imagem), Rua Rio Grande do Norte, 77, Bairro Santa Efigênia, Belo Horizonte, MG CEP: 30130-130, Brazil

Wilson Campos Tavares Jr
Ecoar Diagnostic Medicine (Ecoar Medicina Diagnóstica), Avenida do Contorno, 6760, Bairro Santo Antônio, Belo Horizonte, MG CEP: 30110-044, Brazil

Tae Hyub Lee
College of Medicine, Chung-Ang University, 84 Heukseouk-ro, Donjak-gu, Seoul 06974, South Korea

Gwan Gyu Song
Korea University College of Medicine, 73 Inchon-ro, Seongbuk-gu, Seoul 02841, South Korea
Department of Rheumatology, Korea University Guro Hospital, 148 Gurodong-ro, Guro-gu, Seoul 08308, South Korea

Sung Jae Choi
Korea University College of Medicine, 73 Inchon-ro, Seongbuk-gu, Seoul 02841, South Korea
Division of Rheumatology, Department of Internal Medicine, Korea University Ansan Hospital, 123 Jeokgeum-ro, Danwon-gu, Ansan-si, Gyeonggi-do 15355, South Korea

Jae Hyun Jung
College of Medicine, Chung-Ang University, 84 Heukseouk-ro, Donjak-gu, Seoul 06974, South Korea
Division of Rheumatology, Department of Internal Medicine, Korea University Ansan Hospital, 123 Jeokgeum-ro, Danwon-gu, Ansan-si, Gyeonggi-do 15355, South Korea

Hongdeok Seok
Department of Occupational and Environmental Medicine, Busan Adventist Hospital, Sahmyook Medical Center, 170 Daeti-ro, Seo-gu, Busan 49230, South Korea

Nathália de Carvalho Sacilotto
Hospital do ServidorPúblicoEstadual de São Paulo, Rua Pedro de Toledo, 1800, Vila Clementino, São Paulo, SP 04039-000, Brazil

Rina Dalva Neubarth Giorgi
Serviço de Reumatologia, Instituto de Assistência Médica ao Servidor Público Estadual, Hospital do Servidor Público Estadual de São Paulo, São Paulo, Brazil
Hospital do ServidorPúblicoEstadual de São Paulo, Rua Pedro de Toledo, 1800, Vila Clementino, São Paulo, SP 04039-000, Brazil
Instituto de Assistência Médica ao Servidor Público Estadual, Hospital do Servidor Público Estadual de São Paulo, São Paulo, SP, Brazil

Maria Fernanda Brandão Resende Guimarães
Universidade Federal de Minas Gerais, Belo Horizonte, Brazil

Paulo Louzada Jr
Universidade de São Paulo, Ribeirão Preto, Brazil

Katie Tuckwell, Thierry Sornasse and Michael J. Townsend
Genentech, Inc., 1 DNA Way, South San Francisco, CA 94080, USA

Cem Gabay
University Hospital of Geneva, Geneva, Switzerland

Ruediger Paul Laubender
Roche Diagnostics, Penzberg, Germany

Jianmei Wang
Roche Products, Welwyn Garden City, UK

Ricardo Machado Xavier
Universidade Federal do Rio Grande do Sul, Hospital de Clínicas de Porto Alegre, Porto Alegre, Brazil
Universidade Federal do Rio Grande do Sul (UFRGS), Programa de Pós Graduação em Ciências Médicas (PPGCM), Rua Ramiro Barcelos 2400, segundo andar, Porto Alegre 90035-903, Brazil
Department of Rheumatology, Hospital de Clinicas de Porto Alegre, Rua Ramiro Barcelos 2350, sexto andar, Porto Alegre 90035-903, Brazil

Cristiano Augusto Freitas Zerbini
Centro Paulista de Investigações Clínicas (CEPIC), São Paulo, Brazil

Daniel Feldman Pollak
Universidade Federal de São Paulo, São Paulo, Brazil

Jorge Luis Alberto Morales-Torres
Morales Vargas Centro de Investigación, Guanajuato, Mexico

Philippe Chalem
Fundación Instituto de Reumatología Fernando Chalem, Bogotá, Colombia

José Fernando Molina Restrepo
Centro Integral de Reumatología – Reumalab, Medellín, Colombia

Javier Arnaldo Duhau
Centro de Investigaciones en Enfermedades Reumáticas (CIER), Buenos Aires, Argentina.

Jacqueline Rodríguez Amado
Desarrollos Biomédicos y Biotecnológicos, Monterrey, Mexico

Maurício Abello
Circaribe, Barranquilla, Colombia

Maria Celina de la Vega
CEIM Investigaciones Medicas, Buenos Aires, Argentina

Adriana Pérez Dávila
Instituto Médico Especializado (IME), Buenos Aires, Argentina

Priscila Martin Biegun and Maysa Silva Arruda
AbbVie Farmacêutica Ltda, São Paulo, Brazil

Cesar Ramos-Remus
Unidad de Investigación en Enf. Crónico-Degenerativas, Guadalajara, Mexico

Index